Genetics and the Psychology of Motor Performance

T0383669

Despite the prevalence of behavioral research conducted through genetic studies, there is an absence of literature pertaining to the genetics of motor behavior. *Genetics and the Psychology of Motor Performance* is the first book to integrate cutting-edge genetic research into the study of the psychological aspects of motor learning and control.

The book's central line of enquiry revolves around the extent to which psychological factors central to motor proficiency – including personality, emotion, self-regulation, motivation, and perceptual-cognitive skills – are acquired or inherited. It explains how these factors affect motor performance, distilling the latest research into their genetic underpinnings and, in doing so, assessing the magnitude of the role genetics plays in the stages of motor development, from early proficiency through to expertise.

Written by leading experts in the genetics of human performance and exercise psychology, and thoroughly illustrated throughout, *Genetics and the Psychology of Motor Performance* is a crucial resource for any upper-level student or researcher seeking a deeper understanding of motor learning. It is an important book for anyone studying or working in exercise psychology, motor development, exercise genetics, or exercise physiology more broadly.

Sigal Ben-Zaken is the head of the genetic and molecular biology laboratory at the Wingate Academic College for Physical Education and Sport Sciences, Israel. She obtained her doctoral degree in biomedical engineering from the Technion, the Israeli Institute of Technology. As the head of the genetic and molecular biology laboratory, her main research focus is the genetic basis of athletic performance, trying to combine different aspect of genetics and performance. Sigal has also acted as a lecturer at the Wingate Academic College.

Veronique Richard earned her doctoral degree in sport science from the University of Montreal then went on to complete a postdoctoral fellowship in sport psychology at Florida State University. Her research focuses on the effects of creativity enhancement on motor performance and psychological adaptation. She has a performance psychology practice primarily working as a mental performance consultant with different Canadian national teams and individual elite athletes. Additionally, she is an associate researcher at the National Circus School in Montreal, Canada.

Gershon Tenenbaum is the Benjamin S. Bloom Professor of Educational and Sport Psychology and was the Sport Psychology Graduate Program Director at Florida State University, USA. Gershon was previously the Director of the Ribstein Center for Research and Sport Medicine at the Wingate Institute in Israel, and the Director of the Graduate Program in Sport Psychology at the University of Southern Queensland, Australia. He was also the President of the International Society of Sport Psychology and the Editor of the *International Journal of Sport and Exercise Psychology*. He has published more than 250 articles in peer-reviewed journals and written and edited ten books, handbooks, and encyclopedias. Gershon received several distinguished awards and is a member and fellow of several scientific and professional forums and societies.

Routledge Research in Sport and Exercise Science

The *Routledge Research in Sport and Exercise Science* series is a showcase for cutting-edge research from across the sport and exercise sciences, including physiology, psychology, biomechanics, motor control, physical activity and health, and every core sub-discipline. Featuring the work of established and emerging scientists and practitioners from around the world, and covering the theoretical, investigative and applied dimensions of sport and exercise, this series is an important channel for new and ground-breaking research in the human movement sciences.

Available in this series:

Complex Sport Analytics
Felix Lebed

The Science of Figure Skating
Edited by Jason Vescovi and Jaci VanHeest

The Science of Judo
Edited by Mike Callan

Modelling and Simulation in Sport and Exercise
Edited by Arnold Baca and Jürgen Perl

The Exercising Female
Science and Application
Edited by Jacky J. Forsyth and Claire-Marie Roberts

Genetics and the Psychology of Motor Performance
Sigal Ben-Zaken, Veronique Richard, and Gershon Tenenbaum

For more information about this series, please visit: www.routledge.com/sport/series/RRSES

Genetics and the Psychology of Motor Performance

Sigal Ben-Zaken, Veronique Richard, and Gershon Tenenbaum

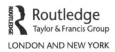
Routledge
Taylor & Francis Group

LONDON AND NEW YORK

First published 2019
by Routledge
2 Park Square, Milton Park, Abingdon, Oxon OX14 4RN

and by Routledge
605 Third Avenue, New York, NY 10017

First issued in paperback 2020

Routledge is an imprint of the Taylor & Francis Group, an informa business

© 2019 Sigal Ben-Zaken, Veronique Richard, and Gershon Tenenbaum

The right of Sigal Ben-Zaken, Veronique Richard, and Gershon
Tenenbaum to be identified as authors of this work has been asserted by
them in accordance with sections 77 and 78 of the Copyright, Designs and
Patents Act 1988.

All rights reserved. No part of this book may be reprinted or reproduced or
utilized in any form or by any electronic, mechanical, or other means, now
known or hereafter invented, including photocopying and recording, or in
any information storage or retrieval system, without permission in writing
from the publishers.

Trademark notice: Product or corporate names may be trademarks or
registered trademarks, and are used only for identification and explanation
without intent to infringe.

British Library Cataloguing-in-Publication Data
A catalogue record for this book is available from the British Library

Library of Congress Cataloging-in-Publication Data
Names: Cohen, Sigal Ben-Zaken, author. | Richard, Vâeronique, author. |
Tenenbaum, Gershon, author.
Title: Genetics and the psychology of motor performance /
Sigal Ben-Zaken Cohen, Veronique Richard, Gershon Tenenbaum.
Description: First edition. | New York : Routledge, [2019] | Includes index.
Identifiers: LCCN 2018046819| ISBN 9781138071360 (hardback) |
ISBN 9781315114682 (ebook)
Subjects: LCSH: Psychophysiology–Genetic aspects. | Motor ability.
Classification: LCC QP360 .C643 2019 | DDC 612.8–dc23
LC record available at https://lccn.loc.gov/2018046819

ISBN 13: 978-0-367-73179-3 (pbk)
ISBN 13: 978-1-138-07136-0 (hbk)

Typeset in Times New Roman
by Wearset Ltd, Boldon, Tyne and Wear

With much love and adoration
To my dear parents, Leah and Avramiko Ben-Zaken; the roots that
enabled me to flourish.
To my beloved children, Nave, Yaari, Doron, and Yogev; the
flowering branches of my life, and to my dearest grandmother,
Rachel Bar-Noy, for her unconditional love.
You are my own personal "perfect storm" of genes and
environment.

Sigal

To Rina, my wife, and to our five children: Ravid, Noam, Sharon,
Yuval, and Dana. You are all intelligent and successful in your life,
and you bring me inspiration, happiness, and motivation to further
explore and contribute.

Gershon

Contents

Figures

Tables

Introduction

Our book is about linking nature with nurture. Specifically, the book introduces to the students the latest scientific progress in the genetic domain, and links it to the psychological constructs required for the development of motor proficiency and expertise. To our knowledge, such a book has not been in the market yet.

Gregor Mendel (1822–84) and Sir Francis Galton (1822–1911) were born in the same year. They were both distinguished researchers trying to explore one of the secrets of the universe – the sources of variability. Unfortunately, they were not aware of the work of the other, though they approached the same issue from different angles. Mendel, without knowing it, put the foundations to what was later known as modern genetics, from which molecular genetics was developed. Galton founded the discipline of behavioral genetics. Ironically, from that point and on, these two domains evolved almost separately, with only a few intersection points. Molecular genetics is the field that studies the structure and function of genes at a molecular level and thus employs methods of both molecular biology and genetics. Molecular genetics provides insight into heredity and genetic variation. Behavioral genetics uses genetic methods to investigate the nature and origins of individual differences in behavior. While the name "behavioral genetics" connotes a focus on genetic influences, the field broadly investigates both genetic and environmental influences, using research designs that allow removal of the confounding of genes and environment, mainly by using twins and families' models. It is only natural to assume that behavioral genetics and molecular genetics will meet at the athletic performance domain. Athletic performance/sport is a field coalescing both psychological and physiological traits influenced by the interrelated relations and interactions of genetic and environmental factors. However, integrating behavioral genetics and molecular genetics in the study of motor performance has not happened. Yet.

The research and publications on the genetic basis of human motor performance have increased dramatically since the early 1990s (see Figure I.1), when the human genome project was completed, and the human genome sequenced. During the human genome project different schools of interest were established around specific interests. The genetic basis of athletic performance and health-related fitness was the center of one such school. The growth of interest in the

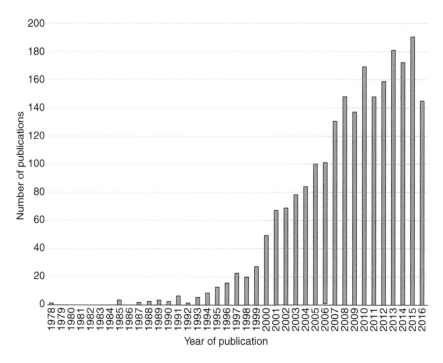

Figure I.1 Number of yearly publications on genetic polymorphism and motor performance.
Source: retrieved from PubMed, August 2018.

genetic basis of motor performance is well documented in the yearly human gene map for performance and health-related fitness phenotypes, which was first published in 2001 and has been published yearly since then (Booth & Vyas, 2001; Booth et al., 2001; Bray et al., 2009; Hagberg et al., 2011; Loos et al., 2015; Perusse et al., 2003, 2013; Rankinen et al., 2002, 2004, 2006, 2010; Roth et al., 2012; Sarzynski et al., 2016; Wolfarth et al., 2005, 2014). Parallel to the extensive research conducted to identify specific genes and genetic variants related to *physiological traits* of motor performance, the study aimed at identifying the genetic basis of *psychological traits* of motor performance is relatively meager. The lack of genetic research in the psychological-behavioral domain of sport and exercise is surprising considering the extensive research into general and clinical psychology. Variables/traits such as motivation, emotion regulation, information processing, decision-making, and other psychological traits are crucial for athletic performance, and yet not sufficiently studied.

The absence of studies on the genetic basis of motor performance-related psychological traits may be attributed to the complexity of defining these traits quantitatively. The identification of the biological mechanism underlying these traits is an inarticulate task; specifically, the continuous inter-relation and interaction of these traits with each other, with physiological traits, and with environmental factors. Therefore, a multidisciplinary approach combining behavioral and molecular genetics must be adopted to study motor behavior and performance. In this book we aim to introduce the main concepts of molecular genetics in simple terms, and, at the same time, to describe the main published findings linking selected psychological traits in the motor/sport domain to genetics. In many cases we stipulated the psychological-genetic links from the general psychological literature when we believed in its conceptual validity and transferability into the motor domain.

To accomplish these aims, we begin by introducing the basic concept of genetics (Chapter 1), which is believed to be the reason for the similarity and variability among peoples' both biological and psychological traits. Specifically, we present the concepts of *heredity* – the study of passing traits from parents to offspring, and *variation*, which centers on the factors for making no two organisms exactly alike (e.g., chromosomes, genes, DNA). In Chapter 2 we provide a short review of the main concepts in developing motor skills and control and summarize the findings which link genetic to motor proficiency. Specifically, heritability and genetic variation in motor learning and control are reviewed and their linkage to the dopaminergic system is introduced.

At this stage we began to review and conceptualize the genetic-psychological trait linkage in the motor and sport domain. *Personality* is the first psychological construct we have selected (Chapter 3) because it is believed to be the most heritable one – a construct that remains relatively stable over the life span. We begin by reviewing the main concepts of personality in sport showing its variability and uniqueness among human beings, and then emphasize its role within the unique sport domain. Genes related to personality traits are shown, and the gene-environment interaction first introduced.

One of the important traits studied in psychology and in sport psychology relates to *emotions* and *emotion regulation*. The effect of emotions and the control over them is crucial for regulating behaviors and achieving personal and team goals. Thus, we begin Chapter 4 by introducing this construct along with its biological-neural foundation, and then link it to the variability among people in both the expression and regulation of emotions. The link between emotion (mainly anxiety) and sport performance is specifically emphasized and linked to genetic variants. Closely related to the construct of emotions is the construct of *self-regulation* and *coping skills*, which enable the biological and psychological system *to adapt* to the changing external and internal conditions. These constructs and their genetic basis are introduced in Chapter 5. Humans tend to first *appraise* the situation they face, which consists of the perceived threat/risk/challenge of the situation and their perceived ability to cope with it. The amygdala along with some genetic variants have a role in this evaluative process. We outline them in this chapter. Because coping skills are required to handle the situation, we explain the term, describe it, and outline the genetic variants related to coping. Of course, self-regulation and control within the adaptational process are clarified and their linkage to the serotonergic, noradrenergic, dopaminergic, neuropeptide Y, and brain-derived neurotrophic factor (BDNF) are summarized.

An additional main construct in psychology and in sport in particular is the energy that drives us to accomplish goals. This energy is called *motivation*. Chapter 6 is devoted to the genetic and environmental determinants of motivation. We first review the theories and concepts of motivation, their relevance to sport and exercise, and their multidimensional and even dynamical features, and then provide a genetic lookout on it – particularly the genetic foundation of motivation to move and exercise. Specifically, we introduce the dopaminergic basis of motivation to take part in physical activity, and the genetic variability in sport participation. We conclude by pointing out the mismatch between the psychological (behavioral and cognitive) foundation of the motivation and the genetic basis for it – behavioral genetics and the concepts and theories underlying human's and athletes' exercise and sport behaviors.

The last psychological construct we review, which is imperative to sport activity, is *perception* and *cognition* (Chapter 7). We introduce the main features of these constructs in sport and provide the genetic foundation for them. We begin by outlining the role of attention, anticipation, memory structures, information processing, and decision-making/alteration to the sport domain and their effect of transferring visual cues into motor actions. Next, we outline the biological mechanisms and genetic factors of the perceptual-cognitive sequence and review the current knowledge on polymorphism in genes associated with the dopaminergic, noradrenergic neurotransmission, serotonergic, and cholinergic systems. We conclude with the current state of the art correlation between genes and environment related to intelligent behavior, outline the role of exercise in developing, maintaining, and changing cognition, and finally summarize the literature and concepts on decision-making under pressure along with providing the neurological foundation of high-level performance.

In Chapter 8, the final chapter of this book, we emphasize the need to expand the scope of the gene-environment paradigm to more reliably capture motor behavior proficiency and development. We return to the immortal debate about the role of nature and nurture in determining human behavior and provide a conceptual framework to study it along with a molecular perspective on the gene-environment relations. By summarizing the knowledge on epigenetic mechanisms in the mental and cognitive domains, we better understand the interpersonal variation in response to the environment. We finalize this chapter and book by presenting a new model which postulates the non-linear relationship of the complex gene-environment interaction to better capture the role of nature and nurture in motor skill development and maintenance as well as in health habits and behaviors.

References

Booth, F. W., & Vyas, D. (2001). The human gene map for performance and health-related fitness phenotypes. *Medicine and Science in Sports and Exercise, 33*(6), 868. Retrieved from www.ncbi.nlm.nih.gov/pubmed/11404648

Booth, F. W., Vyas, D., Rankinen, T., Pérusse, L., Rauramaa, R., Rivera, M. A., ... Bouchard, C. (2001). The human gene map for performance and health-related fitness phenotypes. *Medicine and Science in Sports and Exercise, 33*(6). Retrieved from www.ncbi.nlm.nih.gov/pubmed/11404647

Bray, M. S., Hagberg, J. M., Pérusse, L., Rankinen, T., Roth, S. M., Wolfarth, B., & Bouchard, C. (2009). The human gene map for performance and health-related fitness phenotypes: The 2006–2007 update. *Medicine and Science in Sports and Exercise, 41*(1), 35–73. Retrieved from www.ncbi.nlm.nih.gov/pubmed/19123262

Hagberg, J. M., Rankinen, T., Loos, R. J. F., Pérusse, L., Roth, S. M., Wolfarth, B., & Bouchard, C. (2011). Advances in exercise, fitness, and performance genomics in 2010. *Medicine and Science in Sports and Exercise, 43*(5), 743–52. https://doi.org/10.1249/MSS.0b013e3182155d21

Loos, R. J. F., Hagberg, J. M., Pérusse, L., Roth, S. M., Sarzynski, M. A., Wolfarth, B., ... Bouchard, C. (2015). Advances in exercise, fitness, and performance genomics in 2014. *Medicine and Science in Sports and Exercise, 47*(6), 1105–12. https://doi.org/10.1249/MSS.0000000000000645

Pérusse, L., Rankinen, T., Hagberg, J. M., Loos, R. J. F., Roth, S. M., Sarzynski, M. A., ... Bouchard, C. (2013). Advances in exercise, fitness, and performance genomics in 2012. *Medicine and Science in Sports and Exercise, 45*(5), 824–31. https://doi.org/10.1249/MSS.0b013e31828b28a3

Pérusse, L., Raniken, T., Rauramaa, R., Rivera, M. A., Wolfarth, B., & Bouchard, C. (2003). The human gene map for performance and health-related fitness phenotypes: The 2002 update. *Medicine and Science in Sports and Exercise, 35*(8), 1248–64. https://doi.org/10.1249/01.MSS.0000078938.84161.22

Rankinen, T., Bray, M. S., Hagberg, J. M., Pérusse, L., Roth, S. M., Wolfarth, B., & Bouchard, C. (2006). The human gene map for performance and health-related fitness phenotypes. *Medicine and Science in Sports and Exercise, 38*(11), 1863–88. https://doi.org/10.1249/01.mss.0000233789.01164.4f

Rankinen, T., Pérusse, L., Rauramaa, R., Rivera, M. A., Wolfarth, B., & Bouchard, C. (2002). The human gene map for performance and health-related fitness phenotypes: The 2001 update. *Medicine and Science in Sports and Exercise, 34*(8), 1219–33. Retrieved from www.ncbi.nlm.nih.gov/pubmed/12165675

Rankinen, T., Pérusse, L., Rauramaa, R., Rivera, M. A., Wolfarth, B., & Bouchard, C. (2004). The human gene map for performance and health-related fitness phenotypes: The 2003 update. *Medicine and Science in Sports and Exercise, 36*(9), 1451–69. Retrieved from www.ncbi.nlm.nih.gov/pubmed/15354024

Rankinen, T., Roth, S. M., Bray, M. S., Loos, R., Pérusse, L., Wolfarth, B., ... Bouchard, C. (2010). Advances in exercise, fitness, and performance genomics. *Medicine and Science in Sports and Exercise, 42*(5), 835–46. https://doi.org/10.1249/MSS.0b013e3181d86cec

Roth, S. M., Rankinen, T., Hagberg, J. M., Loos, R. J. F., Pérusse, L., Sarzynski, M. A., ... Bouchard, C. (2012). Advances in exercise, fitness, and performance genomics in 2011. *Medicine and Science in Sports and Exercise, 44*(5), 809–17. https://doi.org/10.1249/MSS.0b013e31824f28b6

Sarzynski, M. A., Loos, R. J. F., Lucia, A., Pérusse, L., Roth, S. M., Wolfarth, B., ... Bouchard, C. (2016). Advances in exercise, fitness, and performance genomics in 2015. *Medicine and Science in Sports and Exercise, 48*(10), 1906–16. https://doi.org/10.1249/MSS.0000000000000982

Wolfarth, B., Bray, M. S., Hagberg, J. M., Pérusse, L., Rauramaa, R., Rivera, M. A., ... Bouchard, C. (2005). The human gene map for performance and health-related fitness phenotypes: The 2004 update. *Medicine and Science in Sports and Exercise, 37*(6), 881–903. Retrieved from www.ncbi.nlm.nih.gov/pubmed/15947712

Wolfarth, B., Rankinen, T., Hagberg, J. M., Loos, R. J. F., Pérusse, L., Roth, S. M., … Bouchard, C. (2014). Advances in exercise, fitness, and performance genomics in 2013. *Medicine and Science in Sports and Exercise, 46*(5), 851–9. https://doi.org/10.1249/MSS.0000000000000300

1 Basic concepts in genetics

Genetics is the study of genes, genetic variation, and heredity in living organisms. Most of the human traits, including psychological and behavioral traits, are, at least in part, heritable, and result from the complex combination of genetic factors, environmental factors, and the interaction between them. Studying the genetic component of complex traits requires the understanding of basic terms and connects: heritability, genes, genetic variability, genetics of multifactorial traits, and gene-environment interaction.

All human beings are similar in some characteristics but different in others. The biological characteristics that define us as a species (e.g., having a backbone, standing upright) are inherited – passed from parents to offspring, but they do not differ from one person to another. However, within the human species, there is also much variation. Traits such as height, athletic ability, and personality characteristics vary substantially from one person to another. Genetics is the study of genes, genetic variation, and heredity in living organisms. It has been derived from the Greek word "gene" (gene = "give birth, beget"). While genetics is relatively new science, questions about heredity and parents-offspring resemblance have occupied the minds of scientists since prehistoric times and have been used to improve crop plants and animals through selective breeding. The modern science of genetics, seeking to understand this process, began with the work of the Augustinian friar Gregor Mendel in the mid-nineteenth century.

Two main constructs compose the field of genetics: (1) heredity – the study of passing traits from parents to offspring, and (2) variation, which centers on the factors responsible for the fact that no two organisms are exactly alike. Other subdomains include: biochemical genetics – focuses on the reactions by which genetic determinants are replicated and produce their effects; developmental genetics – focuses on how the expression of genes controls growth and developmental processes; molecular genetics – studies the structure and the functioning of genes at the molecular level; cytogenetics – deals with the chromosomes that carry those determinants; and population genetics – deals with the statistics properties of genetic transmission in families and populations.

Of this broad diverse field, the most intriguing questions related to motor performance are the ones dealing with the *extent*, the *source*, and the *mechanisms* of genetic influence on motor performance-related psychological traits.

Traits

One of the main concepts of genetics centers on the factors responsible for interpersonal variability. Variability can be seen in various degrees in almost every trait. Trait, or *phenotypic trait*, is a distinct observable and measurable variant of a characteristic of an organism. The term "phenotype" (from the Greek phainein, meaning "to show") means a description of an organism's observable (internal or external) characteristics. Traits may be classified in many ways: physical (e.g., blood type) vs. psychological (e.g., motivation); inherited (transferred from parents to offspring) vs. acquired (developed during lifetime), internal (blood pressure) vs. external (eye color), qualitative (discrete, "yes or no" trait) vs. quantitative (continuous range of variation), and more. The common method to classify traits is through genetic traits (e.g., eye colors), environmental traits (e.g., language), or traits that typically occur as a combination of both genes and environment (e.g., height, fitness, intelligence).

If a single gene or small group of genes controls a trait, it is referred to as a "*single-gene trait*". These traits are often referred to as "simple traits" or "Mendelian traits", since they usually follow a simple/Mendelian pattern of inheritance. Most of the simple traits are qualitative/discrete/"yes or no" traits; but not vice versa. Not all qualitative traits are simple/single-gene traits. For example, being or not being an athlete is a qualitative trait, though it is not a simple/single-gene trait. If multiple genes influence a trait, it is considered a "*polygenic trait*" (e.g., eye color). When multiple genes interact with environmental factors to influence a trait, it is considered a "*multifactorial trait*" (e.g., height). Polygenetic/multifactorial traits are usually quantitative traits and vary on a continuous range. These traits are often referred to as "complex traits" since they usually follow a complex pattern of inheritance. Traits' classification can be seen in Table 1.1. Most of the motor performance-related traits are multifactorial traits, but their location on the gene-environment space varies from one trait to another according to the relative influence of the genes and the environment.

Table 1.1 Traits categorization according to # of genes and environmental influence

# of genes controlling the trait / Environmental influence	Single or few genes	Many genes
Small or none	Simple/discrete/Mendelian trait e.g., cystic fibrosis	Polygenic trait e.g., eye color
Exist	Environmental trait e.g., language	Multi-factorial trait e.g., motivation

Chromosomes, genes, and DNA

Chromosomes, genes, and DNA (deoxyribonucleic acid) are interrelated, connected terms; each one of them explains the others. However, while chromosomes are structures, and DNA is a material, genes are information units or instructions which specify physical, biochemical, and behavioral traits. The genes are arranged one next to another in a linear fashion, on structures called chromosomes, which are made from the biochemical material DNA. We can use the analogy of an encyclopedia to better understand the relationship between DNA molecules, genes, and chromosomes. One DNA subunit represents a letter, a gene equals a single entry, a chromosome represents a volume, and all the human chromosomes represent a complete encyclopedia

A DNA molecule (see Figure 1.1) is made up of a series of sub-units arranged in two strands that resemble a ladder and twist to form a double helix as deduced

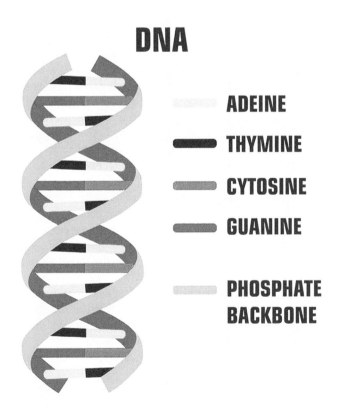

Figure 1.1 The DNA double helix.

by Watson and Crick (1953). Each DNA strand is made of four sub-units, Nitrogenous bases, called nucleotides, which comprise the DNA "alphabet." The bases are adenine (A), thymine (T), guanine (G), and cytosine (C). These bases link in a very specific way: A always pairs with T, and C always pairs with G.

If the two strands are pulled apart, each one can be used to reproduce the other one (and a new DNA molecule). This important property enables the DNA molecule to replicate itself whenever the cell divides.

The order of these nucleotide bases determines the meaning of the information encoded in that part of the DNA. Only a small portion of the DNA molecule contains meaningful information, which can be read as an instruction to synthesize proteins. The information segments are called "genes." Genes are the blueprint for the organism's biology. They contain the instructions for things like the anatomical structures, hormones, neurotransmitters, enzymes, and many more. It is estimated that there are approximately 25,000 different genes in the human genome (the entire set of genes). Since the estimated number of human proteins is 100,000, each gene can code for few proteins (Chin, Boyle, Theile, Parsons, & Coman, 2006); it is not as was previously thought, that one gene encodes to one protein.

Another gene-related term is "allele." Allele is a variant form of a gene. Some genes have different forms, which are located at the same position, named locus (plural loci) on a chromosome. Humans are diploid organisms because they have two pairs of homologue chromosomes, and therefore two alleles at each genetic locus, with one allele inherited from each parent. Each pair of alleles represents the genotype of a specific gene. Genotypes are described as homozygous if the two alleles are identical and as heterozygous if the two alleles differ. Alleles contribute to the organism's phenotype, which is the outward appearance of a trait. Some alleles are dominant or recessive. When an organism is heterozygous at a specific locus and carries one dominant and one recessive allele, the organism will express the dominant phenotype.

The total DNA of a single human cell is approximately 2.5m in length (if stretched out straight) and 3 billion base pairs (though only portions carry meaningful information). The DNA is packaged into a condensed structure, called "*chromatin*" that under a microscope can look like a continuous string of beads. Each long strand of DNA winds around structural protein spools called "*histones*" to form a bead shape unit called "*nucleosome*." The chromatin may further loop and coil, (especially during cells' replication and divisions) to form the tightly condensed chromosome structure (see Figure 1.2). This structure includes: *centromere* (part of the chromosome that pinches inwards), the "*p*" *arm* (the shorter part of the chromosome), the "*q*" *arm* (the longer section of the chromosome), and the *telomeres* (the ends of the chromosomes).

The chromosomes are found in the nucleus of each of our body cells. We have 46 of them, matched up into 23 pairs. Egg and sperm cells, however, have only 23 chromosomes; and when they come together to make a baby, he or she will get 46. The first 22 chromosome pairs (called "autosomes") are the same in men and women. The sex chromosomes make up the twenty-third pair. Generally,

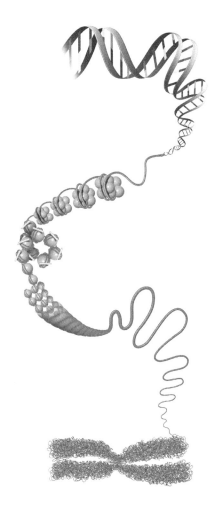

Figure 1.2 Organization of chromosomes.

females have two X chromosomes, while males have one X and one Y chromosome. A picture of chromosomes is called a *karyotype.*

Mendel laws of inheritance

Our modern understanding of how traits are inherited through generations comes from the principles proposed by Gregor Mendel in 1865. Mendel followed the inheritance of seven traits in pea plants (Pisum sativum). He chose traits that had two forms. Mendel began with pure-breeding pea plants, cross-bred them and recorded the traits of their progeny over several generations. Mendel worked on pea plants for eight years before he described his conclusions in a two-part paper, "Experiments on Plant Hybridization," that he read to the Natural History Society of Brünn on February 8 and March 8, 1865 (Mendel, 1865).

Mendel's conclusions were largely ignored and not seen as generally applicable, even by Mendel himself, who thought they only applied to certain categories of species or traits. In 1900, his work was rediscovered by three European scientists, Hugo de Vries, Carl Correns, and Erich von Tschermak, and Mendel was crowned as the founding father of modern genetics (Henig, 2000). Terms derived from his name as "Mendelian trait," "Mendelian inheritance," and 'Mendelism' are commonly used among scientists to this day. A detailed description of his experiments can be found in every genetic textbook, and his three foundational principles of inheritance are: *Law of segregation, Law of independent assortment,* and *Law of dominance*. They apply to traits in both plants and animals.

Mendel did not use the term "genes" that was coined years later, but he did speculate that there were two factors for each basic trait, and that one factor was inherited from each parent. Today, we know that Mendel's inheritance factors are genes, or more specifically alleles – different variants of the same gene. In today's genetic language, a pure-breeding pea plant line is a homozygote – it has two identical copies of the same allele, while heterozygote carry two different alleles. If the different alleles are designated, for example, as A and a, three combinations of alleles, which are actually three genotypes, are possible: AA, Aa, and aa. If AA and aa individuals (homozygotes) show different forms of the trait (phenotypes), and Aa individuals (heterozygotes) show the same phenotype as AA individuals, then allele A is dominant to allele a, and a is said to be recessive to A.

Mendel proposed that during reproduction, the inherited factors (now called alleles) are separated into reproductive cells (gametes: eggs and sperm in animals, pollen and ova in plants) in a process that is now called *meiosis (law of segregation)*, so that each gamete carries only one allele for each gene. Mendel observed that, when peas with more than one trait were crossed, the progeny did not always match the parents. This is because genes for different traits can segregate independently during the formation of gametes (*law of independent assortment*). The *law of dominance* refers to the observation that when pure-bred parent plants were cross-bred, some traits were always seen in the progeny, whereas other traits were hidden until the first-generation hybrid plants were left to self-pollinate. Mendel is also appreciated for his methodical hypothesis testing and careful application of mathematical models. Mendel formed statistical predictions about trait inheritance, and test it with experiments of dihybrid and trihybrid crosses. This method of developing statistical expectations about inheritance data is one of the most significant contributions Mendel made to biology.

Based on Mendel's lows of inheritance, several basic patterns of inheritance exist for single-gene traits (Genetic Alliance, 2009): autosomal dominant, autosomal recessive, X-linked dominant, and X-linked recessive. These patterns are summarized in Table 1.2. However, not all traits follow these patterns, and other forms of inheritance exist, and are discussed later.

Table 1.2 Inheritance patterns of simple traits

		Type of allele carrying the trait	
		Dominant	Recessive
Type of chromosome carrying the allele	Autosomal	*Autosomal dominant* Transmission of the allele causes a trait to be expressed. Males and females are affected with equal frequency. e.g., albinism, Huntington's disease	*Autosomal recessive* An individual must have two copies of a recessive allele (homozygous) to express the trait. e.g., smooth chin, cystic fibrosis
	X chromosome	*X-linked dominant* Both males and females can express the trait, although males may be more severely and less commonly affected e.g., Rett syndrome	*X-linked recessive* Male allele carriers (one X chromosome) will express the trait, but only homozygous females will express it. e.g., color blindness

Complex inheritance

There are some exceptions to Mendel's principles, which have been discovered as the knowledge of genes and inheritance has increased. For example, the principle of independent assortment does not apply if the genes are close together (or linked) on a chromosome. Also, alleles do not always interact in a standard dominant/recessive way, particularly if they are co-dominant or have differences in expressivity or penetrance.

Incomplete dominance (also called partial dominance or semi-dominance) occurs when the phenotype of the heterozygous genotype is distinct from, and often intermediate to, the phenotypes of the homozygous genotypes (Schacherer, 2016). In quantitative genetics, where phenotypes are measured numerically, if a heterozygote's phenotype is exactly between (numerically) that of the two homozygotes, the phenotype is said to exhibit no dominance at all, i.e., dominance exists only when the heterozygote's phenotype measure lies closer to one homozygote than the other.

Co-dominance occurs when the contributions of both alleles are visible in the phenotype. For example, in the ABO blood group system (Yoshida, 1981), chemical modifications to a glycoprotein on the surfaces of blood cells are controlled by three alleles, two of which are co-dominant to each other (I^A, I^B) and dominant over the recessive i at the ABO locus. Thus, I^AI^A and I^Ai individuals both have type A blood, but I^AI^B individuals have both modifications on their blood cells, and thus have type AB blood, so the I^A and I^B alleles are said to be co-dominant

Multiple alleles are a type of non-Mendelian inheritance pattern that involves more than just the typical two alleles that usually code for a certain characteristic in a species (Schacherer, 2016). Therefore, there are more than two phenotypes available depending on the dominant or recessive alleles that are available in the trait and the dominance pattern the individual alleles follow when combined. The human ABO blood type is an example of multiple alleles – co-dominance inheritance.

Polygenic inheritance describes the inheritance of traits that are determined by more than one gene (Schacherer, 2016). Polygenic traits exhibit incomplete dominance, and the genes contributing to a trait have equal influence and the alleles for the gene have an additive effect. The phenotype is a mixture of the phenotypes inherited from the parent alleles. Environmental factors can also influence polygenic traits. Polygenic traits have many possible phenotypes, and usually the variation in the population follows a bell-shaped distribution. Most individuals inherit various combinations of dominant and recessive alleles, and fall in the middle range of the curve, which represents the average range for a particular trait. Individuals at the ends of the curve represent those who either inherit all dominant alleles (on one end) or those who inherit all recessive alleles (on the opposite end).

Eye color, as well as skin color, hair color, body shape, height, and weight are examples of polygenic inheritance. This trait is thought to be influenced by up to 16 different genes (White & Rabago-Smith, 2011). Eye color is determined by the amount of the brown color pigment melanin that a person has in the front part of the iris. Black and dark brown eyes have more melanin than hazel or green eyes. Blue eyes have no melanin in the iris. Several other genes that determine eye color also influence skin color and hair color. For simplifying the explanation, let us assume that two genes determine eye color. In this case, a cross between two individuals with light brown eyes (BbGg) would produce several different phenotype possibilities. In this example, the allele for black color (B) is dominant to the recessive blue color (b) for gene 1. For gene 2, the dark hue (G) is dominant and produces a green color. The lighter hue (g) is recessive and produces a light color. This cross would result in five basic phenotypes and nine genotypes (see Figure 1.3): black eyes (BBGG), dark brown eyes (BBGg, BbGG), light brown eyes (BbGg, BBgg, bbGG), green eyes (Bbgg, bbGg), and blue eyes (bbgg). Having all dominant alleles results in black eye color. The presence of at least two dominant alleles produces the black or brown color. The presence of one dominant allele produces the green color, while having no dominant alleles results in blue eye color. In polygenic inheritance pattern, the more genes control the trait, the more phenotypes there are.

Epistasis describes a relationship between genes where an allele of one gene (the epistatic gene) hides or masks the visible output, or phenotype, of other genes. The system of genes that determines skin color in man, for example, is independent of the gene responsible for albinism (lack of pigment) or the development of skin color (Jablonski & Chaplin, 2017). This gene is an epistatic gene. When the albino condition occurs, the genes that determine skin color are present but not expressed. Figure 1.4 presents epistasis effect on hair color. The gene for total baldness is epistatic to those for blond hair or red hair. The baldness phenotype supersedes genes for hair color.

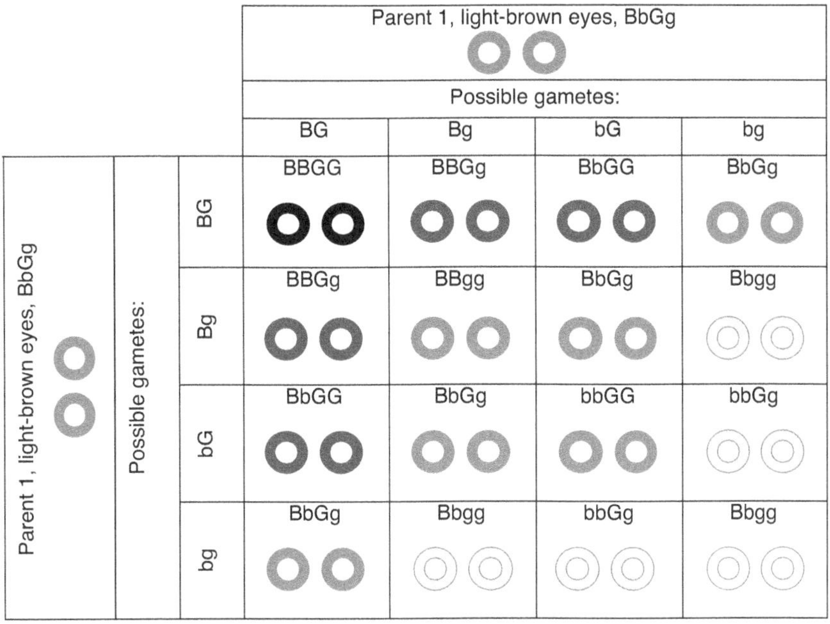

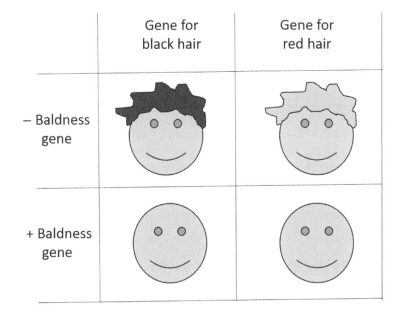

			Parent 1, light-brown eyes, BbGg			
			Possible gametes:			
			BG	Bg	bG	bg
Parent 1, light-brown eyes, BbGg	Possible gametes:	BG	BBGG	BBGg	BbGG	BbGg
		Bg	BBGg	BBgg	BbGg	Bbgg
		bG	BbGG	BbGg	bbGG	bbGg
		bg	BbGg	Bbgg	bbGg	Bbgg

Figure 1.3 Eye color inheritance in polygenic model of two genes with dominant-recessive relations.

Figure 1.4 Epistatic effect.

Heritability

A central question in biology and psychology is whether observed variation in a specific trait is related to genetic variation or environmental variation, known also as the "nature vs. nurture" debate. This is not the same as asking whether genes play a role in the trait. Take the ability to speak as an example of a trait; it is definitely controlled by genes, since genes carry the information for the anatomical, neurological, and biochemical structures and mechanisms of speaking. There is no variation in the ability to speak (except in some medical conditions); therefore, heritability cannot be defined. However, the particular spoken language varies from nation to nation, and that variation is not genetic (Griffiths, Miller, Suzuki, Lewontin, & Gelbart, 2000).

Heritability is a statistic measure defined as the proportion of phenotypic variation attributable to genetic variation (Wray & Visscher, 2008). Any phenotype can be valued as the sum of genetic and environmental effects:

Phenotype (P) = Genotype (G) + Environment (E).

Likewise, the phenotypic variance in the trait – Var (P) – is the sum of effects as follows:

Var (P) = Var (G) + Var (E) + Var (GxE) + Var (e)

Var (P) is the total variance in the population, Var (G) is the genetic variance in the population, Var (E) is the variance associated with shared environmental variation within the population, Var (GxE) is the variance associated with gene by environment interactions, and Var (E) is everything else (variance associated with "unique" environments, developmental "noise," independent epigenetic effects, and errors).

Heritability is defined as:

$$H^2 = \frac{\text{Var(G)}}{\text{Var(P)}}$$

H^2 is the broad-sense heritability. This reflects all the genetic contributions to a population's phenotypic variance. However, genetic variation can be attributed to additive, dominant, epistatic (multi-genic interactions), and parental (where individuals are directly affected by their parents' phenotype) effects.

In psychology and behavioral genetics the definition of Var (P) is slightly different, and composed of the following components (Dochtermann, Schwab, & Sih, 2015):

Var (P) = Var (A) + Var (D) + Var (PE) + Var (TE)

Where Var (A) represents the effects of additive genetic variation, Var (D) represents dominance genetic effects, Var (PE) represents permanent environmental effects, and Var (TE) represents temporary environmental like temporary variation in state (e.g., motivation, energy reserves etc.). Var (PE) includes parental effects, epigenetic effects and other contributors that have long-term impacts on phenotypes (e.g., nutritional state during development).

According to these contributors, repeatability (τ), the variability among individuals relative to total phenotypic variability, is defined as:

$$(\tau = (\text{Var (A)} + \text{Var (D)} + \text{Var (PE)})/(\text{Var(P)})$$

Repeatability is often used to describe personality variation, which is defined as consistent individual differences in behaviors (Bell, Hankison, & Laskowski, 2009; Dingemanse & Dochtermann, 2013).

A particularly important component of the genetic variance is the additive variance, Var (A), which is the variance due to the average effects (additive effects) of the alleles. Since each parent passes a single allele per locus to each offspring, parent-offspring resemblance depends upon the average effect of single alleles. Additive variance represents, therefore, the genetic component of variance responsible for parent-offspring resemblance. It has been suggested that for many complex traits, much of the phenotypic variance is due to additive genetic variance (Polderman et al., 2015). The additive genetic portion of the phenotypic variance is known as narrow-sense heritability and is defined as (Evans et al., 2017):

$$h^2 = \frac{\text{Var(A)}}{\text{Var(P)}}$$

Giving heritability definition (either broad-sense or narrow sense) as a ratio of variance components, the value of heritability always lies between 0 (phenotypic variation is completely attributed to environmental variation) to 1 (phenotypic variation is completely attributed to genetic variation). For instance, for height in humans, narrow-sense heritability is approximately 0.8 (Macgregor, Cornes, Martin, & Visscher, 2006), which means that ~80 percent of height variation observed is attributed to genetic variation.

There are two basic models for estimating heritability: *reaction to selection* and *family studies*. The *reaction to selection* model is often used in animal and crops studies and is based on calculating the strength of selection S (the difference in mean trait between the population as a whole and the selected parents of the next generation) and response to selection R (the difference in offspring and whole parental generation mean trait) (Falconer & Mackay, 1996). Heritability is calculated as the response to selection relative to the strength of selection, $h^2 = R/S$ as illustrated in Figure 1.5.

Traditionally, the heritability of most human traits is estimated from family studies such as family relatives' resemblance, siblings' comparisons, and twin studies. The most prevalent model of heritability estimation by *family relatives' resemblance* is using parent-offspring regression. To estimate heritability using parent-offspring regression, the trait of interest is measured in one or both of the

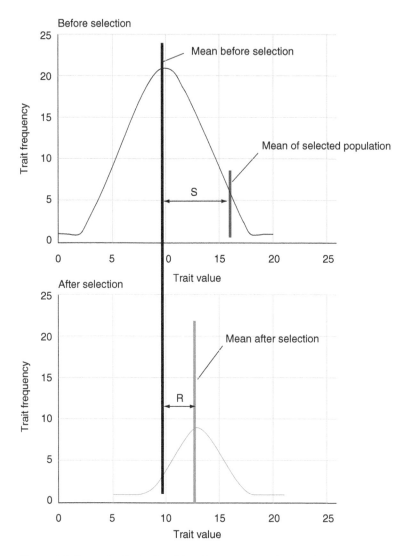

Figure 1.5 Strength of selection (S) and response to selection (R) in an artificial selection experiment, $h^2 = R/S$.

parents and in their raised offspring (Fernandez & Miller, 1985). When the off-spring reach the same developmental stage at which the parents were measured, the same trait is measured in the offspring and the average is taken over all the offspring measured in each family. This offspring average is then regressed on the measurements of the fathers, mothers, and/or the average of the two parents (each point represents one family). Comparing parent and offspring traits may estimate heritability. The slope of the line approximates the heritability of the

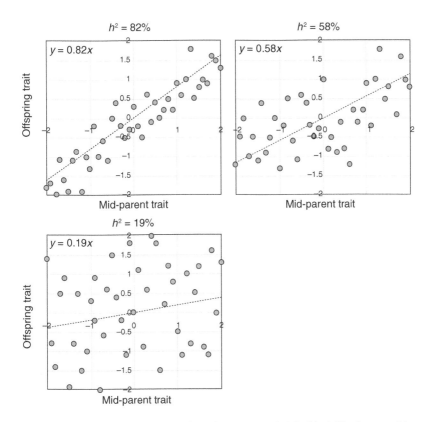

Figure 1.6 Estimation of heritability of 0.2 (a) and 0.8 (b) (offspring – mid-parent regression).

trait (see Figure 1.6). If only one parent's value is used, then heritability is twice the slope.

Parent-offspring regression for estimating heritability can be expanded to regression between other family relatives. In general:

$$h^2 = \frac{b}{r}$$

Where b is the coefficient of relatedness, and r is the coefficient of correlation (Wright, 1942). The main constraint of this model is that for humans, people that share similar genes (e.g., family members) also tend to share similar environments.

Another approach to heritability estimation is the *full-Sibling comparison* designs: comparing similarity between siblings who share both a biological mother and father (Falconer & Mackay, 1996). When there is only additive gene action, this sibling phenotypic correlation is an index of familiarity – the sum of half the additive genetic variance plus the full effect of the common environment. It thus places an upper-limit on additive heritability of twice the full-Sib phenotypic correlation. Half-Sib designs compare phenotypic traits of siblings that share one parent with other sibling groups.

Heritability for many human traits is frequently estimated by using *twin studies*. The basic idea of twin studies (as reviewed in Polderman et al., 2015) is to compare identical/monozygotic twins (MZ) to fraternal/dizygotic same-sex twins (DZ). The classic twin study assesses the variance of a trait and attempts to estimate how much of this is due to: genetic effects (*heritability*), environmental factors that affect both twins in the same way *(shared/common environment, C)*, and environmental factors that affect only one twin, or that affect either twin in a different way (unshared/unique environment, E). If the estimated genetic effect is additive effect (A) than this model is named ACE, and if the estimated genetic effect is dominant effect (D), than this model is named ADE.

The core logic of the twin design is based on that MZ raised in a family that share both 100 percent of their genes, and the entire shared environment. Any differences arising between them in these circumstances are random (unique). If r is correlation, then r_{MZ} and r_{DZ} are the correlations of the trait in MZ and DZ twins respectively. The correlation between identical twins provides an estimate of A+C. DZ twins also share C, but share on average 50 percent of their genes, so the correlation between DZ twins is a direct estimate of ½ A+C. Since MZ twins differ only due to unique environments, E is $1-r_{MZ}$. In summary, the solution of ACE model, is therefore (Falconer & Mackay, 1996; Martin, Boomsma, & Machin, 1997):

$$A\ (H^2)=2\ (r_{MZ}-r_{DZ})\ \text{(known also as Falconer formula)}$$

$$C=r_{MZ}-A$$

$$E=1-r_{MZ}$$

There are a number of limitations regarding the reliability of the heritability estimates generated by twin models. MZ twins usually share a placenta while DZ twins never do, and MZ twins might be treated differently to DZ twins. Aside from these issues, there are other concerns regarding the proper interpretation of twin studies. Should we regard the estimate of heritability as an estimate of the broad-sense heritability (H^2), the narrow-sense heritability (h^2), something between the two, or something else entirely? Should we expect DZ twins to share none of the gene-gene interactions that influence the trait, or some fraction of those shared by MZ twins? It is sometimes said that DZ twins share half the genes shared by MZ twins; this is true in a sense, but it is of course also possible (in fact, it seems rather likely) that the alternative alleles available from each parent are not representative of the alleles available in the population as a whole.

Though twin studies are still popular, new models for heritability estimation were suggested during more recent years, such as the identity-by-descent (IBD) model, where additive genetic variance is estimated from expected genome-wide IBD sharing between relatives. These studies are based on strong assumptions about the covariance between individuals within and between families (Guo, 1995). Another model is the Single Nucleotide Polymorphism (SNP) – genome-wide association study (GWAS) in individuals (Yang, Zeng, Goddard, Wray, & Visscher, 2017). The recent development of efficient genotyping and sequencing technology has led researchers to identify the genetic variants responsible for the genetic component of phenotype directly via GWAS. Since 2005 GWAS has identified thousands of SNPs associated with hundreds of different phenotypes (Hindorff et al., 2009). But, the fraction of the phenotypic variation explained for most phenotypes remains small relative to the published heritability estimates, which are estimated using the trait covariance among relatives (Eichler et al., 2010; Manolio et al., 2009; Zuk, Hechter, Sunyaev, & Lander, 2012). This "missing heritability problem" raises questions about the methods used to estimate heritability as well as the genetic architecture of complex phenotype (for review of the design, limitation and precision of various heritability estimation models, see: Frazer, Murray, Schork, & Topol, 2009; Pasaniuc & Price, 2016; Peters & Musunuru, 2012; Robinson, Wray, & Visscher, 2014; Speed & Balding, 2014; Vinkhuyzen, Wray, Yang, Goddard, & Visscher, 2013).

Genetic variation

Human genetic variation is the genetic difference both within and among populations. No two humans are genetically identical. On average, in terms of DNA sequence, each human is 99.5 percent similar to any other human (Venter et al., 2001). Even MZ twins, who develop from one zygote, have infrequent genetic differences due to mutations occurring during their development (Bruder et al., 2008). Causes of genetic differences among individuals include independent assortment, the exchange of genes (crossing over and recombination) during meiosis, and various mutational events. There are at least two reasons for genetic variation existing between populations. Natural selection may confer an adaptive advantage to individuals in a specific environment if an allele provides a competitive advantage. Alleles under selection are likely to occur only in those geographic regions where they confer an advantage. The second main cause of genetic variation is due to the high degree of neutrality of most mutations. Most mutations do not appear to have any selective effect one way or the other on the organism.

Genetic variation among humans occurs on many scales, from single nucleotide changes to gross alterations in the human karyotype. Chromosome abnormalities are detected in 1 of 160 live human births (Nielsen & Wohlert, 1991). Apart from sex chromosome disorders, most cases of aneuploidy result in the death of the developing fetus (miscarriage); or in post-natal morbidity at various degrees. On the other hand, DNA sequence variations do not necessarily end in disease or disability, but also account for normal inter-personal variability.

The main DNA sequence variations include SNPs (Single Nucleotide Poly-morphism), insertion-deletion (INDEL), and structural variants (including copy number variation, CNV). SNP is a variation in a single nucleotide that occurs at a specific position in the genome, where each variation is present to some appre-ciable degree within a population (e.g., >1 percent). For example, at a specific base position in the human genome, the base C may appear in most individuals, but in a minority of individuals, the position is occupied by base A (see Figure 1.7). There is a SNP at this specific base position, and the two possible nucle-otide variations – C or A – are said to be alleles for this base position.

SNP may fall within coding sequences of genes, non-coding regions of genes, or in the intergenic regions (regions between genes). SNPs within a coding sequence do not necessarily change the amino acid sequence of the protein that is produced due to degeneracy of the genetic code. SNPs in the coding region are of two types, synonymous and nonsynonymous SNPs. Synonymous SNPs do not affect the protein sequence while nonsynonymous SNPs change the amino acid sequence of protein. The nonsynonymous SNPs are of two types: missense and nonsense. SNPs that are not in protein-coding regions may still affect gene splicing, transcription factor binding, messenger RNA degradation, or the sequence of non-coding RNA. Gene expression affected by this type of SNP is referred to as an eSNP (expression SNP) and may be upstream or downstream from the gene.

Structural variation is variation in the structure of an organism's chromo-some, which usually includes microscopic and submicroscopic types, such as deletions, duplications, copy number variants, insertions, inversions, and translo-cations (Feuk, Carson, & Scherer, 2006). Typically, a structure variation affects a sequence length about 1Kb to 3Mb, which is larger than SNPs and smaller than chromosome abnormality, though the definitions have some overlap (Sudmant et al., 2015). Many structural variants are associated with genetic diseases, but many are likely to make an important contribution to human diversity and disease susceptibility. These structural variants include deletions, tandem dupli-cations, inversions, mobile element insertions, and more.

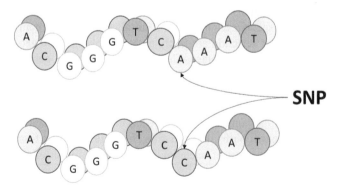

Figure 1.7 Single nucleotide polymorphism.

CNV is the most common structure variation, in which sections of the genome are repeated (see Figure 1.8) and the number of repeats in the genome varies among individuals (McCarroll & Altshuler, 2007; Sudmant et al., 2015).

CNVs can be generally categorized into two main groups: short repeats and long repeats. However, there are no clear boundaries between the two groups and the classification depends on the nature of the loci of interest. Short repeats include mainly bi-nucleotide repeats (two repeating nucleotides; e.g., A-C-A-C-A-C…) and tri-nucleotide repeats. Long repeats include repeats of entire genes. The classification based on the size of the repeat is the most obvious type of classification as size is an important factor in examining the types of mechanisms that most likely give rise to the repeats (Hastings, Lupski, Rosenberg, & Ira, 2009), hence the likely effects of these repeats on phenotype.

The 1000 Genomes Project was set out to provide a comprehensive description of common human genetic variation by applying whole-genome sequencing

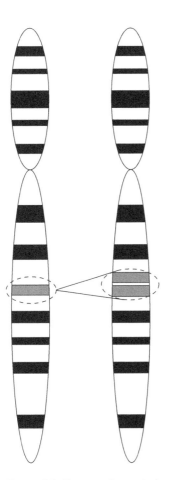

Figure 1.8 Copy number variation (CNV) in gene duplication.

to a diverse set of individuals from multiple populations. Having reconstructed genomes of 2,504 individuals from 26 populations by using low-coverage whole-genome sequencing, deep exome sequencing, and dense microarray genotyping, a broad spectrum of genetic variation totaling over 88 million variants (84.7 million SNPs, 3.6 million short insertions/deletions (indels), and 60,000 structural variants) were mapped (Auton et al., 2015).

The main finding of this project is that typical human genome differs from the reference human genome at 4.1 to 5.0 million sites. Although >99.9 percent of variants consist of SNPs and short indels, structural variants affect more bases: the typical genome contains an estimated 2,100 to 2,500 structural variants affecting ~20 million bases of sequence. The majority of variants in the data set are rare: ~64 million autosomal variants have a frequency <0.5 percent, ~12 million have a frequency between 0.5 percent and 5 percent, and only ~8 million have a frequency >5 percent. Nevertheless, the majority of variants observed in a single genome are common: just 40,000 to 200,000 of the variants in a typical genome (1–4 percent) have a frequency <0.5 percent.

Gene expression and epigenetics

Gene expression is the processes by which information from a gene is used in the synthesis of a functional gene product, mainly protein. These processes consist of two main mechanisms: protein synthesis and protein synthesis regulation and control. Briefly, the process of protein synthesis includes several steps (see Figure 1.9):

*   **Transcription** – the step in which a particular segment of DNA is copied into mRNA, which in turn serves as a template for the protein's synthesis
*   **RNA processing** – the several modifications which the RNA has to undergo to become a mature mRNA
*   **Translation** – the step in which the mRNA is decoded by a ribosome, outside the nucleus, to produce a specific amino acid chain
*   **Post-translational modification** – physical process by which a protein chain acquires its native 3-dimensional structure necessary for biological functioning.

Gene regulation gives the cell control over structure and function, and is the basis for cellular differentiation, morphogenesis, and the versatility and adaptability of any organism. Also, it depends on the state of activator RNA. Gene regulation may also serve as a substrate for evolutionary change, since control of the timing, location, and amount of gene expression can have a profound effect on the functions (actions) of the gene in a cell or in a multicellular organism.

Epigenetics is the study of heritable changes in gene expression (active versus inactive genes) that does not involve changes to the underlying DNA sequence –

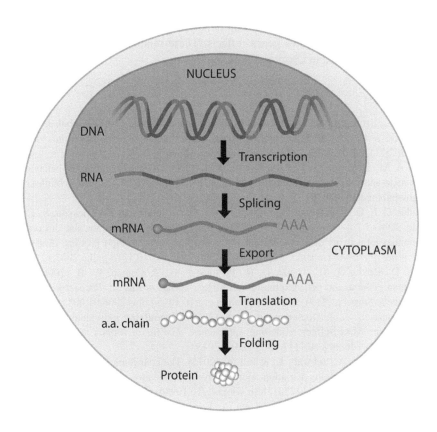

Figure 1.9 From gene to protein.

a change in phenotype without a change in genotype, which in turn affects how cells read the genes (Gibney & Nolan, 2010). Epigenetic change is a regular and natural occurrence but can also be influenced by several factors including age, the environment/lifestyle, and disease state. Epigenetic modifications can manifest as commonly as the manner in which cells terminally differentiate to end up as skin cells, liver cells, brain cells, etc. Or, epigenetic change can have more damaging effects that can result in diseases like cancer. At least three systems including DNA methylation, histone modification, and non-coding RNA (ncRNA)-associated gene silencing are currently considered to initiate and sustain epigenetic change. New and ongoing research is continuously uncovering the role of epigenetics in a variety of human disorders and fatal diseases. All these complex mechanisms are described in detail in biology/genetics text books and reviews.

Gene-environment relations

Gene-environment interactions usually refer to a situation in which the effect of environmental factors is dependent on genotype and vice versa, when environmental exposure moderates genes' effects. These relations are thoroughly presented and discussed in Chapter 8.

References

Auton, A., Brooks, L. D., Durbin, R. M., Garrison, E. P., Kang, H. M., Korbel, J. O., … Abecasis, G. R. (2015). A global reference for human genetic variation. *Nature, 526*(7571), 68–74. http://doi.org/10.1038/nature15393

Bell, A. M., Hankison, S. J., & Laskowski, K. L. (2009). The repeatability of behaviour: A meta-analysis. *Animal Behaviour, 77*(4), 771–83. Retrieved from www.ncbi.nlm.nih.gov/pubmed/24707058

Bruder, C. E. G., Piotrowski, A., Gijsbers, A. A. C. J., Andersson, R., Erickson, S., Diaz de Ståhl, T., … Dumanski, J. P. (2008). Phenotypically concordant and discordant monozygotic twins display different DNA copy-number-variation profiles. *American Journal of Human Genetics, 82*(3), 763–71. http://doi.org/10.1016/j.ajhg.2007.12.011

Chin, D., Boyle, G. M., Theile, D. R., Parsons, P. G., & Coman, W. B. (2006). The human genome and gene expression profiling. *Journal of Plastic, Reconstructive and Aesthetic Surgery, 59*(9), 902–11. http://doi.org/10.1016/j.bjps.2006.01.008

Dingemanse, N. J., & Dochtermann, N. A. (2013). Quantifying individual variation in behaviour: Mixed-effect modelling approaches. *Journal of Animal Ecology, 82*(1), 39–54. http://doi.org/10.1111/1365-2656.12013

Dochtermann, N. A., Schwab, T., & Sih, A. (2015). The contribution of additive genetic variation to personality variation: Heritability of personality. *Proceedings. Biological Sciences, 282*(1798), 20142201. http://doi.org/10.1098/rspb.2014.2201

Eichler, E. E., Flint, J., Gibson, G., Kong, A., Leal, S. M., Moore, J. H., & Nadeau, J. H. (2010). Missing heritability and strategies for finding the underlying causes of complex disease. *Nature Reviews Genetics, 11*(6), 446–50. http://doi.org/10.1038/nrg2809

Evans, L., Tahmasbi, R., Jones, M., Vrieze, S., Abecasis, G., Das, S., … Keller, M. (2017). Narrow-sense heritability estimation of complex traits using identity-by-descent information. *bioRxiv, 164848*. http://doi.org/10.1101/164848

Falconer, D. S., & Mackay, T. F. C. (1996). *Introduction to quantitative genetics*. Harlow, England: Longman.

Fernandez, G. C. J., & Miller, J. C. (1985). Estimation of heritability by parent-offspring regression. *Theoretical and Applied Genetics, 70*(6), 650–4. http://doi.org/10.1007/BF00252291

Feuk, L., Carson, A. R., & Scherer, S. W. (2006). Structural variation in the human genome. *Nature Reviews Genetics, 7*(2), 85–97. http://doi.org/10.1038/nrg1767

Frazer, K. A., Murray, S. S., Schork, N. J., & Topol, E. J. (2009). Human genetic variation and its contribution to complex traits. *Nature Reviews Genetics, 10*(4), 241–51. http://doi.org/10.1038/nrg2554

Genetic Alliance. (2009). *Inheritance patterns*. Washington, DC: Genetic Alliance. Retrieved from www.ncbi.nlm.nih.gov/books/NBK115561/

Gibney, E. R., & Nolan, C. M. (2010). Epigenetics and gene expression. *Heredity, 105*(1), 4–13. http://doi.org/10.1038/hdy.2010.54

Griffiths, A. J., Miller, J. H., Suzuki, D. T., Lewontin, R. C., & Gelbart, W. M. (2000). *Heritability of a trait*. New York, NY: W. H. Freeman. Retrieved from www.ncbi.nlm.nih.gov/books/NBK22001/

Guo, S. W. (1995). Proportion of genome shared identical by descent by relatives: Concept, computation, and applications. *American Journal of Human Genetics, 56*(6), 1468–76. Retrieved from www.ncbi.nlm.nih.gov/pubmed/7762570

Hastings, P. J., Lupski, J. R., Rosenberg, S. M., & Ira, G. (2009). Mechanisms of change in gene copy number. *Nature Reviews Genetics, 10*(8), 551–64. http://doi.org/10.1038/nrg2593

Henig, R. M. (2000). *The monk in the garden: The lost and found genius of Gregor Mendel, the father of genetics*. Boston, MA; New York, NY: Houghton Mifflin.

Hindorff, L. A., Sethupathy, P., Junkins, H. A., Ramos, E. M., Mehta, J. P., Collins, F. S., & Manolio, T. A. (2009). Potential etiologic and functional implications of genome-wide association loci for human diseases and traits. *Proceedings of the National Academy of Sciences, 106*(23), 9362–7. http://doi.org/10.1073/pnas.0903103106

Jablonski, N. G., & Chaplin, G. (2017). The colours of humanity: The evolution of pigmentation in the human lineage. *Philosophical Transactions of the Royal Society B: Biological Sciences, 372*(1724), 20160349. http://doi.org/10.1098/rstb.2016.0349

Macgregor, S., Cornes, B. K., Martin, N. G., & Visscher, P. M. (2006). Bias, precision and heritability of self-reported and clinically measured height in Australian twins. *Human Genetics, 120*(4), 571–80. http://doi.org/10.1007/s00439-006-0240-z

Manolio, T. A., Collins, F. S., Cox, N. J., Goldstein, D. B., Hindorff, L. A., Hunter, D. J., … Visscher, P. M. (2009). Finding the missing heritability of complex diseases. *Nature, 461*(7265), 747–53. http://doi.org/10.1038/nature08494

Martin, N., Boomsma, D., & Machin, G. (1997). A twin-pronged attack on complex traits. *Nature Genetics, 17*(4), 387–92. http://doi.org/10.1038/ng1297-387

McCarroll, S. A., & Altshuler, D. M. (2007). Copy-number variation and association studies of human disease. *Nature Genetics, 39*(Suppl. 7), S37–42. http://doi.org/10.1038/ng2080

Mendel, G. (1865). Experiments in plant hybridization (1865). *Meetings of the Brünn Natural History Society*. Retrieved from www.netspace.org./MendelWeb/

Nielsen, J., & Wohlert, M. (1991). Chromosome abnormalities found among 34910 newborn children: Results from a 13-year incidence study in Århus, Denmark. *Human Genetics, 87*(1), 81–3. http://doi.org/10.1007/BF01213097

Pasaniuc, B., & Price, A. L. (2016). Dissecting the genetics of complex traits using summary association statistics. *Nature Reviews Genetics, 18*(2), 117–27. http://doi.org/10.1038/nrg.2016.142

Peters, D. T., & Musunuru, K. (2012). Functional evaluation of genetic variation in complex human traits. *Human Molecular Genetics, 21*(R1), R18–23. http://doi.org/10.1093/hmg/dds363

Polderman, T. J. C., Benyamin, B., de Leeuw, C. A., Sullivan, P. F., van Bochoven, A., Visscher, P. M., & Posthuma, D. (2015). Meta-analysis of the heritability of human traits based on fifty years of twin studies. *Nature Genetics, 47*(7), 702–9. http://doi.org/10.1038/ng.3285

Robinson, M. R., Wray, N. R., & Visscher, P. M. (2014). Explaining additional genetic variation in complex traits. *Trends in Genetics, 30*(4), 124–32. http://doi.org/10.1016/j.tig.2014.02.003

Schacherer, J. (2016). Beyond the simplicity of Mendelian inheritance. *Comptes Rendus Biologies, 339*(7–8), 284–8. http://doi.org/10.1016/j.crvi.2016.04.006

Speed, D., & Balding, D. J. (2014). Relatedness in the post-genomic era: Is it still useful? *Nature Reviews Genetics, 16*(1), 33–44. http://doi.org/10.1038/nrg3821

Sudmant, P. H., Rausch, T., Gardner, E. J., Handsaker, R. E., Abyzov, A., Huddleston, J., … Korbel, J. O. (2015). An integrated map of structural variation in 2,504 human genomes. *Nature, 526*(7571), 75–81. http://doi.org/10.1038/nature15394

Venter, J. C., Adams, M. D., Myers, E. W., Li, P. W., Mural, R. J., Sutton, G. G., … Zhu, X. (2001). The sequence of the human genome. *Science, 291*(5507), 1304–51. http://doi.org/10.1126/science.1058040

Vinkhuyzen, A. A. E., Wray, N. R., Yang, J., Goddard, M. E., & Visscher, P. M. (2013). Estimation and partition of heritability in human populations using whole-genome analysis methods. *Annual Review of Genetics, 47*, 75–95. http://doi.org/10.1146/annurev-genet-111212-133258

Watson, J. D., & Crick, F. H. (1953). The structure of DNA. *Cold Spring Harbor Symposia on Quantitative Biology, 18*, 123–31. Retrieved from www.ncbi.nlm.nih.gov/pubmed/13168976

White, D., & Rabago-Smith, M. (2011). Genotype–phenotype associations and human eye color. *Journal of Human Genetics, 56*(1), 5–7. http://doi.org/10.1038/jhg.2010.126

Wray, N., & Visscher, P. (2008). Estimating trait heritability. *Nature Education, 1*(1), 29.

Wright, S. (1942). Statistical genetics and evolution. *Bulletin of the American Mathematical Society, 48*(4), 223–47. http://doi.org/10.1090/S0002-9904-1942-07641-5

Yang, J., Zeng, J., Goddard, M. E., Wray, N. R., & Visscher, P. M. (2017). Concepts, estimation and interpretation of SNP-based heritability. *Nature Genetics, 49*(9), 1304–10. http://doi.org/10.1038/ng.3941

Yoshida, A. (1981). Genetic mechanism of blood group (ABO)-expression. *Acta Biologica et Medica Germanica, 40*(7–8), 927–41. Retrieved from www.ncbi.nlm.nih.gov/pubmed/6800172

Zuk, O., Hechter, E., Sunyaev, S. R., & Lander, E. S. (2012). The mystery of missing heritability: Genetic interactions create phantom heritability. *Proceedings of the National Academy of Sciences, 109*(4), 1193–8. http://doi.org/10.1073/pnas.1119675109

2   Genetics and motor proficiency

Motor skills are defined by their complexity and the motor proficiency of the actor. Throughout the skills continuum from novice to expert, performers face different motor challenges requiring essential psychological assets. The question of whether these psychological assets, useful to reach motor proficiency, are acquired or inherited is one of great interest. Practice is a fundamental variable that influences the acquisition of motor skills, but though everyone improves, some improve more than others. This simple fact has led to frequent debate over the relative importance of genetic and environmental influences on motor learning. In principle, these factors could influence subjects' initial level of proficiency, their rate of improvement, or their final level of attainment.

An overview of basic concepts and terms in motor learning and control

Motor skills are essential to human existence as they enable people to move, communicate, interact, and develop. Performing skills such as walking, driving, and jumping, require motor coordination along with perceptual-cognitive proficiency. Motor skills vary in complexity and the motor proficiency of the actor. Because motor skill acquisition and skilled performance share similar underlying perceptual-cognitive and motor mechanisms (Proctor & Dutta, 1995), skill development and acquisition must be viewed via an integrated conceptual framework. In this chapter, we briefly describe the main terms and concepts of skill acquisition and development, relate *skills* to *abilities*, and provide the genetic basis for the perceptual-motor domain.

Skill acquisition was a subject of research interest for many years. Attempts were made to determine the number of trials, duration, time-intervals, mode of delivery, and intensities needed for acquiring a skill to a given proficiency – Power Law of Practice (PLP; Newell & Rosenbloom, 1981). Since the beginning of the twentieth century, the study of *skill-transfer* of motor skill has captured the attention of many researchers. The theory of identical elements, transfer surface, negative and positive transfers were used to describe the extent to which motor and cognitive skills can be transferred from one learning skill to the other non-learned skills. It is obvious that skills vary in complexity, and thus require different amounts of practice time and duration to be acquired (see Proctor & Dutta, 1995; Schmidt & Lee, 2014 for extensive reviews). Among the most accepted theories of motor learning are the three-stage sequential development – *cognitive, associative*, and *autonmous* (Fitts & Posner, 1967), Anderson's (1983) cognitive framework, which distinguishes between *declarative* and *procedural knowledge types* and the *knowledge of compilation* where a declarative operation is converted into a procedural one, and Rasmussen's (1986) modes of perform-ance – *knowledge base, rule base*, and *skill-base*. Skill acquisition is viewed as a sequential process classified within different knowledge compartments, and is consciously controlled at first and becomes automated at last. The motor learning-control-development concepts describe general rules of skill acquisi-tion. However, people vary in the rate and pace they learn and acquire motor skills until reaching a certain level of proficiency, even given similar environ-ments, conditions, and deliberate practice.

Motor skills, like cognitive skills, develop through practice and training, whether *intended* or *incidental*. Coordinated movement patterns become organ-ized and need less conscious attention, freeing mental resources to other activ-ities. Motor skills vary in *complexity* and are viewed as ranging from simple to complex where more attention and perceptual-cognitive resources are gradually needed for their acquisition. Motor skills are also viewed in terms of their *degree of certainty* – *closed skills* are performed in a stable and less complex environ-ment (e.g., rifle shooting) while *open skills* are performed in uncertain environ-ments, not always under the full control of the performer, and thus require anticipatory capabilities (see Proctor & Dutta, 1995; Schmidt & Lee, 2014 for detailed information). We argue that the more complex is the motor skill, and the more it requires mental, perceptual, and cognitive resources, the more is the learning and acquisition of motor skills dependent on the availability of specific genes' expression.

"*Motor abilities*" and "*motor skills*" are two related, yet distinguished, terms. In general, motor abilities such as strength, endurance, and flexibility are vital characteristics to produce motor activity (Schmidt & Lee, 2014). These abilities are shaped by biological, physiological, and environmental factors. Motor abilities are partially inherited, and are considered prerequisites and predictors for motor performance, in the same way that intelligence is for academic performance.

Motor skills refer to the capability of performing with maximum certainty, and minimum energy and time. Typically, motor skills are categorized into *gross motor skills* and *fine motor skills*. Gross motor skills refer to actions such as movement and coordination of the arms, legs, and other large body parts. Gross motor skills require muscles which produce actions such as running, crawling, and swimming. Fine motor skills are involved in refined movements ensuing in the wrists, hands, fingers, feet, and toes. They rely on smaller muscles which control actions such as picking up objects between the thumb and finger, writing carefully, and even blinking. Gross and fine motor skills work together to produce coordinated actions and movements (Schmidt & Lee, 2014).

Three pivotal interrelated terms determine *motor behavior*: *motor control, motor learning*, and *motor development*. Motor learning refers to the process of motor skills enhancement through practice (Schmidt & Lee, 2014). Learning involves changes in behaviors that arise from the interaction with the environment, and is a consequence of the co-adaptation of the neural machinery and structural anatomy (Wolpert, Ghahramani, & Flanagan, 2001). Motor control is defined as the process of initiating, directing, and grading purposeful voluntary movement (Latash, Levin, Scholz, & Schöner, 2010). Motor development refers to the development of the child's bones, muscles, and the ability to move around and manipulate one's environment. Motor development is further divided into two sections: *gross motor development* and *fine motor development* (Adolph & Robinson, 2011).

Several theories and concepts were introduced to capture how the learning of motor skills develops. The most prominent ones are the *schema theory* (i.e., motor programming), and the *perception-action coupling* (i.e., dynamic approach). The role of extrinsic and intrinsic feedback, and practice modes (blocked vs. random), have all been studied extensively, assuming variability among participants is a given fact. Variability in the rate of learning was of less concern to the researchers.

The development of motor skills is closely associated with the use and implementation of perceptual capabilities. Perceptual capabilities enable efficient use of the senses and provide us with environmental information within which we must function and survive. The senses, mainly vision, enable us to *select* and *integrate* the environmental stimuli to produce *perceptual and meaningful patterns* of the environment. Signal detection methods were developed which allow us to determine how we *identify* and *discriminate* among features which vary in shape, color, sound, organization, and other entities. The development of perceptual skills along with cognitive skills (e.g., attention, anticipation, memory – short, working, long, long-term-working, response selection, and decision-making) are strong determinants of the development of motor skills. Specifically, essential is the shift from a fully conscious step-by-step control over the movement to full automaticity, and the intentional back and forth control over this shift upon environmental demands (Schmidt & Lee, 2014).

Reaction time (RT) was used as the core measure of *information processing*, while *accuracy, error-rate*, and the *speed-error rate trade-off* were used to measure performance outcomes. The RT measure was further developed into measures where more choices were given for response, and thus termed *choice reaction time* (CRT). RT is believed to be fixed and ranged within 300ms depending on the type of stimulus presented. In contrast, CRT is alterable and depends on the number of trails, experiences, and familiarity with the task (see Schmidt & Lee, 2014). In recent years, the study of expertise and the implementation of the novice-expert paradigm to study expert development has explored the dependence of performance on anticipatory capabilities, such as attention allocation (*context* vs. *targe control*), *visual focus, gaze fixations and duration, anticipation of upcoming events, long-term-working memory, response selection, quiet-eye duration*; all are governed by mental representations stored in long-term memory and accessible and retrieved upon demand (see Starkes & Ericsson, 2003). Thus, motor expertise is very much dependent on the specific perceptual-cognitive capabilities required for each specific task, rather than fixed perceptual-cognitive capabilities, such as RT (Tenenbaum et al., 2009). Perceptual skills also enable the performer to *chunk* essential stimuli in the environment, which eases the selection of vital cues required for response retrieval and response execution. Moreover, the entire perceptual-cognitive-motor linkage can collapse under pressure, where attentional processes are interfered with and are no longer functional (Tenenbaum et al., 2009). Thus, performance becomes dependent on a multi-array of simultaneous operations, such as the operation of declarative and procedural knowledge structures via the use of perceptual-cognitive processes along with the use of appropriate coping strategies which secure the emotional-affective mode within which perceptual-motor skills must be optimally operative to secure the best response selection and execution (Tenenbaum et al., 2009).

Genetic basis for motor skills

Practice is fundamental to the acquisition of motor skills, but although everyone can improve with practice, some improve more than others. Moreover, people without previous experience perform certain activities better than others who have been practicing for years (i.e., natural variance). Even in people showing similar attainment, retrospective studies revealed individual differences in accumulated practice (Starkes, Deakin, Allard, Hodges, & Hayes, 1996). Individual variations in motor control and learning capabilities have become an important focus in movement science research. This approach recognizes that understanding personal differences in motor performance and skill acquisition can illuminate the broader mechanisms of human motor control and learning (Seidler & Carson, 2017). Such individual differences serve as natural experiments that help reveal how motor skills are acquired, controlled, and refined.

The natural variability of skills and abilities led to frequent debates over the relative importance of genetic and environmental influences on motor learning and development. Differences in motor skills might arise from various intrinsic and extrinsic factors affecting both initial motor abilities and response to practice (Yarrow, Brown, & Krakauer, 2009), and, therefore, they represent complex multi-factorial traits influenced by genes, environment, and the interaction between them (see Figure 2.1).

Taking into consideration the complexity of the mechanisms underlying motor skills, and the involvement of other biological and behavioral factors (e.g., balance, power, proprioception, rhythm, perception), identifying the genetic basis of motor skills become an entangled task. Indeed, compared to physiological and psychological traits, there is merely no data regarding the heritability of motor skills, and genetic variants related to motor skills variation.

Heritability of motor control and motor learning

Early scientific attempts to determine the genetic basis of motor performance and motor skills acquisition failed to link heritability during the earliest stages of

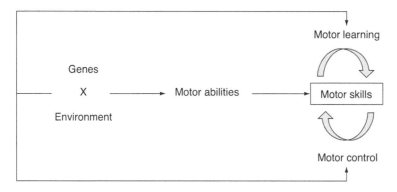

Figure 2.1 Gene-environment interaction affects motor abilities and motor skills.

learning, but it was found to be increasingly influential later in practice (Williams & Gross, 1980). Later research findings maintained that the heritability of motor control and motor learning, assessed in various motor tasks, ranged from 0.56–0.86, depending on the task (Fox, Herschberger, & Bouchard, 1996; Maes et al., 1996; Missitzi, Gentner, Misitzi, Geladas, et al., 2013; Williams & Gross, 1980). High heritability was also found for neuromuscular coordination (0.85) (Missitzi, Geladas, & Klissouras, 2004), motor cortex plasticity (0.68) (Missitzi, Gentner, Misitzi, Nickos, et al., 2013), intra-cortical inhibition (0.80), and intra-cortical facilitation (0.92) (Pellicciari et al., 2009), mean reaction time (0.60), and reaction-time variability (0.50) (Kuntsi et al., 2006).

Findings from twin studies have also demonstrated that the acquisition of motor skills is significantly heritable (Fox et al., 1996; Missitzi, Gentner, Misitzi, Geladas, et al., 2013). Fox et al., (1996) studied learning in a sample of monozygotic and dizygotic twins who had been reared apart, and found that heritability of performance at a rotary pursuit task, in which subjects learned to track a rotating target with a stylus, was high even at baseline (0.66) and increased with practice (0.74), and concluded that the effect of practice is to decrease the effect of environmental variation (i.e., previous learning). However, while twin studies can estimate the overall contribution of genetic factors to a given phenotype (or common genetic paths between phenotypes), they do not provide an indication of biological mechanism. For this, we turn to molecular genetic studies.

Genetic variation in motor control and motor learning

The relatively high proportion of heritability found in various variables related to motor performance and motor learning implies that individual differences found in motor control and motor learning might be attributed to genetic differences.

The past 20 years have brought tremendous progress in the field of genetic variation, starting with the establishment of the first human gene map (Schuler et al., 1996), through the human genome project (Lander et al., 2001; Venter et al.,

2001) to the Map of Human Genetic Variation (HapMap) (Belmont et al., 2005), and the Encyclopedia of DNA Elements (ENCODE) project aimed to construct an exhaustive catalogue of operationally significant genomic elements within the human genetic code (Dunham et al., 2012). Despite these important developments in genetic research, the application of this knowledge to understanding motor control and learning processes remains limited, and as noted in recent reviews, there is still considerable potential to better integrate genetic insights into theories of motor skill acquisition and control (Seidler & Carson, 2017).

When trying to identify genetic variation related to phenotype variation, there are two main approaches: "*hypothesis- based genetic studies*," also known as *candidate genes/genetic variants studies*, and the "*hypothesis- free genetic studies*," mainly represented by *GWAS* and *genome-wide complex trait analysis (GCTA)*. GWAS uses thousands to millions of SNPs genotyped in DNA microarrays to examine the association between common variants across the genome and a phenotype of interest. GCTA estimates the proportion of phenotypic variance due to additive genetic effects from all common SNPs. These approaches are characterized by extremely large (often multi- centered) samples which at times may also lead to het-erogeneity in phenotype measurement. GWAS and GCTA are less applicative in the domain of motor control due to the typically small sample sizes in this field, and the low levels of replication (Colhoun, McKeigue, & Davey Smith, 2003).

The candidate gene model examines the association between specific pheno-types and genetic variants of known function (or genetic variants that lie in or near genes of known function) relevant to the biological systems hypothesized to play a role in the studied phenotype (e.g., motor control and motor learning). Therefore, the focus of candidate gene/genetic variants studies of motor control and motor learning has centered on common genetic variation in the dopaminer-gic system. The dopaminergic system is characterized by its important role in executive function, learning, and reward, and therefore carries neurobiological relevance to motor learning and motor control.

The dopaminergic system

The dopaminergic system (see Figure 2.2) is a group of nerve cells, most of which originate in the midbrain. Dopaminergic neurons (dopamine-producing nerve cells) are comparatively few in number (~ around 400,000 in the human brain), but their axons project to different parts of the forebrain, where they plug into particular functions (Arias-Carrión, Stamelou, Murillo-Rodíguez, Menéndez-González, & Pöppel, 2010).

The largest and most important sources of dopamine neurons are the *substantia nigra* and *ventral tegmental area* (VTA), which are components of the basal ganglia. The substantia nigra is a small midbrain area, that has two parts – an input area called *pars compacta* and an output area, the *pars reticulata*. The dopaminergic neurons are found mainly in the pars compacta (Björklund & Dunnett, 2007; Haber, Fudge, & McFarland, 2000). VTA dopaminergic neurons project via the mesolimbic pathway, which play a central role in reward and other aspects of motivation (Malenka, Nestler, & Hyman, 2009).

The dopaminergic neurons produce the enzymes that synthesize dopamine (3,4-dihydroxyphenethylamine, DA), which plays important roles in many

DOPAMINE SYSTEM

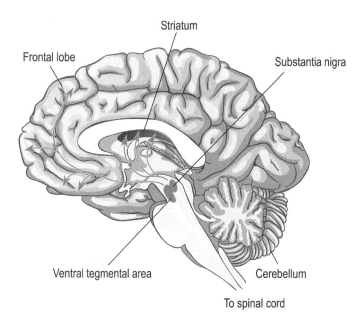

Figure 2.2 Dopaminergic system.

central functions including reward, learning, motivation, response to stimuli, and movement (Smythies, 2005), arousal, reinforcement, reward, and more (Arias-Carrión & Pöppel, 2007; Björklund & Dunnett, 2007; Malenka et al., 2009; McAllister, 2009).

In the central nervous system, DA is synthesized from the aromatic amino acid tyrosine, in the presynaptic neuron. Two reactions transform tyrosine into DA: the first is catalyzed by the enzyme tyrosine hydroxylase, which converts tyrosine into l-3,4-dihydroxyphenylalanine (l-DOPA) (Vallone, Picetti, & Borrelli, 2000). The second process is the decarboxylation of DOPA to DA by the enzyme aromatic l-amino acid decarboxylase (AADC) (Vallone et al., 2000). Dopamine action is mediated by dopamine receptors. There are at least five sub-types of dopamine receptors, D1, D2, D3, D4, and D5. The D1 and D5 receptors are members of the D1-like family of dopamine receptors, whereas the D2, D3, and D4 receptors are members of the D2-like family (Velasco et al., 2002). The two dopamine receptor families interact with each other (Dziedzicka-Wasylewska, 2004; Seeman & Tallerico, 2003) and with other neuro transmitters such as gamma-amino-butyric acid (GABA) (Acosta-García et al., 2009), glutamate (Sesack, Carr, Omelchenko, & Pinto, 2003), GABA (González-Hernández & Rodríguez, 2000), acetylcholine (Sanz, Badia, & Clos, 2000), and serotonin (Esposito, Di Matteo, & Di Giovanni, 2008). Dopamine receptors are found in nearly all areas of the brain, but are most expressed in nigrostriatal and mesolimbic regions (Dearry et al., 1990; Hurley & Jenner, 2006). The dopamine receptors differ in their affinity for dopamine, natural ligands, receptor activity, anatomical locations, genetic sequence, and thus, physiological activity (Callier et al., 2003). Dopamine receptor expression can be affected by the levels of dopamine in the system (Giros, Jaber, Jones, Wightman, & Caron, 1996), pharmacological agents (Buckland, O'Donovan, & McGuffin, 1992), and other external stimuli mediated through rewarding behavior such as sexual activity (Melis & Argiolas, 1995), or exercise (Foley et al., 2006). DA is degraded through several mechanisms (Meiser, Weindl, & Hiller, 2013): neuronal reuptake by dopamine transporter (DAT), oxidative deamination by monoamine oxidase (MAO), and by catechol-O methyl transferase (COMT). A summary of DA metabolic pathways is presented in Figure 2.3.

Based on the dopamine metabolic pathways, several dopaminergic genes are identified (see Figure 2.4). The identification of dopaminergic system transfers them into natural candidates in any study of the genetic basis of motor performance.

The dopaminergic genetic basis of motor skills

Signals of midbrain dopaminergic neurons play a pivotal role in the induction of long-term synaptic plasticity and motor skill acquisition (Kawashima et al., 2012; Molina-Luna et al., 2009; Wickens, Reynolds, & Hyland, 2003). In

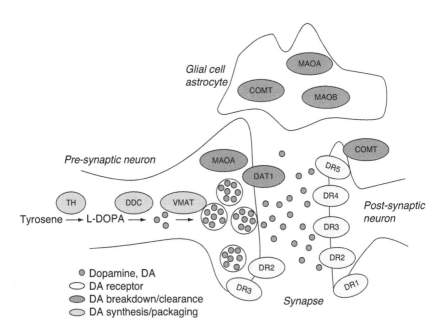

Figure 2.3 Dopamine metabolic pathways.

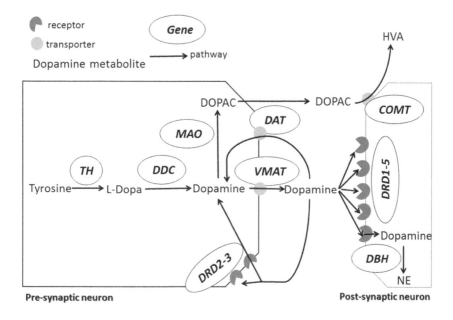

Figure 2.4 Genes related to dopaminergic system.

humans, the respective cortico-striatal circuit contributes to the encoding and consolidation of motor sequence memory, thereby providing the basis for the learning and automatization of motor skills. Automatization is associated with task control that shifts from an initially attentional to a predominantly non-attentional control as practice proceeds and the respective skill representation is consolidated (Doyon et al., 2009; Keele, Ivry, Mayr, Hazeltine, & Heuer, 2003).

Nigrostriatal DA is critical for motor learning (Malenka et al., 2009; Miyachi, Hikosaka, & Lu, 2002; Packard & Knowlton, 2002), presumably through modulation of synaptic plasticity in the striatum (Reynolds & Wickens, 2000). Despite considerable evidence that DA mediates both motor performance and learning, isolating these separate functions of DA, and the relationship between them, remains challenging.

Dopamine genetic polymorphism and motor skills

Identifying genetic variants related to motor skills variation via the candidate genes approach requires prior knowledge about gene function. The candidate gene approach begins with selection of a putative candidate gene based on its relevance in the mechanism of the trait being investigated. This is followed by assessing and selecting polymorphisms, usually the tag SNPs, and/or having a functional consequence, either by affecting gene regulation or its protein product. Finally, the gene variant is verified for trait association by observing its occurrence in random test subjects caring the trait and the selected control subjects, which do not carry the trait (Kwon & Goate, 2000; Patnala, Clements, & Batra, 2013).

Polymorphisms in the genes encoding for dopamine receptors and degradation enzymes contribute to inter-individual differences in learning (Doll, Hutchinson, & Frank, 2011) and performance variation in factors ranging from neuroanatomical phenotypes such as cortical size or integrity of gray/white matter (Rimol et al., 2010) to the function and availability of various neurochemicals; mainly, polymorphisms that reduce dopamine neurotransmission thought to impair learning and cognitive performance, and those that increase dopamine neurotransmission improving these behaviors (Egan et al., 2001; McAllister et al., 2008).

Pioneering results suggest the possibility that variation in the genetics of dopamine neurotransmission might affect motor learning and motor cortex plasticity. Abundant evidence supports the role of dopamine in learning and cortical plasticity in the motor system (Hosp, Pekanovic, Rioult-Pedotti, & Luft, 2011; Luft & Schwarz, 2009; Molina-Luna et al., 2009). Furthermore, the principle that genetic variability can influence motor learning and motor cortex plasticity in humans has been established, mainly with polymorphism in the *BDNF* (Kleim et al., 2006; McHughen, Pearson-Fuhrhop, Ngo, & Cramer, 2011). However, little is known regarding the influence that dopamine-related gene variants have on learning and cortical plasticity in the healthy motor system.

Substitution of the α-amino acids valine (val) and methionine (met) in *COMT* gene encoding to COMT (rs4680 Val158Met polymorphism) affects the activity of the COMT enzyme, with the met allele being associated with increased availability of intrasynaptic dopamine (Matsumoto et al., 2003). As a result, met-carriers exhibit higher prefrontal dopamine levels (i.e., more baseline synaptic dopamine). The number of met-alleles has also been found to be associated with enhanced performance in tasks which demand active manipulation and maintenance of information; these features are related to prefrontal mediated cognition, working memory, and executive functioning (Dickinson & Elvevåg, 2009).

Motor skill acquisition is extensively dependent on reinforcement, and on the provision of error information. In this context, processing of reward signals obviously plays a crucial role. These processes are also closely linked to the dopaminergic system and are afforded by the prevalence of specific *COMT* genotypes: neural activities in the primate orbitofrontal cortex (OFC), striatum (caudate, putamen, and ventral striatum including nucleus accumbens), and midbrain (VTA and substantia nigra) dopaminergic neurons related to the expectation and delivery of reward (particularly if unexpected). Activities in the respective striatal neurons are also related to the preparation, initiation, and execution of movements, which reflect the expected rewards (Schultz, Tremblay, & Hollerman, 2000). These findings gave rise to the hypothesis that phasic DA cell activity encodes a reward prediction error, which is critical for reinforcement-dependent learning (Dayan & Niv, 2008; Glimcher, 2011).

Moreover, Dreher, Kohn, Kolachana, Weinberger, and Berman, (2009) found interactions of neural activation during reward processing and *COMT* genotype, with met-carriers exhibiting higher bilateral activations in the OFC, which may have important functions for discriminating the relative value of rewards and maintaining recent reward information experiences in an "active working memory-like state" (Frank & Fossella, 2011). *COMT* val-val carriers demonstrated poorer performance in the sequence learning task compared with the met-met carriers and showed a learning deficit in the visuo-motor adaptation task compared with both met-met and val-met carriers (Noohi et al., 2014)

A significant body of research, comprehensively reviewed by Noohi et al. (2014), has examined how the DRD2 G>T polymorphism affects motor performance through its influence on dopamine systems. Their review highlighted that this genetic variation plays a crucial role in regulating dopamine receptor expression in the striatum. Building on previous findings (Doll et al., 2011; Xu et al., 2007), they emphasized the importance of D2 receptor activity for motor control, coordination, and error avoidance processes.Research has shown that carriers of the T allele variant of the DRD2 gene (rs 1076560) exhibit reduced D2 expression patterns. As Noohi and colleagues (2014) discussed, this reduction appears to result in decreased cognitive processing abilities and impaired motor performance, as initially reported by Bertolino et al. (2009). Furthermore, neuroimaging studies have revealed that T allele carriers show more extensive brain activation patterns during working memory tasks while achieving lower performance levels, suggesting less efficient neural processing (Zhang et al., 2007; as cited in Noohi et al., 2014).Seidler and Carson (2017) provided an important analysis of findings from Noohi et al.'s (2014) research on genetic variations in motor learning. Their review highlighted a particularly interesting observation: while COMT variations influenced how quickly individuals adapted to visuomotor tasks, these same genetic differences did not affect their ability to learn motor sequences. Based on this finding, Seidler and Carson (2017) proposed that different types of motor tasks may be influenced by distinct genetic mechanisms, suggesting a more complex relationship between genetic factors and motor learning than previously thought

Taken together, these findings concerning increased prefrontal dopamine availability and enhanced dopamine-dependent reward processing in met-carriers might bear relevance to motor automatization, in that met-carriers are liable to establish and consolidate a sufficient skill representation – and thereby reduce the need of a predominantly cognitive mode of control – considerably sooner than val-carriers. Several met-alleles indicated a tendency toward enhanced motor automatization. Thus, due to an increased prefrontal dopamine level, met-carriers may be able to develop a well formed and stable, spatially coded movement representation early in practice, thereby supporting the formation of a representation in motor coordinates during extended practice, which later enables automatic movement execution. This process might also be enhanced by a prevalence of met-carriers to functionally evaluate positive feedback information (i.e., rewards), and to better maintain recent reward information in active working memory (Krause, Beck, Agetjen, & Blischke, 2014).

In their comprehensive review of genetic influences on motor control and learning, Seidler and Carson (2017) identified BDNF as one of the most extensively studied dopaminergic genetic variants. The protein, which begins as proBDNF before being cleaved into its mature form (Seidah et al., 1996), plays crucial roles in multiple neural processes including neurogenesis, synaptogenesis, synaptic transmission, and various cognitive functions. Research has particularly focused on the Val66Met polymorphism, where valine is substituted with methionine at position 66 in the prodomain. As discussed by Seidler and Carson (2017), studies have shown that Val-val carriers demonstrate enhanced motor potentials (MEPs) following movement repetition, with both larger scalp areas producing MEPs and higher MEP amplitudes compared to met allele carriers (Kleim et al., 2006). However, while numerous studies have examined this polymorphism's effects on short-term motor performance, longitudinal research examining retention and transfer effects on motor learning remains limited (McHughen et al., 2010; Nooshabadi et al., 2016).

Seidler and Carson (2017) identified several key methodological challenges in studying BDNF's role in motor learning. Despite strong evidence of BDNF's influence on neural processes from animal studies, its impact on human motor learning remains unclear. They highlighted two major issues: (1) Sample size requirements: Adequate statistical power for testing single SNPs typically requires at least 248 cases (Hong & Park, 2012), making many existing studies underpowered (Button et al., 2013). They noted that researchers often face a trade-off between high-reliability measures with small samples and lower-reliability measures with larger samples, with the latter potentially being more valuable for genetic analyses (Chabris et al., 2013); (2) Replication challenges: As Seidler and Carson (2017) emphasized, determining whether associations between genotypes and motor function represent true effects or false positives remains difficult. They noted that meta-analyses in related fields have shown diminishing effect sizes in follow-up studies (Gyekis et al., 2013; Kavvoura et al., 2008; Molendijk et al., 2012), a common issue in candidate gene studies across various domains (Duncan & Keller, 2011).

Another constraint is the polygenic nature of most of the motor proficiency traits. Since probably large number of genes and genetic variants are involved in motor control and motor learning, each of which makes only a small contribution to a person's motor proficiency, the genotype space creates many possible pathways toward the phenotype space as described in Figure 2.5.

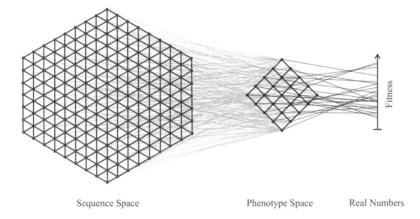

Sequence Space   Phenotype Space   Real Numbers

Figure 2.5 Genotype-phenotype space.

Source: reprinted with permission from Schuster (2002). From https://en.paperblog.com/genotype-phenotype-maps-and-mathy-biology-317240/.

In reviewing approaches to studying genetic influences on motor learning, Seidler and Carson (2017) discussed a notable study by Pearson-Fuhrhop et al. (2013). This research took an innovative approach by developing a combined genetic score based on five polymorphisms known to affect dopamine neurotransmission. The researchers examined variations in multiple dopamine-related genes: three dopamine receptor genes (DRD1, DRD2, and DRD3) and two genes encoding dopamine degradation enzymes (COMT and DAT).The study assessed motor learning using a manual dexterity sequencing task. By incorporating prior knowledge about how these genetic variations affect dopamine neurotransmission in cognitive and learning contexts, the researchers created a comprehensive gene score. Their results showed that participants with higher gene scores, indicating greater endogenous dopaminergic neurotransmission, performed better after two weeks of training.However, as Seidler and Carson (2017) critically noted in their analysis, while these findings confirmed the dopaminergic system's involvement in motor learning, they did not substantially advance our understanding of the specific mechanisms through which these genetic variations influence motor learning processes.

Moving forward to more sophisticated approaches, such as gene pathway association analyses, and gene expression studies, is necessary for uncovering genetic architectures and gene-environment interaction of complex traits (Xiong, Ancona, Hauser, Mukherjee, & Furey, 2012) such as motor proficiency (Rama-samy et al., 2014).

Summary

Motor skills are multifactorial traits, hence influenced by both genes and environment, as well as the interaction between them. Identifying genetic variants related to motor skills, motor learning, and motor control variation is complicated since each genetic variant might have a small contribution to the overall phenotype, and due to methodological constraints dictated by the nature of motor proficiency study. Therefore, other approaches such as gene expression studies must be considered. The field of genetic analysis in motor proficiency, though relatively new, shows considerable promise for future research. According to Seidler and Carson's (2017) assessment, this developing area has the potential to significantly advance our knowledge of how humans control and learn motor skills.

References

Acosta-García, J., Hernández-Chan, N., Paz-Bermúdez, F., Sierra, A., Erlij, D., Aceves,

J., & Florán, B. (2009). D4 and D1 dopamine receptors modulate [3H]GABA release in the substantia nigra pars reticulata of the rat. *Neuropharmacology, 57*(7–8), 725–30. https://doi.org/10.1016/j.neuropharm.2009.08.010

Adolph, K. E., & Robinson, S. R. (2011). *Motor development.* New York, NY: Schmuckler Smitsman and Corbetta Vollmer and Forssberg. Retrieved from www.psych.nyu. edu/adolph/publications/AdolphRobinson-inpress-MussenMotorDev.pdf

Anderson, J. R. (1983). *The architecture of cognition.* Cambridge, MA: Harvard University Press.

Arias-Carrión, O., & Pöppel, E. (2007). Dopamine, learning, and reward-seeking behavior. *Acta Neurobiologiae Experimentalis, 67*(4), 481–8. Retrieved from www. ncbi.nlm.nih.gov/pubmed/18320725

Arias-Carrión, O., Stamelou, M., Murillo-Rodríguez, E., Menéndez-González, M., & Pöppel, E. (2010). Dopaminergic reward system: A short integrative review. *International Archives of Medicine, 3*, 24. https://doi.org/10.1186/1755-7682-3-24

Belmont, J. W., Boudreau, A., Leal, S. M., Hardenbol, P., Pasternak, S., Wheeler, D. A., … Stewart, J. (2005). A haplotype map of the human genome. *Nature, 437*(7063), 1299–320. https://doi.org/10.1038/nature04226

Bertolino, A., Fazio, L., Caforio, G., Blasi, G., Rampino, A., Romano, R., … Sadee, W. (2009). Functional variants of the dopamine receptor D2 gene modulate prefronto-striatal phenotypes in schizophrenia. *Brain, 132*(2), 417–25. https://doi.org/10.1093/brain/awn248

Björklund, A., & Dunnett, S. B. (2007). Dopamine neuron systems in the brain: An update. *Trends in Neurosciences, 30*(5), 194–202. https://doi.org/10.1016/j.tins.2007.03.006

Buckland, P. R., O'Donovan, M. C., & McGuffin, P. (1992). Changes in dopamine D1, D2 and D3 receptor mRNA levels in rat brain following antipsychotic treatment. *Psychopharmacology, 106*(4), 479–83. Retrieved from www.ncbi.nlm.nih.gov/pubmed/1349752

Button, K. S., Ioannidis, J. P. A., Mokrysz, C., Nosek, B. A., Flint, J., Robinson, E. S. J., & Munafò, M. R. (2013). Power failure: Why small sample size undermines the reliability of neuroscience. *Nature Reviews Neuroscience, 14*(5), 365–76. https://doi.org/10.1038/nrn3475

Callier, S., Snapyan, M., Le Crom, S., Prou, D., Vincent, J.-D., & Vernier, P. (2003). Evolution and cell biology of dopamine receptors in vertebrates. *Biology of the Cell, 95*(7), 489–502. Retrieved from www.ncbi.nlm.nih.gov/pubmed/14597267

Chabris, C. F., Lee, J. J., Benjamin, D. J., Beauchamp, J. P., Glaeser, E. L., Borst, G., … Laibson, D. I. (2013). Why it is hard to find genes associated with social science traits:

Theoretical and empirical considerations. *American Journal of Public Health, 103*(Suppl. 1), S152–66. https://doi.org/10.2105/AJPH.2013.301327

Colhoun, H. M., McKeigue, P. M., & Davey Smith, G. (2003). Problems of reporting genetic associations with complex outcomes. *Lancet, 361*(9360), 865–72. Retrieved from www.ncbi.nlm.nih.gov/pubmed/12642066

Dayan, P., & Niv, Y. (2008). Reinforcement learning: The good, the bad and the ugly. *Current Opinion in Neurobiology, 18*(2), 185–96. https://doi.org/10.1016/j.conb.2008.08.003

Dearry, A., Gingrich, J. A., Falardeau, P., Fremeau, R. T., Bates, M. D., & Caron, M. G. (1990). Molecular cloning and expression of the gene for a human D1 dopamine receptor. *Nature, 347*(6288), 72–6. https://doi.org/10.1038/347072a0

Dickinson, D., & Elvevåg, B. (2009). Genes, cognition and brain through a COMT lens. *Neuroscience, 164*(1), 72–87. https://doi.org/10.1016/j.neuroscience.2009.05.014

Doll, B. B., Hutchison, K. E., & Frank, M. J. (2011). Dopaminergic genes predict individual differences in susceptibility to confirmation bias. *The Journal of Neuroscience: The Official Journal of the Society for Neuroscience, 31*(16), 6188–98. https://doi.org/10.1523/JNEUROSCI.6486-10.2011

Doyon, J., Bellec, P., Amsel, R., Penhune, V., Monchi, O., Carrier, J., … Benali, H. (2009). Contributions of the basal ganglia and functionally related brain structures to motor learning. *Behavioural Brain Research, 199*(1), 61–75. https://doi.org/10.1016/j.bbr.2008.11.012

Dreher, J.-C., Kohn, P., Kolachana, B., Weinberger, D. R., & Berman, K. F. (2009). Variation in dopamine genes influences responsivity of the human reward system. *Proceedings of the National Academy of Sciences of the United States of America, 106*(2), 617–22. https://doi.org/10.1073/pnas.0805517106

Duncan, L. E., & Keller, M. C. (2011). A critical review of the first 10 years of candidate gene-by-environment interaction research in psychiatry. *American Journal of Psychiatry, 168*(10), 1041–9. https://doi.org/10.1176/appi.ajp. 2011.11020191

Dunham, I., Kundaje, A., Aldred, S. F., Collins, P. J., Davis, C. A., Doyle, F., … Birney, E. (2012). An integrated encyclopedia of DNA elements in the human genome. *Nature, 489*(7414), 57–74. https://doi.org/10.1038/nature11247

Dziedzicka-Wasylewska, M. (2004). Brain dopamine receptors–research perspectives and potential sites of regulation. *Polish Journal of Pharmacology, 56*(6), 659–71. Retrieved from www.ncbi.nlm.nih.gov/pubmed/15662079

Egan, M. F., Goldberg, T. E., Kolachana, B. S., Callicott, J. H., Mazzanti, C. M., Straub, R. E., … Weinberger, D. R. (2001). Effect of COMT Val108/158 Met genotype on frontal lobe function and risk for schizophrenia. *Proceedings of the National Academy of Sciences of the United States of America, 98*(12), 6917–22. https://doi.org/10.1073/pnas.111134598

Esposito, E., Di Matteo, V., & Di Giovanni, G. (2008). Serotonin–dopamine interaction: An overview. In E. Esposito, V. Di Matteo, & G. Di Giovanni (Eds.), *Serotonin–dopamine interaction: Experimental evidence and therapeutic relevance* (Vol. 172, pp. 3–6). Amsterdam, the Netherlands: Elsevier. https://doi.org/10.1016/S0079-6123(08)00901-1

Fitts, P. M., & Posner, M. I. (1967). *Human performance*. Belomont, CA: Brooks/Cole.

Foley, T., Greenwood, B., Day, H., Koch, L., Britton, S., & Fleshner, M. (2006). Elevated central monoamine receptor mRNA in rats bred for high endurance capacity: Implications for central fatigue. *Behavioural Brain Research, 174*(1), 132–42. https://doi.org/10.1016/j.bbr.2006.07.018

Fox, P. W., Hershberger, S. L., & Bouchard, T. J. (1996). Genetic and environmental contributions to the acquisition of a motor skill. *Nature, 384*(6607), 356–8. https://doi. org/10.1038/384356a0

Frank, M. J., & Fossella, J. A. (2011). Neurogenetics and pharmacology of learning, motivation, and cognition. *Neuropsychopharmacology: Official Publication of the American College of Neuropsychopharmacology, 36*(1), 133–52. https://doi. org/10.1038/npp. 2010.96

Giros, B., Jaber, M., Jones, S. R., Wightman, R. M., & Caron, M. G. (1996). Hyperloco-motion and indifference to cocaine and amphetamine in mice lacking the dopamine transporter. *Nature, 379*(6566), 606–12. https://doi.org/10.1038/379606a0

Glimcher, P. W. (2011). Understanding dopamine and reinforcement learning: The dopamine reward prediction error hypothesis. *Proceedings of the National Academy of Sciences, 108*(Suppl. 3), S15647–54. https://doi.org/10.1073/pnas.1014269108

González-Hernández, T., & Rodríguez, M. (2000). Compartmental organization and chemical profile of dopaminergic and GABAergic neurons in the substantia nigra of the rat. *The Journal of Comparative Neurology, 421*(1), 107–35. Retrieved from www. ncbi.nlm.nih.gov/pubmed/10813775

Gyekis, J. P., Yu, W., Dong, S., Wang, H., Qian, J., Kota, P., & Yang, J. (2013). No association of genetic variants in *BDNF* with major depression: A meta- and gene-based analysis. *American Journal of Medical Genetics Part B: Neuropsychiatric Genetics, 162*(1), 61–70. https://doi.org/10.1002/ajmg.b.32122

Haber, S. N., Fudge, J. L., & McFarland, N. R. (2000). Striatonigrostriatal pathways in primates form an ascending spiral from the shell to the dorsolateral striatum. *The Journal of Neuroscience: The Official Journal of the Society for Neuroscience, 20*(6), 2369–82. Retrieved from www.ncbi.nlm.nih.gov/pubmed/10704511

Hong, E. P., & Park, J. W. (2012). Sample size and statistical power calculation in genetic association studies. *Genomics and Informatics, 10*(2), 117. https://doi.org/10.5808/ GI.2012.10.2.117

Hosp, J. A., Pekanovic, A., Rioult-Pedotti, M. S., & Luft, A. R. (2011). Dopaminergic projections from midbrain to primary motor cortex mediate motor skill learning. *The Journal of Neuroscience: The Official Journal of the Society for Neuroscience, 31*(7), 2481–7. https://doi.org/10.1523/JNEUROSCI.5411-10.2011

Hurley, M. J., & Jenner, P. (2006). What has been learnt from study of dopamine receptors in Parkinson's disease? *Pharmacology and Therapeutics, 111*(3), 715–28. https://doi.org/10.1016/j.pharmthera.2005.12.001

Kavvoura, F. K., McQueen, M. B., Khoury, M. J., Tanzi, R. E., Bertram, L., & Ioannidis, J. P. A. (2008). Evaluation of the potential excess of statistically significant findings in published genetic association studies: Application to Alzheimer's disease. *American Journal of Epidemiology, 168*(8), 855–65. https://doi.org/10.1093/aje/kwn206

Kawashima, S., Ueki, Y., Kato, T., Matsukawa, N., Mima, T., Hallett, M., … Ojika, K. (2012). Changes in striatal dopamine release associated with human motor-skill acquisition. *PloS One, 7*(2), e31728. https://doi.org/10.1371/journal.pone.0031728

Keele, S. W., Ivry, R., Mayr, U., Hazeltine, E., & Heuer, H. (2003). The cognitive and neural architecture of sequence representation. *Psychological Review, 110*(2), 316–39. Retrieved from www.ncbi.nlm.nih.gov/pubmed/12747526

Kleim, J. A., Chan, S., Pringle, E., Schallert, K., Procaccio, V., Jimenez, R., & Cramer, S. C. (2006). BDNF val66met polymorphism is associated with modified experience-dependent plasticity in human motor cortex. *Nature Neuroscience, 9*(6), 735–7. https:// doi.org/10.1038/nn1699

Krause, D., Beck, F., Agethen, M., & Blischke, K. (2014). Effect of catechol-O-methyltransferase-val158met-polymorphism on the automatization of motor skills – A post hoc view on an experimental data. *Behavioural Brain Research, 266*, 169–73. https://doi.org/10.1016/j.bbr.2014.02.037

Kuntsi, J., Rogers, H., Swinard, G., Börger, N., van der Meere, J., Rijsdijk, F., & Asherson, P. (2006). Reaction time, inhibition, working memory and "delay aversion" performance: Genetic influences and their interpretation. *Psychological Medicine, 36*(11), 1613–24. https://doi.org/10.1017/S0033291706008580

Kwon, J. M., & Goate, A. M. (2000). The candidate gene approach. *Alcohol Research and Health: The Journal of the National Institute on Alcohol Abuse and Alcoholism, 24*(3), 164–8. Retrieved from www.ncbi.nlm.nih.gov/pubmed/11199286

Lander, E. S., Linton, L. M., Birren, B., Nusbaum, C., Zody, M. C., Baldwin, J., … International Human Genome Sequencing Consortium. (2001). Initial sequencing and analysis of the human genome. *Nature, 409*(6822), 860–921. https://doi.org/10.1038/35057062

Latash, M. L., Levin, M. F., Scholz, J. P., & Schöner, G. (2010). Motor control theories and their applications. *Medicina, 46*(6), 382–92. Retrieved from www.ncbi.nlm.nih.gov/pubmed/20944446

Luft, A. R., & Schwarz, S. (2009). Dopaminergic signals in primary motor cortex. *International Journal of Developmental Neuroscience: The Official Journal of the International Society for Developmental Neuroscience, 27*(5), 415–21. https://doi.org/10.1016/j.ijdevneu.2009.05.004

Maes, H. H., Beunen, G. P., Vlietinck, R. F., Neale, M. C., Thomis, M., Vanden Eynde, B., … Derom, R. (1996). Inheritance of physical fitness in 10-yr-old twins and their parents. *Medicine and Science in Sports and Exercise, 28*(12), 1479–91. Retrieved from www.ncbi.nlm.nih.gov/pubmed/8970142

Malenka, R., Nestler, E., & Hyman, S. (2009). Widely projecting systems: Monoamines, acetylcholine, and orexin. In A. Sydor & R. Brown (Eds.), *Molecular neuropharmacology: A foundation for clinical neuroscience* (2nd ed., pp. 147–57). New York, NY: McGraw-Hill Medical.

Matsumoto, M., Weickert, C. S., Akil, M., Lipska, B. K., Hyde, T. M., Herman, M. M., … Weinberger, D. R. (2003). Catechol O-methyltransferase mRNA expression in human and rat brain: Evidence for a role in cortical neuronal function. *Neuroscience, 116*(1), 127–37. Retrieved from www.ncbi.nlm.nih.gov/pubmed/12535946

McAllister, T. W. (2009). Polymorphisms in genes modulating the dopamine system. *Journal of Head Trauma Rehabilitation, 24*(1), 65–8. https://doi.org/10.1097/HTR.0b013e3181996e6b

McAllister, T. W., Flashman, L. A., Harker Rhodes, C., Tyler, A. L., Moore, J. H., Saykin, A. J., … Tsongalis, G. J. (2008). Single nucleotide polymorphisms in ANKK1 and the dopamine D2 receptor gene affect cognitive outcome shortly after traumatic brain injury: A replication and extension study. *Brain Injury, 22*(9), 705–14. https://doi.org/10.1080/02699050802263019

McHughen, S. A., Pearson-Fuhrhop, K., Ngo, V. K., & Cramer, S. C. (2011). Intense training overcomes effects of the Val66Met BDNF polymorphism on short-term plasticity. *Experimental Brain Research, 213*(4), 415–22. https://doi.org/10.1007/s00221-011-2791-z

McHughen, S. A., Rodriguez, P. F., Kleim, J. A., Kleim, E. D., Crespo, L. M., Procaccio, V., & Cramer, S. C. (2010). BDNF val66met polymorphism influences motor system function in the human brain. *Cerebral Cortex, 20*(5), 1254–62. https://doi.org/10.1093/cercor/bhp189

Meiser, J., Weindl, D., & Hiller, K. (2013). Complexity of dopamine metabolism. *Cell Communication and Signaling: CCS, 11*(1), 34. https://doi.org/10.1186/1478-811X-11-34

Melis, M. R., & Argiolas, A. (1995). Dopamine and sexual behavior. *Neuroscience and Biobehavioral Reviews, 19*(1), 19–38. Retrieved from www.ncbi.nlm.nih.gov/pubmed/7770195

Missitzi, J., Geladas, N., & Klissouras, V. (2004). Heritability in neuromuscular coordination: Implications for motor control strategies. *Medicine and Science in Sports and Exercise, 36*(2), 233–40. https://doi.org/10.1249/01.MSS.0000113479.98631.C4

Missitzi, J., Gentner, R., Misitzi, A., Geladas, N., Politis, P., Klissouras, V., & Classen, J. (2013). Heritability of motor control and motor learning. *Physiological Reports, 1*(7), e00188. https://doi.org/10.1002/phy2.188

Missitzi, J., Gentner, R., Misitzi, A., Nickos, G., Panagiotis, P., Klissouras, V., & Classen, J. (2013). Heritability of motor control and motor learning. *Physiological Reports, 1*(17), e00188.

Miyachi, S., Hikosaka, O., & Lu, X. (2002). Differential activation of monkey striatal neurons in the early and late stages of procedural learning. *Experimental Brain Research, 146*(1), 122–6. https://doi.org/10.1007/s00221-002-1213-7

Molendijk, M. L., Bus, B. A. A., Spinhoven, P., Kaimatzoglou, A., Voshaar, R. C. O., Penninx, B. W. J. H., … Elzinga, B. M. (2012). A systematic review and meta-analysis on the association between BDNF val66met and hippocampal volume – A genuine effect or a winners curse? *American Journal of Medical Genetics Part B: Neuropsychiatric Genetics, 159B*(6), 731–40. https://doi.org/10.1002/ajmg.b.32078

Molina-Luna, K., Pekanovic, A., Röhrich, S., Hertler, B., Schubring-Giese, M., Rioult-Pedotti, M.-S., & Luft, A. R. (2009). Dopamine in motor cortex is necessary for skill learning and synaptic plasticity. *PloS One, 4*(9), e7082. https://doi.org/10.1371/journal.pone.0007082

Newell, A., & Rosenbloom, P. S. (1981). Mechanisms of skill acquisition and the law of practice. In J. R. Anderson (Ed.), *Cognitive skills and their acquisition* (pp. 1–55). Hillsdale, NJ: Laurence Erlbaum.

Nikolova, Y. S., Ferrell, R. E., Manuck, S. B., & Hariri, A. R. (2011). Multilocus genetic profile for dopamine signaling predicts ventral striatum reactivity. *Neuropsychopharmacology, 36*(9), 1940–7. https://doi.org/10.1038/npp. 2011.82

Noohi, F., Boyden, N. B., Kwak, Y., Humfleet, J., Burke, D. T., Müller, M. L. T. M., … Seidler, R. D. (2014). Association of COMT val158met and DRD2 Gandgt; T genetic polymorphisms with individual differences in motor learning and performance in female young adults. *Journal of Neurophysiology, 111*(3), 628–40. https://doi.org/10.1152/jn.00457.2013

Nooshabadi, A. S., Kakhki, A. S., Sohrabi, M., & Dowlati, M. A. (2016). Do environmental factors (practice and feedback) moderate the effect of the val66met BDNF polymorphism on motor learning? *Biosciences, Biotechnology Research Asia, 13*(2), 1037–44. https://doi.org/10.13005/bbra/2130

Packard, M. G., & Knowlton, B. J. (2002). Learning and memory functions of the basal ganglia. *Annual Review of Neuroscience, 25*(1), 563–93. https://doi.org/10.1146/annurev.neuro.112701.142937

Patnala, R., Clements, J., & Batra, J. (2013). Candidate gene association studies: A comprehensive guide to useful in silico tools. *BMC Genetics, 14*, 39. https://doi.org/10.1186/1471-2156-14-39

Pearson-Fuhrhop, K. M., Minton, B., Acevedo, D., Shahbaba, B., & Cramer, S. C. (2013). Genetic variation in the human brain dopamine system influences motor learning and its modulation by l-dopa. *PloS One, 8*(4), e61197. https://doi.org/10.1371/journal.pone.0061197

Pellicciari, M. C., Veniero, D., Marzano, C., Moroni, F., Pirulli, C., Curcio, G., … De Gennaro, L. (2009). Heritability of intracortical inhibition and facilitation. *Journal of Neuroscience, 29*(28), 8897–900. https://doi.org/10.1523/JNEUROSCI.2112-09.2009

Proctor, R. W., & Dutta, A. (1995). *Skill acquisition and human performance.* Thousand Oaks, CA: Sage.

Ramasamy, A., Trabzuni, D., Guelfi, S., Varghese, V., Smith, C., Walker, R., … Weale, M. E. (2014). Genetic variability in the regulation of gene expression in ten regions of the human brain. *Nature Neuroscience, 17*(10), 1418–28. https://doi.org/10.1038/nn.3801

Rasmussen, J. (1986). *Information processing and human-machine interaction: An approach to cognitive engineering* (North-Holland Series in System Science and Engineering, 12). Amsterdam, the Netherlands: North-Holland.

Reynolds, J. N., & Wickens, J. R. (2000). Substantia nigra dopamine regulates synaptic plasticity and membrane potential fluctuations in the rat neostriatum, in vivo. *Neuroscience, 99*(2), 199–203. Retrieved from www.ncbi.nlm.nih.gov/pubmed/10938425

Rimol, L. M., Panizzon, M. S., Fennema-Notestine, C., Eyler, L. T., Fischl, B., Franz, C. E., … Dale, A. M. (2010). Cortical thickness is influenced by regionally specific genetic factors. *Biological Psychiatry, 67*(5), 493–9.

Sanz, A. G., Badia, A., & Clos, M. V. (2000). Role of calcium on the modulation of spontaneous acetylcholine efflux by the D2 dopamine receptor subtype in rat striatal synaptosomes. *Brain Research, 854*(1–2), 42–7. Retrieved from www.ncbi.nlm.nih.gov/pubmed/10784105

Schmidt, R. A., & Lee, T. D. (2014). *Motor learning and performance* (5th ed.). Champaign, IL: Human Kinetics.

Schuler, G. D., Boguski, M. S., Stewart, E. A., Stein, L. D., Gyapay, G., Rice, K., … Hudson, T. J. (1996). A gene map of the human genome. *Science, 274*(5287), 540–6. Retrieved from www.ncbi.nlm.nih.gov/pubmed/8849440

Schultz, W., Tremblay, L., & Hollerman, J. R. (2000). Reward processing in primate orbitofrontal cortex and basal ganglia. *Cerebral Cortex, 10*(3), 272–84. Retrieved from www.ncbi.nlm.nih.gov/pubmed/10731222

Schuster, P. (2002). A testable genotype-phenotype map: Modeling evolution of RNA molecules. In M. Lässig & A. Valleriani (Eds.), *Biological evolution and statistical physics. Lecture notes in physics* (Vol. 585, pp. 55–81). Berlin; Heidelberg, Germany: Springer.

Seeman, P., & Tallerico, T. (2003). Link between dopamine D1 and D2 receptors in rat and human striatal tissues. *Synapse, 47*(4), 250–4. https://doi.org/10.1002/syn.10171

Seidah, N. G., Benjannet, S., Pareek, S., Chrétien, M., & Murphy, R. A. (1996). Cellular processing of the neurotrophin precursors of NT3 and BDNF by the mammalian pro-protein convertases. *FEBS Letters, 379*(3), 247–50. Retrieved from www.ncbi.nlm.nih.gov/pubmed/8603699

Seidler, R. D., & Carson, R. G. (2017). Sensorimotor learning: Neurocognitive mechanisms and individual differences. *Journal of Neuroengineering and Rehabilitation, 14*(1), 74. https://doi.org/10.1186/s12984-017-0279-1

Sesack, S. R., Carr, D. B., Omelchenko, N., & Pinto, A. (2003). Anatomical substrates for glutamate-dopamine interactions: Evidence for specificity of connections and extra-synaptic actions. *Annals of the New York Academy of Sciences, 1003*, 36–52. Retrieved from www.ncbi.nlm.nih.gov/pubmed/14684434

Smythies, J. (2005). The dopamine system. In *International review of neurobiology* (Vol. 64, Section II, pp. 123–72). https://doi.org/10.1016/S0074-7742(05)64002-0

Starkes, J. L., Deakin, J., Allard, F., Hodges, N., & Hayes, A. (1996). Deliberate practice in sports: What is it anyway? In K. Ericsson (Ed.), *The road to excellence: The acquisition of expert performance in the arts and sciences, sports and games* (pp. 81–106). Mahwah, NJ: Lawrence Erlbaum Associates.

Starkes, J. L., & Ericsson, K. A. (2003). *Expert performance in sport.* Champaign, IL: Human Kinetics.

Stice, E., Yokum, S., Burger, K., Epstein, L., & Smolen, A. (2012). Multilocus genetic composite reflecting dopamine signaling capacity predicts reward circuitry responsivity. *Journal of Neuroscience, 32*(29), 10093–100. https://doi.org/10.1523/JNEUROSCI.1506-12.2012

Tenenbaum, G., Hatfield, B., Eklund, R. C., Land, W., Camielo, L., Razon, S., & Schack, K. A. (2009). Conceptual framework for studying emotions-cognitions-performance linkage under conditions which vary in perceived pressure. In M. Raab., J. G. Johnson., & H. Heekeren (Eds.), *Progress in brain research: Mind and motion – The bidirectional link between thought and action* (pp. 159–78). Amsterdam, the Netherlands: Elsevier.

Vallone, D., Picetti, R., & Borrelli, E. (2000). Structure and function of dopamine receptors. *Neuroscience & Biobehavioral Reviews, 24*(1), 125–32.

Velasco, M., Contreras, F., Cabezas, G. A., Bolívar, A., Fouillioux, C., & Hernández, R. (2002). Dopaminergic receptors: A new antihypertensive mechanism. *Journal of Hypertension. Supplement: Official Journal of the International Society of Hypertension, 20*(Suppl. 3), S55–8. Retrieved from www.ncbi.nlm.nih.gov/pubmed/12184056

Venter, J. C., Adams, M. D., Myers, E. W., Li, P. W., Mural, R. J., Sutton, G. G., … Zhu, X. (2001). The sequence of the human genome. *Science, 291*(5507), 1304–51. https://doi.org/10.1126/science.1058040

Wickens, J. R., Reynolds, J. N. J., & Hyland, B. I. (2003). Neural mechanisms of reward-related motor learning. *Current Opinion in Neurobiology, 13*(6), 685–90. Retrieved from www.ncbi.nlm.nih.gov/pubmed/14662369

Williams, L. R., & Gross, J. B. (1980). Heritability of motor skill. *Acta Geneticae Medicae et Gemellologiae, 29*(2), 127–36. Retrieved from www.ncbi.nlm.nih.gov/pubmed/7196128

Wolpert, D. M., Ghahramani, Z., & Flanagan, J. R. (2001). Perspectives and problems in motor learning. *Trends in Cognitive Sciences, 5*(11), 487–94.

Xiong, Q., Ancona, N., Hauser, E. R., Mukherjee, S., & Furey, T. S. (2012). Integrating genetic and gene expression evidence into genome-wide association analysis of gene sets. *Genome Research, 22*(2), 386–97. https://doi.org/10.1101/gr.124370.111

Xu, H., Kellendonk, C., Simpson, E., Keilp, J., Bruder, G., Polan, H., … Gilliam, T. (2007). DRD2 C957T polymorphism interacts with the COMT Val158Met polymorphism in human working memory ability. *Schizophrenia Research, 90*(1–3), 104–7. https://doi.org/10.1016/j.schres.2006.10.001

Yarrow, K., Brown, P., & Krakauer, J. W. (2009). Inside the brain of an elite athlete: The neural processes that support high achievement in sports. *Nature Reviews Neuroscience, 10*(8), 585–96. https://doi.org/10.1038/nrn2672

Zhang, Y., Bertolino, A., Fazio, L., Blasi, G., Rampino, A., Romano, R., … Sadee, W. (2007). Polymorphisms in human dopamine D2 receptor gene affect gene expression, splicing, and neuronal activity during working memory. *Proceedings of the National Academy of Sciences, 104*(51), 20552–7. https://doi.org/10.1073/pnas.0707106104

3   Genetics and personality

Many personality traits have been associated with optimal performance such as determination, commitment, exertion and pain tolerance, grit, and so on. As personality contributes to an individual's enduring and distinctive patterns of feeling, thinking, and behaving, it can influence in many ways the performer's pathway toward excellence. It is generally accepted that both nature and nurture play an important role in the development of personality, but to what extent each affects us is still a point of major controversy. The field of study which is dedicated to understanding the genetic components of personality is called behavioral genetics. The goal of behavioral genetics is to uncover the genes that affect behavior.

Among the different psychological factors linked to motor proficiency, personality is one that is intuitively associated to genetics. This assumption relies on the consistent and enduring conceptualization that personality is not likely to change regardless of environmental conditions (Mosley & Laborde, 2015a). Consistent with this view, most of the researchers emphasize the role of genetic factors in maintaining personality stability throughout the lifespan, and the unique environmental factors acting to promote personality change (Allen, Greenlees, & Jones, 2013). Before exploring more in-depth the role of genetics in the expression of personality traits linked to motor proficiency, the state of the literature regarding the relationship between personality and motor performance is reviewed.

Definition and historical background

Personality is defined as "psychological qualities that contribute to an individual's enduring and distinctive patterns of feeling, thinking, and behaving" (Pervin & Cervone, 2010, p. 8). Since the first sport and exercise psychology laboratories were developed early in the twentieth century, personality was considered a dominant area of inquiry, and believed to significantly predict success in sport (Griffith, 1930). Between 1930 and 1960, personality research dominated the field of sport psychology. Most prominent works have established personality profiles of successful athletes, noted personality differences among different groups of athletes, and pointed to personality predictors of sport and exercise participation (see Allen et al., 2013 for a review). This line of research continued to grow exponentially during the next decades leading to more than 1000 published studies related to personality in sport alone (Fisher, 1984). It is noteworthy that whereas contemporary theories of personality gained recognition around the turn of the 1990s, research related to personality in the motor domain declined suddenly (Allen et al., 2013). Consequently, the last 20 years were marked by few attempts to advance our understanding of the relationship between personality and motor proficiency. On one hand, some argue that the absence of integrative perspectives presented potential difficulties preventing the discipline to grow (Coulter, Mallett, Singer, & Gucciardi, 2015). On the other hand, some explain this decline by the fact that sport scientists shifted their attention toward more specific performance-related traits such as anxiety, optimism, hardiness, and mental toughness (Vanden Auweele, Nys, Rzewnicki, & Van Mele, 2001). The following section aims to clarify and integrate the conceptual frameworks of personality research, and present the related empirical evidence for them.

Personality: theoretical framework and related research in sport

Linking people's feelings, thoughts, and behaviors to personality's types is a challenging research goal. Nevertheless, some scientists introduced integrative theories of personality to promote a holistic understanding of people. Among the different existing models, McAdams' three-layered framework of personality (1995, 2013) presents a simple and modern take on personality integrating both trait-state continuum and contrasting personality paradigm. In this framework, each layer represents a branch of personality theory, namely (a) dispositional traits, (b) characteristic adaptations, and (c) personal narratives (see Figure 3.1). Also known as the *actor–agent–author* framework (McAdams, 2013), this

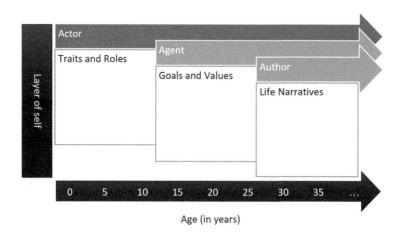

Figure 3.1 Three layers of self developing over time (McAdams, 2013).

model first describes an individual as a *social actor* with stable traits that define what kind of person he/she is. Then, the next layer considers the individual as a *motivated agent* with distinct goals and values allowing him/her to adapt to motivational, social-cognitive, and developmental challenges and tasks contextualized in time, place, situation, or social role. Finally, the third layer looks at who a person considers themselves to be. The last layer illustrates the person as an *autobiographical author* who gives life a sense of unity, purpose, and meaning by integrating the past, present, and future. Widely endorsed in the field of personality psychology, McAdams' three-layered framework has recently gained popularity in the field of sport and exercise psychology because of its potential in explaining the complex nature of athletes and exercisers (Coulter et al., 2015). Similarly, this model presents a good potential in explaining the influence of personality on motor proficiency from a genetic standpoint. To meet our purpose, we focus our attention on the first and second layers of McAdams's model.

Layer 1: A trait perspective

Five-factor theory of personality

Traits are largely based on the transaction between genes and early life experiences influencing broadly people's behavioral signature (McAdams, 2013). Perhaps the most significant and accepted conceptualization of personality traits is the so-called "Big Five" and by extension the *5-factor theory of personality* (McCrae & Costa, 2008; McCrae & John, 1992). This model of personality consists of hierarchical organization of personality traits in terms of five basic dimensions: *extraversion, neuroticism, openness, agreeableness, and conscientiousness* (McCrae & John, 1992). Each dimension encompasses several specific traits termed facets (see Table 3.1) (Allen et al., 2013). The value of the 5-factor model is that it conveys order to an otherwise chaotic description of personality measures by positioning a person on a series of bipolar, linear continua that describe the basic dimensions upon which he or she is typically perceived to differ (Coulter et al., 2015). This approach decontextualized, and is a non-conditional indicator of, overall behavioral trends (Allen et al., 2013). Typically assessed via self-report questionnaires or observer ratings, personality traits have been explored by sport scientists to compare and distinguish trait patterns in athletes and exercisers. Several conclusions drawn from this line of research are presented next.

The first concern related to the role of personality in the motor domain is whether there is such an entity as *athletic personality*. According to Rhodes and Smith's (2006) meta-analysis, physical activity involvement has a moderate positive association with extraversion as well as with conscientiousness, and a small negative correlation with neuroticism. It should be noted, however, that similar personality traits of people that choose to invest seriously in organized sport tend to slightly differ from those who simply exercise. Notably, whereas exercisers benefit from being conscientious to maintain

Table 3.1 Big five personality traits and the associated specific facets

Dimensions	Specific facets	
Extraversion	**Introverted** Unsociable, quiet, passive	**Extraverted** Sociable, outgoing, active
Neuroticism	**Emotional stability** Calm, controlled, even-tempered	**Emotionally unstable** Anxious, hostile, irritable
Openness	**Open to new experiences** Curious, creative, imaginative	**Closed to new experiences** Conventional, uncreative, unimaginative
Agreeableness	**Compassionate** Good-natured, unselfish, forgiving	**Antagonize** Cynical, rude, uncooperative
Conscientiousness	**Conscientious** Organized, punctual, hardworking	**Lackadaisical** Unreliable, lazy, careless

Source: based on McCrae and John (1992).

their healthy life discipline, openness to experience is a common characteristic in athletes as it allows them to seek out new and exciting experiences to progress in their sport. This discrepancy between exercisers and athletes' personality traits can be attributed to the different motives that drive people toward one activity or the other (Allen et al., 2013).

What about sport performance? Do high-level athletes unveil some different personality traits to low-level athletes? Although contentious, results from early studies revealed that elite athletes tend to be more extraverted and emotionally stable than recreational-level athletes (Egloff & Jan Gruhn, 1996; Kirkcaldy, 1982). The need for stimulation through bodily activity of extraverted individuals, and the higher capacity to tolerate anxiety by emotionally stable people can, in parts, account for these personality differences associated with skill-level (Egloff & Jan Gruhn, 1996). Other research findings point toward high level of conscientiousness as a determining trait of successful athletes (Piedmont, Hill, & Blanco, 1999). In this vein, more recent research indicates that athletes competing in national or international competitions possess a lower level of neuroticism and higher level of conscientiousness and agreeableness than athletes competing in club or regional competitions. High levels of conscientiousness might act as a control or suppressor of tough-mindedness, explaining the relationship between this characteristic and athletic success (Allen, Greenlees, & Jones, 2011).

Significant effects have also been observed between athletes' personality and their selection in the highest level of competition (Aidman, 2007; Gee, Marshall, & King, 2010; Martin, Malone, & Hilyer, 2011). For instance, Martin et al. (2011) found that personality traits were important factors differentiating the top 12 athletes composing the 2004 US women's Paralympic basketball gold-medal team from the 13 athletes who did not make the team. The best athletes scored lower in neuroticism (anxiety) and higher on openness to experience (tough-mindedness). On the other hand, comparing personality profiles of starting athletes versus non-starting athletes, non-significant personality differences were noted (Evans & Quarterman, 1983; Garland & Barry, 1990). Similarly, person-ality measures have not been found to be a reliable predictor of single-match success (Morgan, 1968; Rogulj et al., 2006).

In summary, higher levels of extraversion, conscientiousness and openness to experience, and lower levels of neuroticism have been identified as potential pre-dictors of long-term athletic success. However, it seems that short-term perform-ance, such as winning a competition or being in the starting line-up, is not directly associated to personality traits (Allen & Laborde, 2014). Although the Five-Factor model has been the dominant theoretical framework for sport and exercise psych-ology (Allen & Laborde, 2014), other characteristics such as *perfectionism, optimism, mental toughness, trait anger, trait anxiety, emotional intelligence, hardiness, reinvestment*, and *narcissism* can potentially explain individual achieve-ment differences, and thus deserve further attention (Laborde & Allen, 2016).

Personality-trait-like individual differences

An "umbrella" termed *personality-trait-like individual differences* (PTLID) has been developed to designate psychological differences among athletes. The PTLIDs are not directly related to the Big Five but are located at the trait level (Laborde, Breuer-Weissborn, & Dosseville, 2013). The PTLIDs offer a practical framework for investigating unique patterns, or combinations, of individual differ-ences, which correspond to sport-specific environmental demands (Laborde & Allen, 2016). This conceptual framework highlights a range of traits that have been associated with psychological functioning (Mosley & Laborde, 2015a), and neuro-physiological processes (Mosley & Laborde, 2015b) under pressure conditions. Table 3.2 defines the characteristics that have initially been identified as PTLIDs linked to performance in sport. Interestingly, although some similarities were noted among the studies using this framework regarding the positive PTLID com-ponents, the specific dimensions of this umbrella concept have not yet reached a consensus (Laborde, Guillén, Dosseville, & Allen, 2015). Instead, researchers designate the characteristics that best suit the aim of their research according to the scientific literature. This allows researchers to explore the "global picture" of the sport-related personality phenomenon (Laborde & Allen, 2016).

The first study to use a combination of positive individual characteristics to explore the difference between athletes and non-athletes had grouped *hope, optimism, perseverance*, and *resilience* under the umbrella term "mental toughness" (Guillén & Laborde, 2014). Hope was defined as an expectation of success relative to designated goals (Snyder et al., 1991), whereas perseverance as the propensity of being eager to work hard when facing challenges, in spite of fatigue or frustration (Cloninger, Przybeck, Svrakic, & Wetzel, 1994). Findings revealed that athletes exhibited a higher level of mental toughness than non-athletes. Although a

Table 3.2 Definitions of personality-trait-like individual differences linked to performance in sport

Psychological individual differences	Definition
Competitive aggressiveness and anger	Propensity to engage in acts of aggression during sporting competitions
Competitive trait anxiety	Tendency to perceive competitive situations as threatening and to respond to these situations with (increased state)-anxiety
Emotional intelligence	The propensity to behave in a certain way in emotional situations
Hardiness	Multidimensional disposition that combines the three attitudes of commitment, control, and challenge resulting in enhanced performance under stressful circumstances
Mental toughness	"Collection of values, attitudes, emotions, and cognitions that influence the way in which an individual approaches, responds to, and appraises demanding events to consistently achieve his or her goals" (Gucciardi, Gordon, & Dimmock, 2009, p. 54)
Optimism	Tendency to expect the best possible outcome or dwell on the most hopeful aspects of a situation
Perfectionism	A strive for "flawlessness and setting exceedingly high standards for performance, accompanied by tendencies for overly critical evaluations"
Reinvestment	Tendency of individuals to the manipulation of conscious, explicit, rule-based knowledge, by working memory, to control the mechanics of one's movements during motor output
Risk-taking/sensation seeking	"the need for varied, novel, and complex sensations and experiences and the willingness to take physical and social risks for the sake of such experience"
Coping-trait	Actions that people usually perform under stressful circumstances
Self-concept (self-esteem)	The awareness of good possessed by the self
Resilience	The ability to master a crisis with the aid of personally and socially mediated resources

Source: based on Laborde et al. (2013).

multidimensional conceptualization of mental toughness initially prevails in scientific literature, recent research suggests that a unidimensional model may be more
appropriate (Gucciardi, Hanton, Gordon, Mallett, & Temby, 2015). Consequently,
PTLID seemed more suitable to study several individual characteristics linked to
optimal performance than the term mental toughness (Laborde et al., 2015).

Laborde et al. (2015) grouped *self-efficacy, hope, optimism, perseverance, resilience,* and *trait emotional intelligence* under the umbrella-term *positive PTLID* to investigate whether these characteristics were linked to sport participation. Self-efficacy is one's belief that one maintains the power to produce effects by one's actions (Bandura, 2000). Using structural equation modeling, a positive association was found between sport participation and PTLID. In another study, positive PTLID was composed of *perseverance, positivity* (i.e., tendency to view life and experiences with a positive outlook), *resilience, self-esteem,* and *self-efficacy* to explore the difference between 600 athletes and 600 non-athletes. Findings revealed that athletes scored systematically higher than non-athletes on positive PTLID and athletes from individual sports scored higher than athletes from team sports (Laborde, Guillén, & Mosley, 2016).

Initially listed as an influential PTLID (Laborde et al., 2013), *hardiness* is another stable personality disposition that has been associated with performance. The underlying psychological factors, namely *commitment, control,* and *challenge,* allow athletes to think, feel, and behave in ways conducive to high-level performance in sport. Using a sample composed of international, national, county/provincial, and club/regional athletes, Sheard and Golby (2010) supported the notion by showing that international competitors scored significantly higher in commitment and total hardiness than their lower level counterparts.

Finally, although not included in the PTLID, *grit* is a personality trait that has been of interest in recent times. Defined as *perseverance and passion for long-term goals,* it has initially been associated to successful outcomes in Ivy League undergraduates, United States Military Academy, and the National Spelling Bee contest (Duckworth, Peterson, Matthews, & Kelly, 2007). In a study investigating the influence of grit in youth elite soccer players, findings revealed that grittier players accumulated significantly more time in soccer-specific activities, and performed better on perceptual-cognitive skills tests than their less gritty counterparts (Larkin, O'Connor, & Williams, 2016). In this vein, grit has been found to be a good predictor of exercise behaviors (Reed, 2014).

To conclude, many PTLID appear to influence performance in the motor domain. Using mostly cross-sectional design, research findings revealed that athletes tend to score higher on positive individual characteristics than non-athletes. It may thus be that these personality traits are leading to a higher interest in sport activities, or that sport participation is a relevant route to express these traits (Laborde et al., 2016). It is important to keep in mind that every individual differs in PTLID patterns and magnitude. A good understanding of the various PTLID, and their influence on performance, is thus a key to help athletes unleash their potential. PTLID grouped multiple individual characteristics together to globally explore the impact of these characteristics on motor proficiency. Yet it is not clear whether these characteristics come from the same set of genes and are truly related. A deeper exploration of the genetic basis of positive individual characteristics in the next section of this chapter sheds light on this question.

Layer 2: Characteristic adaptations

The three layers of McAdams's (2013) model being interconnected, the type of person somebody is (traits) may influence how they might respond to events in given contexts, periods, or roles (characteristic adaptations). Therefore, researchers have attempted to overcome some of the challenges related to the establishment of a direct link between personality traits and athletic performance (e.g., bad luck or unexpected events) by exploring how personality dimensions relate to behaviors associated with success (Allen et al., 2013).

Because it has been identified as being pivotal to achieving peak performance in sport (Schinke, Tenenbaum, Lidor, & Battochio, 2010), significant attention was devoted to the link between personality and coping – cognitive and behavioral strategies employed to manage specific external and internal demands (Lazarus & Folkman, 1984). Using the Five-Factor model, research has shown that *conscientiousness, extraversion* and *openness to experience* were associated with more efficient *coping strategies* (Allen, Frings, & Hunter, 2012; Allen et al., 2011). Similarly, another study pertained to the extent to which personality influences each aspect of the stress-coping process (i.e., type, frequency, and intensity of the stressors, and coping selection). Findings revealed that *agreeableness* was linked to lower stressor intensity and *conscientiousness* to a higher perceived stressor control (Kaiseler, Polman, & Nicholls, 2012). Psychological *resilience* has also been identified as a protective factor to the potential negative effect of stressors through its positive influence on *challenge appraisal* and *metacognitions* (Fletcher & Sarkar, 2012). Being *optimistic* also led to a more efficient use of coping strategies, which secure *goal attainment* and maintain *positive emotional states* (Gaudreau & Blondin, 2004). Finally, *mentally tough* athletes frequently used strategies such as *mental imagery, effort expenditure, thought control, logical analysis* and seldom strategies such as *distancing, mental distraction*, and *resignation* (Nicholls, Polman, Levy, & Backhouse, 2008).

Risk taking is another behavior that has been shown to be influenced by personality traits. Results of a study showed that athletes expressing low *conscientiousness* combined with high *extraversion* and/or high *neuroticism* were greater risk-takers than those exhibiting high conscientiousness combined with low extraversion and/or high extraversion (Castanier, Le Scanff, & Woodman, 2010). Surprisingly, Klinar, Burnik, and Kajtna, (2017) demonstrated that high-risk sports' athletes were less *open to experience* than recreational athletes. This contradicts previous findings showing a positive association between openness to experience and risk taking (Kajtna, 2013).

In addition to the direct effects observed of personality on various performance outcomes, traits also have important moderating effects upon the athletic population (Allen et al., 2013). The impact of different genes on these moderators is presented in more depth in the following chapters. Yet it is important to keep in mind that traits may not only influence athletic success, but the whole process leading to such accomplishment.

Heritability of personality

Heritability of personality relies on the estimation of the degree of variation in peoples' personalities that is due to genetic variation among them within the population. Heritability of personality is studied extensively in *behavior genetics*. *Behavior genetics* is a scientific field focusing on identifying the genetic and environmental sources of individual differences in behavioral phenotypes. Therefore, behavior genetic studies of personality focus mainly on the trait theory, described previously. The trait theory is based on the concepts of individual differences and has valid measures and normal distribution in the population.

According to the basic assumption of the behavioral genetic theory, personality variations might gush from genetic and environmental factors. Environmental factors can be further divided to *common/shared environment* (environmental influences that have the effect of making twins/family members more similar to one another), and *non-shared environment* (environmental influences that are unique to each and every of the twins/family members). Environmental influences that contribute to the personality variability are almost exclusively non-shared between family members. Thus, family members are similar due to their shared genes – not due to their shared family environment (Plomin, DeFries, McClearn, & McGuffin, 2008). Genetic factors can be further divided to *dominance effect* and *additive effect*. Some other types of interplay between genes and environment (gene-environment interaction and correlation, moderation of third variable, etc.) also exist and are studied.

The basic approach for testing the genetic hypothesis and estimating heritability is to relate interpersonal variation in personality traits with genetic variability by measuring phenotypic similarity of individuals who share genes or environment to a known degree (see Figure 3.2). The classic study designs include: twin studies, family studies, and adoption studies. Other designs, such as extended families, pedigree studies, twin/family, or twin/adoption studies also exist.

Though these classical designs carry some serious limitations (Sahu & Prasuna, 2016), they still play a pivotal role in behavioral genetics. Overall, heritability estimation from behavioral genetic studies range between 0.2 to 0.5, depending on the study design (Bratko, Butković, & Vukasović Hlupić, 2017). The average estimation converges around 0.40, meaning that 40 percent of individual differences are due to the genetic differences in the population (Krueger & Johnson, 2008; Turkheimer, Pettersson, & Horn, 2014; Vukasović & Bratko, 2015). Therefore, non-shared environments have a substantial effect on personality traits (Krueger & Johnson, 2008; Krueger, South, Johnson, & Iacono, 2008). Findings from behavioral studies on personality heritability can be summarized into three main observations (Bratko et al., 2017; Vukasović & Bratko, 2015): (1) identical twins are more similar in personality than fraternal twins, (2) adopted children are more similar in personality to their biological parents than to their adoptive parents, and (3) identical twins reared apart are more similar in personality than are dizygotic twins reared together. It seems that findings in the

	Twin studies		Family studies		
	Identical twins	Fraternal twins	Parent & offspring	Parent & adoptee	Parent & adopted away offspring
Genes, G	100%	50%	50%	0%	50%
Shared Environment, C	100%	100%	100%	100%	0%
Non-shared Environment, E	0%	0%	0%	0%	0%
Source of differences	E	E+0.5G	E+0.5G	E+G	0.5G+C+A

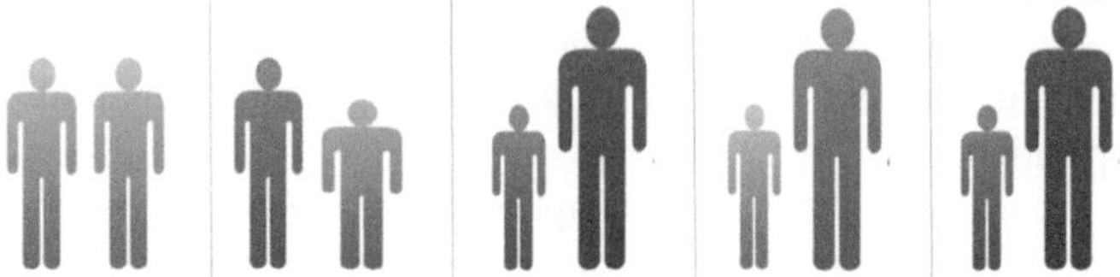

Figure 3.2 Genes and environment in twins and family study.

personality domain follow the universal pattern of other behavioral traits, formulated in a form of behavioral genetic laws (Turkheimer, 2000): (1) all behavioral traits are heritable, (2) the effect of the family environment is smaller than the effect of genes, and (3) a substantial portion of the variance is not accounted for by the effect of genes or family environment (see also Turkheimer & Gottesman, 1991).

What is the relevance of *personality heritability* to *athletic-personality heritability*? Do the same forces and interplays between genetic and environmental factors that exist in the general population exist in the athletic population? It must be noted that heritability is defined for a particular population in a specific moment in time. The genetic variance in one population may be (somewhat) different from that in another population and should not be used to make predictions about mean changes in the population over time or about differences between groups. Theoretically, if one intends to study the heritability of athletic personality, study design must include athletic twins and/or athletic family members. However, this study design is not applicable, and conclusions must be drawn indirectly from the heritability of specific personality traits or dimensions that are of particular importance to athletic performance, like mental toughness (Nicholls et al., 2008) or from other fields (longitudinal studies, molecular genetic studies, etc.).

Longitudinal studies

Longitudinal studies contribute to the understanding of the interplay between gene and environment in personality. In general, genetic factors maintain personality stability throughout the lifespan, and unique environmental factors act to promote personality change (Krueger & Johnson, 2008). This principle was supported by studies' findings indicating that personality is more variable during childhood and adolescence (Briley & Tucker-Drob, 2014; Roberts & DelVecchio, 2000), and probably plateaus around early adulthood (Briley & Tucker-Drob, 2014; Terracciano, McCrae, & Costa, 2010). Longitudinal studies indicate that as people progress from adolescence through late midlife, they become more agreeable, conscientious, and emotionally stable (Caspi, Roberts, & Shiner, 2005; McAdams & Olson, 2010). This has become known as the *maturity principle* (Roberts, Walton, & Viechtbauer, 2006). Of note is that the maturity principle or developmental pattern has not been shown in all people, and some people have been shown to change more than others. Those individuals that show greater consistency in personality traits appear to be those who already display a personality profile associated with maturity – low neuroticism and high agreeableness and conscientiousness (McAdams & Olson, 2010).

Molecular genetics of personality

Advances in molecular genetics have made the collection of DNA and resultant genotyping cheap and straightforward. The genetic contribution to human personality has been studied through associations between personality traits and common genetic variants. Two relationships have received the greatest attention from personality researchers: the association between the dopamine D4 receptor gene (*DRD4*) and extraversion/novelty seeking traits, and the association between the serotonin transporter gene (*5-HTT*) and neuroticism/anxiety-related traits (Bratko et al., 2017). Generally, results from "genetic polymorphism" – "personality traits" association studies are contradicting, and while some have found association between genetic variants and personality traits, others failed to find any association (Munafò et al., 2003). A meta-analyses showed a non-significant effect for DRD4 on extraversion (Munafò et al., 2008; Schinka, Letsch, & Crawford, 2002), and a small but significant effect for *5-HTT* on neuroticism (Clarke, Flint, Attwood, & Munafò, 2010; Munafò, Yalcin, Willis-Owen, & Flint, 2009; Schinka, Busch, & Robichaux-Keene, 2004). These contradicting results are not surprising, since personality traits are multifactorial-polygenic traits, influenced by multiple genes (each makes only a small contribution), as well as the interactions between them. Several other candidate genes have been identified in GWAS. A summary of the main genes associated with personality traits is given in Table 3.3.

Though molecular genetic studies carry significant potential for sport psychology, data regarding genetic variants associated with personality traits among athletes are scare.

Table 3.3 Genes related to personality traits

Gene	Personality trait	Remarks	Reference
Serotonin and dopamine genes			
Serotonin transporter 5-HTTLPR	Neuroticism	Meta-analysis	(Sen, Burmeister, & Ghosh, 2004) (Munafò et al., 2009)
	Harm avoidance		(Schinka et al., 2004)
	Anxiety		(Troisi, Carola, & Gross, 2017)
	Insecure attachment		
MAOA	Extraversion	Age dependant	(Xu et al., 2017)
DRD4	Extraversion	Meta-analysis	(Munafò et al., 2008; Schinka et al., 2002)
	Novelty seeking		(Lee et al., 2003; Noble et al., 1998)
DRD2	Reward dependence		(Lee et al., 2003)
	Novelty seeking		(Noble et al., 1998)
BDNF	Introversion		(Terracciano, Tanaka, et al., 2010)
	Neuroticism		
DBH	Reward dependence		(Plieger et al., 2018)
Other genes			
RASA1	Openness to experience	GWAS	(de Moor et al., 2012)
KATNAL2	Conscientiousness		
PER3	Extraversion		(Jiménez, Pereira-Morales, & Forero, 2017)
A1AT	Extraversion	Women, marginal effect	(Golimbet et al., 2017)
	Neuroticism		

Gene-environment interactions in personality

Classic study designs of personality are based on quantitative models of human individual differences that estimate genetic and environmental contributions as constants, and assume that their influences act independently and additively. However, genes and environmental factors may have complex interplays and relationships (see Chapter 8 for elaboration and discussion). These relationships can be divided into two main contrasts: "gene-environment correlation" and "gene-environment interaction." Gene-environment correlation refers to the situations in which genes and environment are correlated, or interdependent. Gene-environment interaction refers to situations in which the effect of genes depends on the environment, and/or the effect of the environment depends on genotype (Halldorsdottir & Binder, 2017; Krueger et al., 2008; Manuck & McCaffery, 2014).

Gene-environment (GxE) interaction can be assessed by various study designs ranging from the traditional behavior genetic designs to molecular analyses. GxE interactions in behavior genetics are explored via family, twin, and adoption studies. These study designs are extensively used in clinical psychology (Dick, 2011), but are not applicable in sport psychology. Studies examining GxE interaction using latent models have yielded mixed results in relation to impulsivity, neuroticism (see Burt, 2008 for review), and extraversion (Krueger et al., 2008; Lemery-Chalfant, Kao, Swann, & Goldsmith, 2013).

On the other hand, molecular analyses, which study the outcome of the interactions between specific genetic make-ups and environment carry serious potential for the study of GxE interactions in sport psychology. In 2002 Caspi et al. reported that a functional polymorphism in the gene encoding the neurotransmitter-metabolizing enzyme *MAOA* moderated the effect of maltreatment: males who carried the genotype conferring high levels of *MAOA* expression were less likely to develop antisocial problems when exposed to maltreatment (Caspi et al., 2002). In 2003, Caspi's group reported that a functional polymorphism in the promoter region of the serotonin transporter gene (*5-HTT*) was found to moderate the influence of stressful life events on depression. Individuals carrying the short allele of the *5-HTT* promoter polymorphism exhibited more depressive symptoms, diagnosable depression, and suicidality in relation to stressful life events than did individuals homozygous for the long allele (Caspi et al., 2003). These pioneer studies followed by many others aimed to replicate, extend, and explore the findings of the original papers. But, findings were controverting (Risch et al., 2009), implying that these interactions are complicated, and not easy to capture.

In 2017, Leighton, Botto, Silva, Jiménez, and Luyten reviewed 315 papers related to GxE interactions on behavior that have been published since Caspi's study in 2002, and found that polymorphisms of 34 different genes, most of them related to the serotonin and dopamine systems, have been studied using 160 original samples (Leighton et al., 2017). Personality traits were included as an effect of GxE studies in 21 of the 315 papers, with studies focusing on *5HTTLPR* interaction with impulsivity, neuroticism, emotional dysregulation, and self-esteem; *DRD4, BDNF,* and *NPSR* (Neuropeptide S Receptor) interaction with anxiety sensitivity; *TPH1* (Tryptophan Hydroxylase 1)/*TPH2* (Tryptophan Hydroxylase 2) interaction with harm avoidance and impulsivity; and *COMT* interaction with impulsivity.

Clinical psychology had taken the study of GxE interactions one step forward by testing the *susceptibility hypothesis* in experimental models by environmental manipulation. According to the susceptibility hypothesis, in positive environments vulnerable children may outperform their peers, who turn out to be less susceptible not only to bad environments, but also to optimal environments (Bakermans-Kranenburg & van IJzendoorn, 2007). Recent meta-analysis of randomized GxE experiments has shown support for the differential susceptibility model with dopamine-related genes emerging as susceptibility markers. The effects of experimental manipulation of the environment for the better were much stronger in the susceptible genotypes than in the non-susceptible genotypes (Bakermans-Kranenburg & van IJzendoorn, 2015). Though this experimental model is feasible in sport psychology, as in the whole field of behavioral genetic, the sport domain is far behind the clinical domain.

Insights for sport

When discussing the relationship between genetics, personality, and sport, it is necessary to distinguish between *sport participation* and *sport performance*. Sport participation is a fundamental environmental factor that may act on personality, interact with personality, or become an outcome of personality. Sport participation might have a role in the maturity principle. Through sport participation children and adolescents are subjected to adult concepts such as organization, discipline, fair-play, sportsmanship, and teamwork that may facilitate maturational development and personality traits more commonly observed in adults (low neuroticism, and high agreeableness and conscientiousness). There may also be an important GxE interaction effect in the context of sport participation facilitating maturity, but only for those with particular genetic traits. Indeed, research in national level swimmers (aged 10–24 years) has demonstrated that variability in the *5-HTT* gene is associated with positive psychological development in the context of sport (Golby & Sheard, 2006).

Moreover, sport participation cannot be considered as a "pure" environmental factor. Genetic variation contributes substantially to sport and exercise participation (De Geus & De Moor, 2011; Stubbe & De Geus, 2009). Genes associated with sport participation might also influence personality (Stubbe et al., 2006). The most promising genes in this context are probably genes related to the dopaminergic system since they are associated with both personality (Lee et al., 2003; Munafò et al., 2008; Noble et al., 1998) and sport participation (Knab & Lightfoot, 2010; Lightfoot, 2011). The observed GxE interaction in adolescent sport might also be related to personality. Stubbe, Boomsma, and De Geus (2005) observed that between ages 13 and 16 genetic factors have little effect on sport participation (between 0.16 and 0.22), at age 17–18 genetic factors have a slightly greater role (0.36), and after 18 years genetics largely explain individual differences in sport participation (0.85). Further studies have supported the notion that environmental factors have a greater role in adolescence and genetics has a greater role in adulthood (Stubbe & De Geus, 2009), and personality may have an important role in this developmental change.

As for sport performance, it is well established that genetics contribute substantially to sport performance (Davids & Baker, 2007; Klissouras, 2001; Lippi, Longo, & Maffulli, 2010; Macarthur & North, 2005; Ostrander, Huson, & Ostrander, 2009; Pitsiladis et al., 2013; Santos et al., 2016; Schoenfelder, 2010). Most of the genes studied in association to sport performance are related to physiological traits (see for example: Sarzynski et al., 2016), and studies on genes associated with psychological traits are scarce. Research into the interplay between genes and personality might strengthen our understanding of both sport participation and performance. However, the traditional categorization of "genes" and "environment" are challenged when dealing with sport and personality, since they are not separate independent entities, and they maintain interaction and correlation relationships, as schematically described in Figure 3.3.

Summary

To facilitate the investigation of the impact of genes on personality traits leading to motor proficiency, the current introduction followed the assumption that personality traits cause some individuals to perform better or worse than others in the athletic domain. Yet, athletic success and the environmental changes that come with

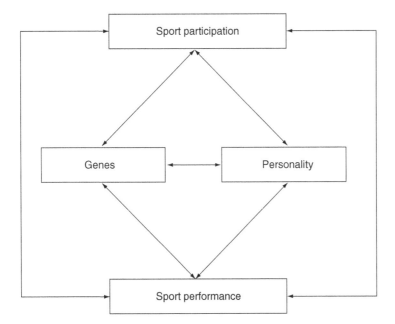

Figure 3.3 Genes-personality inter-relationship in sport.

it may also be responsible for personality alterations (Allen & Laborde, 2014). As illustrated by the third layer of McAdams' model, people can draw meaning and purpose from life events that define their identity (Coulter et al., 2015; McAdams, 2013). This last layer of personality is thus strongly influenced by environmental conditions. Keeping this in mind, the current chapter was aimed at identifying the different genes associated with performance-related personality traits.

References

Aidman, E. V. (2007). Attribute-based selection for success: The role of personality attributes in long-term predictions of achievement in sport. *The Journal of the American Board of Sport Psychology, 3,* 1–18. Retrieved from www.americanboard ofsportpsychology.org/Portals/24/absp-journalaidman1.pdf

Allen, M. S., Frings, D., & Hunter, S. (2012). Personality, coping, and challenge and threat states in athletes. *International Journal of Sport and Exercise Psychology, 10*(4), 264–75. http://dx.doi.org/10.1080/1612197X.2012.682375

Allen, M. S., Greenlees, I., & Jones, M. (2011). An investigation of the five-factor model of personality and coping behaviour in sport. *Journal of Sports Sciences, 29*(8), 841–50.

Allen, M. S., Greenlees, I., & Jones, M. (2013). Personality in sport: A comprehensive review. *International Review of Sport and Exercise Psychology, 6*(1), 184–208. doi:10. 1080/1750984X.2013.769614

Allen, M. S., & Laborde, S. (2014). The role of personality in sport and physical activity. *Current Directions in Psychological Science, 23,* 460–5. http://dx.doi.org/10.1177/ 0963721414550705

Bakermans-Kranenburg, M. J., & van IJzendoorn, M. H. (2007). Research review: Genetic vulnerability or differential susceptibility in child development: The case of attachment. *Journal of Child Psychology and Psychiatry, 48*(12), 1160–73. https://doi. org/10.1111/j.1469-7610.2007.01801.x

Bakermans-Kranenburg, M. J., & van IJzendoorn, M. H. (2015). The hidden efficacy of interventions: Gene × environment experiments from a differential susceptibility perspective. *Annual Review of Psychology, 66*(1), 381–409. https://doi.org/10.1146/ annurev-psych-010814-015407

Bandura, A. (2000). Self-efficacy. In Alan E. Kazdin (Ed.), *Encyclopedia of psychology.* New York, NY: Oxford University Press.

Bratko, D., Butković, A., & Vukasović Hlupić, T. (2017). Heritability of personality. *Psychological Topics, 1,* 1–24.

Briley, D. A., & Tucker-Drob, E. M. (2014). Genetic and environmental continuity in personality development: A meta-analysis. *Psychological Bulletin, 140*(5), 1303–31. https://doi.org/10.1037/a0037091

Burt, S. A. (2008). Gene–environment interactions and their impact on the development of personality traits. *Psychiatry, 7*(12), 507–10. https://doi.org/10.1016/j. mppsy.2008.10.005

Caspi, A., McClay, J., Moffitt, T. E., Mill, J., Martin, J., Craig, I. W., … Poulton, R. (2002). Role of genotype in the cycle of violence in maltreated children. *Science, 297*(5582), 851–4. https://doi.org/10.1126/science.1072290

Caspi, A., Roberts, B. W., & Shiner, R. L. (2005). Personality development: Stability and change. *Annual Review of Psychology, 56*(1), 453–84. https://doi.org/10.1146/annurev. psych.55.090902.141913

Caspi, A., Sugden, K., Moffitt, T. E., Taylor, A., Craig, I. W., Harrington, H., ... Poulton, R. (2003). Influence of life stress on depression: Moderation by a polymorphism in the 5-HTT gene. *Science, 301*(5631), 386–9. https://doi.org/10.1126/science.1083968

Castanier, C., Le Scanff, C., & Woodman, T. (2010). Who takes risks in high-risk sports? A typological personality approach. *Research Quarterly for Exercise and Sport, 81*(4), 478–84.

Clarke, H., Flint, J., Attwood, A. S., & Munafò, M. R. (2010). Association of the 5-HTTLPR genotype and unipolar depression: A meta-analysis. *Psychological Medicine, 40*(11), 1767–78. https://doi.org/10.1017/S0033291710000516

Cloninger, C. R., Przybeck, T. R., Svrakic, D. M., & Wetzel, R. D. (1994). *The temperament and character inventory (TCI): A guide to its development and use.* St Louis, MO: Center for Psychobiology of Personality.

Coulter, T. J., Mallett, C. J., Singer, J. A., & Gucciardi, D. F. (2015). Personality in sport and exercise psychology: Integrating a whole person perspective. *International Journal of Sport and Exercise Psychology, 14*(1), 23–41. http://dx.doi.org/10.1080/1612197x.2015.1016085

Davids, K., & Baker, J. (2007). Genes, environment and sport performance: Why the nature-nurture dualism is no longer relevant. *Sports Medicine, 37*(11), 961–80. Retrieved from www.ncbi.nlm.nih.gov/pubmed/17953467

De Geus, E. J. C., & De Moor, M. H. M. (2011). Genes, exercise, and psychological factors. In C. Bouchard & E. Hoffman (Eds.), *Genetic and molecular aspects of sport performance* (pp. 294–305). Oxford, England: Wiley-Blackwell.

de Moor, M. H. M., Costa, P. T., Terracciano, A., Krueger, R. F., de Geus, E. J. C., Toshiko, T., ... Boomsma, D. I. (2012). Meta-analysis of genome-wide association studies for personality. *Molecular Psychiatry, 17*(3), 337–49. https://doi.org/10.1038/mp.2010.128

Dick, D. M. (2011). Gene-environment interaction in psychological traits and disorders. *Annual Review of Clinical Psychology, 7*, 383–409. https://doi.org/10.1146/annurev-clinpsy-032210-104518

Duckworth, A. L., Peterson, C., Matthews, M. D., & Kelly, D. R. (2007). Grit: Perseverance and passion for long term goals. *Journal of Personality and Social Psychology, 92*, 1087–101.

Egloff, B., & Jan Gruhn, A. (1996). Personality and endurance sports. *Personality and Individual Differences, 21*(2), 223–9. http://dx.doi.org/10.1016/0191-8869(96)00048-7

Evans, V., & Quarterman, J. (1983). Personality characteristics of successful and unsuccessful Black female basketball players. *International Journal of Sport Psychology, 14*(2), 105–15.

Fisher, A. C. (1984). New directions in sport personality research. In J. M. Silva & R. S. Weinberg (Eds.), *Psychological foundations of sport* (pp. 70–80). Champaign, IL: Human Kinetics.

Fletcher, D., & Sarkar, M. (2012). A grounded theory of psychological resilience in Olympic champions. *Psychology of Sport and Exercise, 13*(5), 669–78. http://dx.doi.org/10.1016/j.psychsport.2012.04.007

Garland, D. J., & Barry, J. R. (1990). Sport expertise: The cognitive advantage. *Perceptual and Motor Skills, 70*(Suppl. 3), S1299–314. https://doi.org/10.2466/pms.1990.70.3c.1299

Gaudreau, P., & Blondin, J.-P. (2004). Differential associations of dispositional optimism and pessimism with coping, goal attainment, and emotional adjustment during sport competition. *International Journal of Stress Management, 11*(3), 245–69. http://dx.doi.org/10.1037/1072-5245.11.3.245

Gee, C. J., Marshall, J. C., & King, J. F. (2010). Should coaches use personality assessments in the talent identification process? A 15-year predictive study on professional hockey players. *International Journal of Coaching Science, 4*, 25–34. Retrieved from www.selfmgmt.com/documents/IJCS%20Manuscript.pdf

Golby, J., & Sheard, M. (2006). The relationship between genotype and positive psychological development in national-level swimmers. *European Psychologist, 11*(2), 143–8. https://doi.org/10.1027/1016-9040.11.2.143

Golimbet, V. E., Alfimova, M. V., Korovaitseva, G. I., Lezheiko, T. V., Kondrat'ev, N. V., Krikova, E. V., ... Kolesina, N. Y. (2017). Studies of the effects of genes for inflammatory factors on basic personality dimensions. *Neuroscience and Behavioral Physiology, 47*(9), 1060–4. https://doi.org/10.1007/s11055-017-0512-1

Griffith, C. R. (1930). A laboratory for research in athletics. *Research Quarterly for Exercise and Sport, 1*, 34–40. Retrieved from www.getcited.org/pub/103378567

Gucciardi, D. F., Gordon, S., & Dimmock, J. A. (2009). Advancing mental toughness research and theory using personal construct psychology. *International Review of Sport and Exercise Psychology, 2*(1), 54–72. doi:10.1080/17509840802705938

Gucciardi, D. F., Hanton, S., Gordon, S., Mallett, C. J., & Temby, P. (2015). The concept of mental toughness: Tests of dimensionality, nomological network, and traitness. *Journal of Personality, 1*, 26. doi:10.1111/jopy.12079

Guillén, F., & Laborde, S. (2014). Higher-order structure of mental toughness and the analysis of latent mean differences between athletes from 34 disciplines and non-athletes. *Personality and Individual Differences, 60*, 30–5. http://dx.doi.org/10.1016/j.paid.2013.11.019

Halldorsdottir, T., & Binder, E. B. (2017). Gene × environment interactions: From molecular mechanisms to behavior. *Annual Review of Psychology, 68*(1), 215–41. https://doi.org/10.1146/annurev-psych-010416-044053

Jiménez, K. M., Pereira-Morales, A. J., & Forero, D. A. (2017). Higher scores in the extraversion personality trait are associated with a functional polymorphism in the PER3 gene in healthy subjects. *Chronobiology International, 34*(2), 280–6. https://doi.org/10.1080/07420528.2016.1268149

Kaiseler, M., Polman, R. C. J., & Nicholls, A. R. (2012). Effects of the big five personality dimensions on appraisal coping, and coping effectiveness in sport. *European Journal of Sport Science, 12*, 62–72.

Kajtna, T. (2013). *Nekateri psihološki vidiki rizičnih športov (Znanstvena monografija)* [Some psychological aspects of high-risk sports (Scientific monography)]. Ljubljana, Slovenia: University of Ljubljana.

Kirkcaldy, B. D. (1982). Personality profiles at various levels of athletic participation. *Personality and Individual Differences, 3*(3), 321–6. http://dx.doi.org/10.1016/0191-8869(82)90052-6

Klinar, P., Burnik, S., & Kajtna, T. (2017). Personality and sensation seeking in high-risk sports. *Acta Gymnica, 47*(1), 41–8.

Klissouras, V. (2001). The nature and nurture of human performance. *European Journal of Sport Science, 1*(2), 1–10.

Knab, A. M., & Lightfoot, J. T. (2010). Does the difference between physically active and couch potato lie in the dopamine system? *International Journal of Biological Sciences, 6*(2), 133–50. Retrieved from www.ncbi.nlm.nih.gov/pubmed/20224735

Krueger, R. F., & Johnson, W. (2008). Behavioral genetics and personality: A new look at the integration of nature and nurture. In O. P. John, R. W. Robins, & L. A. Pervin (Eds.), *Handbook personality: Theory and research* (3rd ed., pp. 287–310). New York, NY; London, England: The Guilford Press.

Krueger, R. F., South, S., Johnson, W., & Iacono, W. (2008). The heritability of personality is not always 50%: Gene-environment interactions and correlations between personality and parenting. *Journal of Personality, 76*(6), 1485–522. https://doi.org/10.1111/j.1467-6494.2008.00529.x

Laborde, S., & Allen, M. S. (2016). Personality-trait-like individual differences: Much more than noise in the background for sport and exercise psychology. In M. Raab, P. Wylleman, R. Seiler, A.-M. Elbe, & A. Hatzigeorgiadis (Eds.), *Sport and exercise psychology research from theory to practice* (pp. 201–10). Amsterdam, the Netherlands: Elsevier.

Laborde, S., Breuer-Weissborn, J., & Dosseville, F. (2013). Personality-trait-like individual differences in athletes. In C. Mohiyeddini (Ed.), *Advances in the psychology of sports and exercise* (pp. 25–60). New York, NY: Nova.

Laborde, S., Guillén, F., Dosseville, F., & Allen, M. S. (2015). Chronotype, sport participation, and positive personality-trait-like individual differences. *Chronobiology International: The Journal of Biological and Medical Rhythm Research, 32*, 942–51.

Laborde, S., Guillén, F., & Mosley, E. (2016). Positive personality-trait-like individual differences in athletes from individual- and team sports and in non-athletes. *Psychology of Sport and Exercise, 26*, 9–13. https://doi.org/10.1016/j.psychsport.2016.05.009

Larkin, P., O'Connor, D., & Williams, A. M. (2016). Does grit influence sport-specific engagement and perceptual-cognitive expertise in elite youth soccer? *Journal of Applied Sport Psychology, 28*, 129–38. doi:10.1080/10413200.2015.1085922

Lazarus, R. S., & Folkman, S. (1984). *Stress appraisal and coping.* New York, NY: Springer.

Lee, H.-J., Lee, H.-S., Kim, Y.-K., Kim, L., Lee, M. S., Jung, I.-K., … Kim, S. (2003). D2 and D4 dopamine receptor gene polymorphisms and personality traits in a young Korean population. *American Journal of Medical Genetics, 121B*(1), 44–9. https://doi.org/10.1002/ajmg.b.20054

Leighton, C., Botto, A., Silva, J. R., Jiménez, J. P., & Luyten, P. (2017). Vulnerability or sensitivity to the environment? Methodological issues, trends, and recommendations in gene-environment interactions research in human behavior. *Frontiers in Psychiatry, 8*, 106. https://doi.org/10.3389/fpsyt.2017.00106

Lemery-Chalfant, K., Kao, K., Swann, G., & Goldsmith, H. H. (2013). Childhood temperament: Passive gene-environment correlation, gene-environment interaction, and the hidden importance of the family environment. *Development and Psychopathology, 25*(1), 51–63. https://doi.org/10.1017/S0954579412000892

Lightfoot, J. T. (2011). Current understanding of the genetic basis for physical activity. *The Journal of Nutrition, 141*(3), 526–30. https://doi.org/10.3945/jn.110.127290

Lippi, G., Longo, U. G., & Maffulli, N. (2010). Genetics and sports. *British Medical Bulletin, 93*, 27–47. https://doi.org/10.1093/bmb/ldp007

Macarthur, D. G., & North, K. N. (2005). Genes and human elite athletic performance. *Human Genetics, 116*(5), 331–9. https://doi.org/10.1007/s00439-005-1261-8

Manuck, S. B., & McCaffery, J. M. (2014). Gene-environment interaction. *Annual Review of Psychology, 65*(1), 41–70. https://doi.org/10.1146/annurev-psych-010213-115100

Martin, J. J., Malone, L. A., & Hilyer, J. C. (2011). Personality and mood in women's Paralympic basketball champions. *Journal of Clinical Sport Psychology, 5*, 197–210. Retrieved from http://journals.humankinetics.com/jcsp-back-issues/jcsp-volume-5-issue-3-september-/personality-and-mood-in-womens-paralympic-basketball-champions

McAdams, D. P. (1995). What do we know when we know a person? *Journal of Personality, 63*(3), 365–96. doi:10.1111/1467-6494.ep9510042296

McAdams, D. P. (2013). The psychological self as actor, agent, and author. *Perspectives on Psychological Science, 8*(3), 272–95. doi:10.1177/1745691612464657

McAdams, D. P., & Olson, B. D. (2010). Personality development: Continuity and change over the life course. *Annual Review of Psychology, 61*(1), 517–42. https://doi.org/10.1146/annurev.psych.093008.100507

McCrae, R. R., & Costa, P. T., Jr. (2008). The five-factor theory of personality. In O. P. John, R. W. Robins, & L. A. Pervin (Eds.), *Handbook of personality: Theory and research* (3rd ed., pp. 159–81). New York, NY: Guilford Press.

McCrae, R. R., & John, O. P. (1992). An introduction to the five-factor model and its applications. *Journal of Personality, 60*(2), 175–215.

Morgan, W. P. (1968). Personality characteristics of wrestlers participating in the world championships. *Journal of Sports Medicine, 8*, 212–16.

Mosley, E., & Laborde, S. (2015a). Performing under pressure: Influence of personality-trait-like individual differences. In M. Raab, B. Lobinger, S. Hoffmann, A. Pizzera, & S. Laborde (Eds.), *Performance psychology: Perception, action, cognition, and emotion* (pp. 292–314). Amsterdam, the Netherlands: Elsevier.

Mosley, E., & Laborde, S. (2015b). Performing with all my heart: Heart rate variability and its relationship with personality-trait-like-individual-differences (PTLIDs) in pressurized performance situations. In S. Walters (Ed.), *Heart rate variability (HRV): Prognostic significance, risk factors and clinical applications* (pp. 45–60). New York: NY: Nova Publishers.

Munafò, M. R., Clark, T. G., Moore, L. R., Payne, E., Walton, R., & Flint, J. (2003). Genetic polymorphisms and personality in healthy adults: A systematic review and meta-analysis. *Molecular Psychiatry, 8*(5), 471–84. https://doi.org/10.1038/sj.mp. 4001326

Munafò, M. R., Freimer, N. B., Ng, W., Ophoff, R., Veijola, J., Miettunen, J., … Flint, J. (2009). 5-HTTLPR genotype and anxiety-related personality traits: A meta-analysis and new data. *American Journal of Medical Genetics Part B: Neuropsychiatric Genetics, 150B*(2), 271–81. https://doi.org/10.1002/ajmg.b.30808

Munafò, M. R., Yalcin, B., Willis-Owen, S. A., & Flint, J. (2008). Association of the dopamine D4 receptor (DRD4) gene and approach-related personality traits: Meta-analysis and new data. *Biological Psychiatry, 63*(2), 197–206. https://doi.org/10.1016/j.biopsych.2007.04.006

Nicholls, A. R., Polman, R. C. J., Levy, A. R., & Backhouse, S. H. (2008). Mental toughness, optimism, pessimism, and coping among athletes. *Personality and Individual Differences, 44*(5), 1182–92. https://doi.org/10.1016/J.PAID.2007.11.011

Noble, E. P., Ozkaragoz, T. Z., Ritchie, T. L., Zhang, X., Belin, T. R., & Sparkes, R. S. (1998). D2 and D4 dopamine receptor polymorphisms and personality. *American Journal of Medical Genetics, 81*(3), 257–67. Retrieved from www.ncbi.nlm.nih.gov/pubmed/9603615

Ostrander, E. A., Huson, H. J., & Ostrander, G. K. (2009). Genetics of athletic performance. *Annual Review of Genomics and Human Genetics, 10*(1), 407–29. https://doi.org/10.1146/annurev-genom-082908-150058

Pervin, L. A., & Cervone, D. (2010). *Personality: Theory and research* (11th ed.). New York, NY: Wiley.

Piedmont, R. L., Hill, D. C., & Blanco, S. (1999). Predicting athletic performance using the five-factor model of personality. *Personality and Individual Differences, 27*(4), 769–77. http://dx.doi.org/10.1016/S0191-8869(98)00280-3

Pitsiladis, Y., Wang, G., Wolfarth, B., Scott, R., Fuku, N., Mikami, E., … Lucia, A. (2013). Genomics of elite sporting performance: What little we know and necessary advances. *British Journal of Sports Medicine, 47*(9), 550–5. https://doi.org/10.1136/bjsports-2013-092400

Plieger, T., Felten, A., Melchers, M., Markett, S., Montag, C., & Reuter, M. (2018). Association between a functional polymorphism on the dopamine-β-hydroxylase gene and reward dependence in two independent samples. *Personality and Individual Differences, 121,* 218–22. https://doi.org/10.1016/J.PAID.2017.05.050

Plomin, R., DeFries, J. C., McClearn, G. E., & McGuffin, P. (2008). *Behavioral genetics* (5th ed.). New York, NY: Worth Publishers.

Reed, J. (2014). A survey of grit and exercise behavior. *Journal of Sport Behavior, 37,* 390–406.

Rhodes, R. E., & Smith, N. E. (2006). Personality correlates of physical activity: A review and meta-analysis. *British Journal of Sports Medicine, 40,* 958–65. doi:10.1136/bjsm.2006.028860

Risch, N., Herrell, R., Lehner, T., Liang, K.-Y., Eaves, L., Hoh, J., … Merikangas, K. R. (2009). Interaction between the serotonin transporter gene (5-HTTLPR), stressful life events, and risk of depression. *JAMA, 301*(23), 2462. https://doi.org/10.1001/jama.2009.878

Roberts, B. W., & Del Vecchio, W. F. (2000). The rank-order consistency of personality traits from childhood to old age: A quantitative review of longitudinal studies. *Psychological Bulletin, 126*(1), 3–25. Retrieved from www.ncbi.nlm.nih.gov/pubmed/10668348

Roberts, B. W., Walton, K. E., & Viechtbauer, W. (2006). Patterns of mean-level change in personality traits across the life course: A meta-analysis of longitudinal studies. *Psychological Bulletin, 132*(1), 1–25. https://doi.org/10.1037/0033-2909.132.1.1

Rogulj, N., Nazor, M., Srhoj, V., & Božin, D. (2006). Differences between competitively efficient and less efficient junior handball players according to their personality traits. *Kinesiology, 38*(2), 158–63.

Sahu, M., & Prasuna, J. G. (2016). Twin studies: A unique epidemiological tool. *Indian Journal of Community Medicine: Official Publication of Indian Association of Preventive and Social Medicine, 41*(3), 177–82. https://doi.org/10.4103/0970-0218.183593

Santos, C. G. M., Pimentel-Coelho, P. M., Budowle, B., de Moura-Neto, R. S., Dornelas-Ribeiro, M., Pompeu, F. A. M. S., & Silva, R. (2016). The heritable path of human physical performance: From single polymorphisms to the "next generation." *Scandinavian Journal of Medicine and Science in Sports, 26*(6), 600–12. https://doi.org/10.1111/sms.12503

Sarzynski, M. A., Loos, R. J. F., Lucia, A., Pérusse, L., Roth, S. M., Wolfarth, B., … Bouchard, C. (2016). Advances in exercise, fitness, and performance genomics in 2015. *Medicine and Science in Sports and Exercise, 48*(10), 1906–16. https://doi.org/10.1249/MSS.0000000000000982

Schinka, J. A., Busch, R. M., & Robichaux-Keene, N. (2004). A meta-analysis of the association between the serotonin transporter gene polymorphism (5-HTTLPR) and trait anxiety. *Molecular Psychiatry, 9*(2), 197–202. https://doi.org/10.1038/sj.mp.4001405

Schinka, J. A., Letsch, E. A., & Crawford, F. C. (2002). DRD4 and novelty seeking: Results of meta-analyses. *American Journal of Medical Genetics, 114*(6), 643–8. https://doi.org/10.1002/ajmg.10649

Schinke, R. J., Tenenbaum, G., Lidor, R., & Battochio, R. C. (2010). Adaptation in action: The transition from research to intervention. *The Sport Psychologist, 24,* 542–57.

Schoenfelder, M. (2010). Genetics-based performance talent research: Polymorphisms as predictors of endurance performance. *Journal of Applied Physiology, 108*(6), 1454–5. https://doi.org/10.1152/japplphysiol.00331.2010

Sen, S., Burmeister, M., & Ghosh, D. (2004). Meta-analysis of the association between a serotonin transporter promoter polymorphism (5-HTTLPR) and anxiety-related personality traits. *American Journal of Medical Genetics, 127B*(1), 85–9. https://doi.org/10.1002/ajmg.b.20158

Sheard, M., & Golby, J. (2010). Personality hardiness differentiates elite-level sport performers. *International Journal of Sport and Exercise Psychology, 8*(2), 160–9.

Snyder, C., Harris, C., Anderson, J. R., Holleran, S. A., Irving, L. M., Sigmon, S. T., ... Harney, P. (1991). The will and the ways: Development and validation of an individual-differences measure of hope. *Journal of Personality and Social Psychology, 60*(4), 570–85.

Stubbe, J. H., Boomsma, D. I., & De Geus, E. J. C. (2005). Sports participation during adolescence: A shift from environmental to genetic factors. *Medicine and Science in Sports and Exercise, 37*(4), 563–70. Retrieved from www.ncbi.nlm.nih.gov/pubmed/15809553

Stubbe, J. H., Boomsma, D. I., Vink, J. M., Cornes, B. K., Martin, N. G., Skytthe, A., ... de Geus, E. J. C. (2006). Genetic influences on exercise participation in 37,051 twin pairs from seven countries. *PloS One, 1*(1), e22. https://doi.org/10.1371/journal.pone.0000022

Stubbe, J. H., & De Geus, E. J. C. (2009). Genetics of exercise behavior. In Y. K. Kim (Ed.), *Handbook of behavior genetics* (pp. 343–58). Berlin, Germany: Springer.

Terracciano, A., McCrae, R. R., & Costa, P. T. (2010). Intra-individual change in personality stability and age. *Journal of Research in Personality, 44*(1), 31–7. https://doi.org/10.1016/j.jrp.2009.09.006

Terracciano, A., Tanaka, T., Sutin, A. R., Deiana, B., Balaci, L., Sanna, S., ... Costa, P. T. Jr. (2010). BDNF Val66Met is associated with introversion and interacts with 5-HTTLPR to influence neuroticism. *Neuropsychopharmacology: Official Publication of the American College of Neuropsychopharmacology, 35*(5), 1083–9. https://doi.org/10.1038/npp. 2009.213

Troisi, A., Carola, V., & Gross, C. (2017). Genetic variation in the serotonin transporter gene influences adult attachment style. *Neuropsychiatry, 14*(4), 241–6.

Turkheimer, E. (2000). Three laws of behavior genetics and what they mean. *Current Directions in Psychological Science, 9*(5), 160–4. https://doi.org/10.1111/1467-8721.00084

Turkheimer, E., & Gottesman, I. I. (1991). Individual differences and the canalization of human behavior. *Developmental Psychology, 27*(1), 18–22. http://dx.doi.org/10.1037/0012-1649.27.1.18

Turkheimer, E., Pettersson, E., & Horn, E. E. (2014). A phenotypic null hypothesis for the genetics of personality. *Annual Review of Psychology, 65*(1), 515–40. https://doi.org/10.1146/annurev-psych-113011-143752

Vanden Auweele, Y., Nys, K., Rzewnicki, R., & Van Mele, V. (2001). Personality and the athlete. In R. N. Singer, H. A. Hausenblas, & C. M. Janelle (Eds.), *Handbook of sport psychology* (2nd ed., pp. 239–68). New York, NY: Wiley.

Vukasović, T., & Bratko, D. (2015). Heritability of personality: A meta-analysis of behavior genetic studies. *Psychological Bulletin, 141*(4), 769–85. https://doi.org/10.1037/bul0000017

Xu, M. K., Gaysina, D., Tsonaka, R., Morin, A. J. S., Croudace, T. J., Barnett, J. H., ... The L. G. Group (2017). Monoamine Oxidase A (MAOA) gene and personality traits from late adolescence through early adulthood: A latent variable investigation. *Frontiers in Psychology, 8*, 1736. https://doi.org/10.3389/fpsyg.2017.01736

4 Genetics, emotions, and emotions regulation

Emotions play an important part in sport and exercise from both an intra- and interpersonal perspective. Defined as an organized psychophysiological reaction to an environmental stimulus, emotions influence an individual's physiological, cognitive, motivational, and behavioral states which may have a major impact on motor performance. Emotionality varies among and within individuals, depending on the context and life history. This variation may be attribute, at least in part, to genetic variation. Significant progress has been made in identifying genetic variants that modulate inter-individual differences in emotionality processing.

Emotion in sport

Participation in competitive sport triggers a myriad of emotional experiences. Whether it is the pleasure felt after scoring a goal in training, the anxiety provoked by a crucial competition, the pride of winning, or the frustration of losing, emotions are ubiquitous in the context of sport performance (Martinent, Gareau, Lienhart, Nicaise, & Guillet-Descas, 2018; Vallerand & Blanchard, 2000). On one hand, research has revealed that sport involvement offers opportunities to experience various positive emotions (Lundqvist & Kenttä, 2010; Martinent, Campo, & Ferrand, 2012). Yet, given the idiosyncratic nature of emotional states, others argue that the pressure imposed on athletes in competitive sport context can lead to negative emotional experiences (Gaudreau, Amiot, & Vallerand, 2009; Martinent, Guillet-Descas, & Moiret, 2015). Thus, to achieve greatness in the motor domain, the ability to optimize emotional experience is a critical psychological skill to possess (Janelle, Fawver, & Beatty, 2018). But what influences the emotional response of an individual facing various sport situations? Is this ability to optimize emotional experience more a matter of nature or nurture? To answer these questions, the current chapter aims to examine the role that genetics play in the generation of emotional response leading to optimal motor performance. Before answering this question, though, emotion is defined, and the theoretical framework presented.

Definitions

Defining what is an emotion presents many challenges. Since William James first raised this question in 1984, many definitions have been suggested; yet, none have encompassed all the research or considered entirely the categories, dimensions, or components of emotion (Vallerand & Blanchard, 2000). Moreover, terms such as affect, mood, and emotion are used interchangeably which increase the confusion when trying to draw conclusions from the scientific literature. Although the combination of these terms is referred to as an *affective phenomenon*, it is essential to conceptually differentiate emotion from affect and mood.

Emotions are considered a member of the family of terms under the umbrella of affect (Janelle et al., 2018). In contemporary use, affect refers to the mental states that involve judgment and the conscious experience of feeling (Barrett & Russell, 2015; Ekkekakis, 2012). It encompasses a range of general, dispositional, time independent characteristics, to more time constrained concepts (Janelle et al., 2018). Moods and emotions are thus some forms of affect (Janelle & Naugle, 2012). However, moods are typically experienced less intensively and last longer than emotions (Ekkekakis, 2012; Janelle & Naugle, 2012). In fact, emotions are elicited in response to a discrete stimulus or object leading to a cascade of organized psychophysiological changes that prepare the body for immediate action (Janelle et al., 2018; Janelle & Naugle, 2012; Lazarus, 2000; Vallerand & Blanchard, 2000). The current chapter focuses on emotions.

Theoretical approaches

Two theoretical approaches are frequently adopted by researchers to explain emotional reactivity and regulation (Janelle et al., 2018). First, the discrete approach considers that each emotion is unique. Thus, the qualitative aspect of each emotion must be considered to capture the functional consequence of an emotional experience. On the other hand, according to the dimensional approach, discrete emotions can be accurately classified using affective valence and arousal as the two main components of an emotion (P. J. Lang, 1995). Affective valence refers to the relative pleasantness of emotional experience, and arousal is a physiological measure of emotional intensity (Janelle & Naugle, 2012).

As illustrated in Figure 4.1, emotions manifest and can be measured through three primary response systems: *physiological, cognitive*, and *behavioral*. Studying the interactions between these three systems to explore how the physiological attributes of emotional reactions are associated with cognitive representations to result in various behaviors allows a complete understanding of an individual's emotional experience (Janelle et al., 2018). In the sport and exercise domain, performance indicators can be considered as the behavioral outcome, and physiological and cognitive factors as mediators between emotional reaction and performance.

For instance, early theoretical frameworks linking emotions to performance have considered arousal as the most prominent predictor of performance

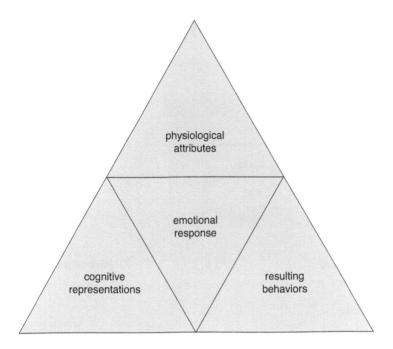

Figure 4.1 Triangulation of the three indices of emotional response
Source: based on Janelle et al. (2018).

(Baumeister & Showers, 1986). Other theories rely on the impact of anxiety, one of the most studied emotions in sport (Janelle & Naugle, 2012), on cognitive processes influencing performance (Beilock & Gray, 2007; Eysenck & Calvo, 1992; Eysenck, Derakshan, Santos, & Calvo, 2007; Masters & Maxwell, 2008). Finally, to go beyond anxiety, researchers have designed idiosyncratic emotion frameworks to examine the impact of various discrete emotions on performance (Hanin, 1995; Martinent, Nicolas, Gaudreau, & Campo, 2013).

Biological basis of emotion

Both physiological attributes and cognitive representations, illustrated in Figure 4.1, rely on biological mechanisms which interact with each other to result in experiencing emotions. The physiological attributes are expressed mainly through the physiological responses to stress, and the cognitive representations through the neural structures.

Neural structures related to emotions. From the biological perspective, emotions are assumed to be the product of neural circuits in the brain. The neural structure that plays a pivotal role in emotion expression and emotion regulation is the limbic system (see Figure 4.2). The limbic system is a complex set of

The Limbic System

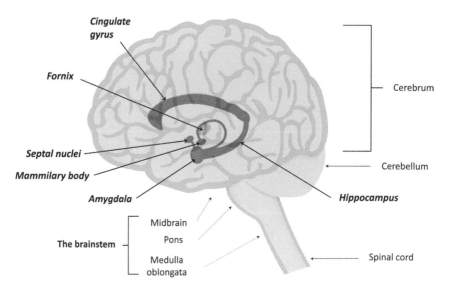

Figure 4.2 The Limbic system.

structures that lies on both sides of the thalamus, just under the cerebrum. It includes the hypothalamus, the hippocampus, the amygdala, and several other nearby areas (Rajmohan & Mohandas, 2007).

The term "limbic" was coined by Paul Pierre Broca in 1878, but its putative role in emotion was elaborated by James Papez in 1937 (Papez, 1937). The limbic lobe, situated at the inferomedial aspect of the cerebral hemispheres, consists of two concentric gyri surrounding the corpus callosum: (a) the limbic gyrus (limbic lobe) which consists of the isthmus of the cingulate gyrus, and the parahippocampal gyrus; both of which are continuous via a bundle of white matter called "cingulum," and (b) the subcallosal area (Hirai et al., 2000). The cingulate gyrus is heavily interconnected with the association areas of the cerebral cortex. The parahippocampal gyrus in the medial temporal lobe contains several distinct regions, the most important being the entorhinal cortex (ERC). The ERC funnels highly processed cortical information to the hippocampal formation, and serves as its major output pathway (Rajmohan & Mohandas, 2007). The hippocampal formation in the temporal lobe has three distinct zones: (a) the dentate gyrus, (b) the hippocampus proper, and (c) the subiculum. The dentate gyrus is composed of three layers: (a) an outer acellular molecular layer, (b) a granular middle layer, and (c) an inner polymorphic layer. The hippocampus is a trilaminate structure with an outer molecular layer, a middle pyramidal layer, and an inner polymorphic layer. Because of differences in cytoarchitecture and connectivity, the hippocampus maintains four fields (named by Lorente de No in 1934): CA1, CA2, CA3, and CA4 (CA: Cornu Ammonis). The hypothalamus plays a role in the activation of the sympathetic nervous system, which takes place in any emotional reaction (McCorry, 2007).

The limbic system's structure plays a major role in emotion expression and emotion regulation. Briefly, the thalamus serves as a sensory relay center; its neurons project signals to both the amygdala and the higher cortical regions for further processing (McCorry, 2007); the hippocampus integrates emotional experience with cognition (Tyng, Amin, Saad, & Malik, 2017); and the amygdala plays a role in processing emotional information and delivering that information to cortical structures (Gallagher & Holland, 1994). The amygdala is an almond-shaped structure deep within the temporal lobe and contains an enormous diversity of nuclei and cell types. It receives projections from most cortical fields and usually returns them (Murray, 2007). The amygdala is related to emotion, processing information, episodic memory encoding, pleasant scene, and face perception (Weymar & Schwabe, 2016). The amygdala is a key structure triggering the organisms' survival circuit that is organized into distinct motivational systems; namely, the appetitive and the defensive motivation systems (P. J. Lang & Bradley, 2013). These systems engage processes that eventually mobilize the organism for appropriate coping actions, such as approach or avoidance (P. J. Lang & Bradley, 2013; Weymar & Schwabe, 2016). The amygdala is activated by emotionally arousing stimuli, regardless of whether they are pleasant or unpleasant evidenced in face and natural scene processing studies (Sabatinelli et al., 2011), and in studies incorporating fMRI (Bonnet et al., 2015). The amygdala links emotional perception and experience (Anderson, 2007), and is also important for tagging salient cues in our environment or assigning values to important cues, which might carry functional significance such as interrupting an ongoing activity and automatically directing attention toward external signal (Weymar & Schwabe, 2016).

The physiological response to stress

The response to stress is set in the Darwinian tradition, whether we relate to the survival and adaptation of species over eons of time, or the ability of individuals to change their behavior in the face of momentarily changing circumstances. The so-called "stress response" represents an integrated reaction to stressors, broadly defined as real or perceived threats to the homeostasis or well-being (Herman et al., 2016). The crucial insights of Claude Bernard, formalized as the concept of homeostasis by Cannon in 1932, provided a critical impetus, especially to the physiological understanding of stress (Cannon, 1932). However, the concept of stress or stress response/reaction is attributed to Hans Selye. Based on his experiments with mice, and his observations on his patients, Selye described the phenomenon of stress response in his first short scientific article a "nonspecific neuroendocrine response of the body" (Selye, 1936). The term "nonspecific" refers to the principle that various agents may cause stress. Later, Selye dropped the "neuroendocrine" because he realized that in addition to the involvement of the neuroendocrine system, almost every other organ system (e.g., especially the cardiovascular, pulmonary, and renal systems) is also affected in one or several stages of stress response (Selye, 1956). According to Selye, the physiological stress response consists of a series of three stages: first, the *alarm reaction*, in which the adrenal medulla releases epinephrine and the adrenal cortex produces glucocorticoids, both of which help to restore homeostasis. Restoration of homeostasis leads to the second stage, that of *resistance*, in which defense and adaptation are sustained at optimal levels. If the stressor persists, the third stage, *exhaustion*, follows, and the *adaptive response* ceases; the consequence may be illness and death. Following the work of Lenard Levi, who distinguished between "positive" and "negative" stress (Levi, 1971), Selye introduced the terms "distress" and "eustress" to distinguish stress response of negative, unpleasant experience from positive emotions (Selye, 1976). Selye's idea of an unspecific stress response to all kinds of stimuli was challenged by Mason (1968a, 1968b, 1971), who underlined the importance of specific emotional reactions that determine a specific endocrine stress response. Mason showed that specific situational characteristics, such as novelty, uncontrollability, unpredictability, ambiguity, anticipation of negative consequences, and high ego involvement lead to specific hormonal stress responses. Two decades later, Henry (1992) distinguished between response to uncontrollability and helplessness, in which the HPA axis is activated to provide a response to a challenging situation, in which the sympathetic-adrenal-medulla (SAM) axis system is activated. The principle of "effort with distress" (HPA axis) versus "effort without distress" (SAM axis) was partially supported by Frankenhaeuser, Lundberg, and Forsman (1980), and Lundberg (1983). The HPA and SAM response to arousal are further discussed in the next section.

Arousal-performance relationship

The pressure coming from situational incentives for optimal, maximal, or superior performance (Baumeister & Showers, 1986) have been shown to influence arousal levels (Cooke, Kavussanu, McIntyre, Boardley, & Ring, 2011). When emotional arousal increases, athletes may experience a range of perceptible physiological changes such as elevated heart rate (e.g., Cooke et al., 2011; Cooke, Kavussanu, McIntyre, Boardley, & Ring, 2010; Cottyn, De Clercq, Pannier, Crombez, & Lenoir, 2006), elevated skin conductance response (e.g., Edmonds, Tenenbaum, Mann, Johnson, & Kamata, 2008; Perkins, Wilson, & Kerr, 2001), and alteration in breathing patterns (e.g., Ritz, George, & Dahme, 2000). The psychophysiological cascade triggered by an emotional episode generally activates the systems to get the body ready to attend, perceive, and react to stimuli in the environment (P. J. Lang & Bradley, 2010).

In this vein, evidence shows that physiological changes partially mediate the relationship between pressure conditions and motor performance (Balk, Adriaanse, De Ridder, & Evers, 2013; Cooke et al., 2011; Cooke et al., 2010). In fact, the "inverted-U" model (Yerkes & Dodson, 1908), stipulates that physiological arousal benefits performance, but only up to a certain threshold. Once athletes' arousal levels exceed that critical point, performance will suffer. By controlling for incentive and directly manipulating the arousal, Arent and Landers (2003) supported the prediction of a curvilinear relationship between arousal and performance.

Several factors may alter the shape, or slope, of the inverted-U curve (Janelle et al., 2018). First, the optimal arousal level for tasks demanding high physical effort such as weightlifting will be higher than for tasks requiring precision such as golf (Parfitt, Hardy, & Pates, 1995; Parfitt, Jones, & Hardy, 1990). Expertise also plays a role in the arousal-performance relationship. While it has been shown that the performance of novice golfers deteriorates under increased arousal (Balk et al., 2013; Cooke et al., 2010), the performance of expert golfers improved under similar physiological states (Cooke et al., 2011). Finally, personality (e.g., trait anxiety) can also interfere with the arousal-performance relationship (Janelle et al., 2018). Although the inverted-U model has been accepted as a guiding framework in sport psychology, it remains largely descriptive and does not account for individual differences or task constraints.

To circumvent these limitations, Kamata, Tenenbaum, and Hanin, (2002) developed the individual arousal-related performance zones (IAPZs). Based on the inverted-U idea that poor and moderate performance can happen both above and below an optimal level, van der Lei, Tenenbaum, and Land, (2016) monitored heart rate during a putting and swinging golf task, and then associated it to each athlete's perceived level of performance (poor, moderate, optimal). Analysis of heart rate during the three self-reported levels of performance allowed the creation of IAPZs. These zones were then used to test whether routine patterns implemented by athletes before putting or swinging are influenced by arousal states. The findings revealed observable changes in temporal and behavioral patterns as the golfers fluctuated in and out of their optimal IAPZs. Importantly, these changes and fluctuations were specific to each golfer. Criticism about the inverted-U model and the IAPZs both highlight the idiosyncratic nature of the arousal-performance relationship. In addition to environmental factors, individual differences account for the variation in people's physiological reaction to stressful situations.

As mentioned above, two biological systems act upon arousal: the hypothalamus–pituitary–adrenal (HPA) axis and the autonomic nervous system. The autonomic nervous system causes the rapid release of (nor)adrenaline from the adrenal medulla into the circulation which – as a hormone – can rapidly regulate the function of peripheral organs. Noradrenaline is also released in various brain areas, including cells in the limbic system, and structures like the amygdala and hippocampus (McGaugh, 2004; Valentino & Van Bockstaele, 2008). Later, the HPA axis is activated, which causes the secretion of corticosteroid hormones from the adrenal cortex. Corticosteroid hormones are very lipophilic and therefore easily pass the blood–brain barrier, in principle reaching all cells but acting only on those carrying receptors (Krugers, Karst, & Joëls, 2012).

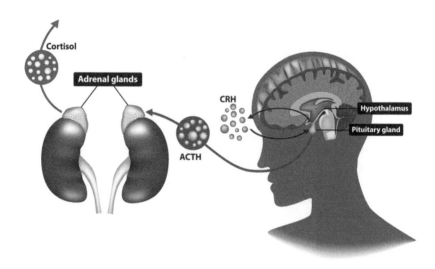

Figure 4.3 The Hypothalamo–Pituitary–Adrenal (HPA) stress axis.

The HPA axis (see Figure 4.3) is a hierarchical hormone system which encompasses the hypothalamus, the pituitary gland, and the adrenal cortex with their respective hormonal secretagogues (Kupfermann, 1991).

Facing internal or external challenge, neural stimulation of the paraventricular nucleus (PVN) of the hypothalamus initiates the secretion of corticotrophin releasing hormone (CRH). Important afferent stimulation or inhibition of the PVN originates from brain areas like the brain stem, specifically, the locus coeruleus and the nucleus tractus solitarius, the amygdala, and the hippocampus. In the pituitary, CRH leads to cleavage of proopiomelanocortin (POMC) into adrenocorticotropin (ACTH), beta-endorphin, and other peptides and to subsequent release of these peptides. CRH is the most potent but not the only trigger of ACTH release (Herman et al., 2016). Other ACTH secretagogues, such as vasopressin, oxytocin, adrenaline, and noradrenaline, significantly modulate the effects of CRH. After release, ACTH is transported via the bloodstream to the adrenal cortex and triggers the secretion of glucocorticoids (predominantly cortisol). Cortisol exerts its effects via genomic as well as nongenomic pathways (McEwen, 1991, 1994). It has a wide range of physiological effects since virtually every nucleated cell in the body has cortisol receptors and significant amounts of glucocorticoids penetrate the blood–brain barrier (de Kloet, Joëls, & Holsboer, 2005; de Kloet, Vreugdenhil, Oitzl, & Joëls, 1998). Under stress, cortisol redirects energy utilization among various organs. (Chrousos & Gold, 1992; McEwen, 2003). Cortisol also impacts on other important physiological systems (Lovallo, 2016), such as the cardiovascular system, the immune system, fluid volume, and cognitive processes (Het, Ramlow, & Wolf, 2005).

One of the key challenges in investigating the effects of sport competition on the cortisol response is separating cortisol secretion due to emotional stress or due to physiological demands of the exercise. Exercise intensity influences blood glucose levels and results in declining levels to elicit the hypothalamus to secrete the corticotrophin releasing CRH. CRH triggers the release of the adrenocortico-tropic hormone, which activates the adrenal cortex to release cortisol, which supports homeostasis of blood glucose levels (Paz & Pare, 2013). Cortisol secretion with the aim of mobilizing energy sources is therefore independent from experiencing psychosocial stressors. Indeed, blood glucose significantly decreased while salivary cortisol significantly increased after high-intensity exercise compared to rest and low-intensity exercise (Engert et al., 2013; Jacks, Sowash, Anning, McGloughlin, & Andres, 2002). The anticipatory cortisol response before sport competition reflects moderate cortisol reactivity that prepares athletes optimally for the demands of sport competition via the influence on cognitive processes and attentional control (van Paridon, Timmis, Nevison, & Bristow, 2017). However, both female athletes and international competitors did not demonstrate a significant anticipatory cortisol response, possibly due to differences in appraisal of the stress of sport competition (van Paridon et al., 2017).

The sympathetic-adrenalmedulla (SAM) axis is not characterized by a hierarchical organization with integrated feedback loops. Sympathetic nerve fibers project to single chromaffin mark cells in the adrenal medulla with cholinergic synapses. The sympathetic nerves, innervated by the CNS, stimulate the adrenal medulla, which in turn secretes adrenaline (~0.80) and noradrenaline (~0.20). In the medulla, the conversion of noradrenaline to adrenalin is mediated by cortisol. Under resting conditions, the adrenal medulla releases only low levels of catecholamines into the blood. During stress, significant amounts may be secreted from the adrenal medulla (up to approximately 0.35 of the total circulating noradrenaline), while the remainder is released from sympathetic nerve endings and may enter the bloodstream from the site of release. Catecholamines are then transported throughout the body and impact the organ systems. Adrenaline and noradrenaline secreted from the adrenal medulla can have the same target organs as the neurotransmitter of postganglionic sympathetic neurons. However, noradrenaline released from sympathetic nerve endings act mainly locally with only a small proportion of released noradrenaline reaching the bloodstream. Although adrenaline has several equivalent effects on the body as direct sympathetic stimulation, the effects last considerably longer and can, via the bloodstream, also reach organs without direct sympathetic innervations (Kudielka & Kirschbaum, 2007). The effect of a sympathetic nerve impulse is short due to a rapid reuptake in postganglionic neurons and fast enzymatic degradation by *COMT* or *MAO* (Linares et al., 1987). Besides extreme heat or cold, pain, blood loss, and lack of oxygen supply, etc., physical effort (e.g., physical labor, exercising like bicycle ergometry and treadmill running) and psychological stress (e.g., parachute jumps, exams, public speeches, cognitive conflict tasks, the Trier Social Stress Test) activate catecholamine release (Axelrod & Reisine, 1984; Mason, 1968b; Schommer, Hellhammer, & Kirschbaum, 2003). Interestingly, under repeated psychosocial stress, the reactivity of the HPA axis and the SAM system dissociates. Although HPA-axis responses quickly habituate, the SAM system shows rather uniform activation patterns with repeated exposure to psychosocial challenge (Schommer et al., 2003). The fundamental role of catecholamine secretion is the rapid mobilization of stored energy depots (e.g., supply of free fatty acids and glucose, glucogenolysis, and lipolysis), and to downregulate less important organ functions (e.g., the gastrointestinal tract, reproduction). With respect to cardiovascular functioning during stress, catecholamines mediate the so-called defense reaction by increasing heart rate, cardiac output, and blood pressure (for reviews, see Hjemdahl, 2000). Central noradrenergic neurons terminate the PVN and synapse on CRH neurons directly activating CRH neurons. Some of these stress-related adaptational processes were identified as the "fight-or-flight" response by Cannon as early as the first half of the last century (Cannon, 1929).

Besides the HPA and SAM axes, several other endocrine systems contribute to a reestablishment of homeostasis under stress (Herman, 2012; Ulrich-Lai & Herman, 2009). Some of these systems show significant alterations during periods of acute stress. These systems act directly by causing changes in the release of endocrine stress mediators or act more indirectly by changing levels of monitored parameters which then in turn provoke homeostatic adjustment.

The marked interpersonal variability in responses to different stressors was interpreted by subjective perception of the situation (Biondi & Picardi, 1999), and by the specific neurochemical "signature" of each stressor (Pacak & McCarty, 2000).

The HPA axis displays extensive variability in reactivity among human subjects. Common gene variants have been associated with several changes in HPA-axis reactivity. These gene variants are identified in the *GABA* receptor, the μ-opioid receptor, *5-HTT*, catechol O-methyltransferase (*COMT*), monoamine oxidase (*MAOA*), the α2-adrenergic receptor, *BDNF*, and the angiotensin-converting enzyme (DeRijk, 2009). Because of these genetic variants, HPA-axis reactivity changes, exposing not only the brain, but the whole body, to suboptimal cortisol levels during challenges. These genetic variants, which modulate HPA-axis reactivity, are part of the genetic make-up that determines individual stress responsivity and coping style, and consequently, affect performance.

Anxiety–performance relationship

Of all emotional responses, anxiety has been the most widely studied in sport psychology because of its potential influence on performance (Janelle & Naugle, 2012). Defined as the fear of the unknown leading to negative thoughts, worries, and concerns in anticipation of future danger (APA, 2000), anxiety can be a trait or a state. According to Spielberger's Anxiety conceptualization (1972), trait-anxiety represents an individual's general tendency to experience elevations in state anxiety when exposed to stressors, and state anxiety refers to the intensity of that emotion at a given time. Another important aspect of anxiety is its multi-dimensionality. For instance Martens, Vealey, & Burton, (1990) recommend that two dimensions, namely somatic anxiety (i.e., perception of physiological arousal), and cognitive anxiety (i.e., degree of negative thoughts, worries and concerns) be considered when studying the relationship between anxiety and performance.

Anxiety is characterized by increased arousal, expectancy, autonomic, and neuroendocrine activation. Several mechanisms are involved in the induction and inhibition of anxious states, including: neurotransmitters (GABA and gluta-mate), adenosine, cannabinoids, numerous neuropeptides, hormones, neuro-trophins, cytokines, and several cellular mediators (Millan, 2003). A genetic predisposition to anxiety is undoubted; however, the nature and extent of that contribution is still unclear (Steimer, 2002). Several SNPs have been reported in relation to trait anxiety (Savage, Sawyers, Roberson-Nay, & Hettema, 2017). Probably the best studied one is a SNP in the promoter of the serotonin trans-porter (frequently abbreviated as 5-HTT or SERT). 5-HTT is encoded by the SLC6A4 gene and its transcription is modulated by a repetitive sequence, the SLC6A4-linked polymorphic region (5-HTTLPR). 5-HTTLPR is either expressed as a short or long allele. The short allele leads to the synthesis of less 5-HTT protein than the long one, leading to higher serotonin concentration in the synaptic cleft (Canli & Lesch, 2007). The lower expressing 5-HTTLPR short variant allele was found to be associated with trait anxiety, and reduced gray matter volume in limbic regions and alterations in neural circuit activation (e.g., amygdala, hypothalamus) during stress and emotional processing (see Weger & Sandi, 2018 for review). Variations in genes from the catecholamine systems, GABAergic system, HPA axis, and brain bioenergetics are also associated with anxiety and neuroticism (Weger & Sandi, 2018).

Following this recommendation, early evidence revealed that when experi-encing high state anxiety, the performance levels of high trait-anxiety athletes deteriorate more sharply than the performance of low and moderate trait-anxiety ones (Sonstroem & Bernardo, 1982). More recent work supports these findings by showing that when under pressure, choking-susceptible athletes (high-trait anxiety) suffered from performance decrements whereas choking-resistant ones (low trait-anxiety) improved their performance (Mesagno & Marchant, 2013). This discrepancy could be explained by the fact that these two opposite person-ality profiles experience substantively different cognitions under pressure.

In line with this assumption, several cognitive frameworks have been developed to explain the anxiety–performance relationship. In the early 1990s, the Cusp Catastrophe Model (CCM) integrated physiological arousal and cog-nitive anxiety to explain how the two interact and impact performance out-comes (Hardy, 1990). First, when cognitive anxiety is low, alterations in physiological arousal result in slight and continuous changes in performance. Yet, at a high level of cognitive anxiety, the impact of physiological arousal on performance follows a curvilinear relationship meaning that performance cata-strophically drops once the optimal arousal level is exceeded. On the other hand, when physiological arousal is low, cognitive anxiety has a positive linear relationship with performance whereas at high levels of physiological arousal cognitive anxiety has a negative influence on performance (Hardy, 1996; Janelle et al., 2018).

Higher trait anxiety can also alter performance through its influence on attentional processes. According to the processing efficiency theory (PET; Eysenck & Calvo, 1992), when performers reach a certain level of anxiety, their executive attentional process is compromised. Specifically, anxiety has two effects on the central executive component of the attentional system. First, worrisome thoughts provoked by elevated state anxiety consume attentional capacity leaving fewer attentional resources for the task at hand. If insufficient resources remain to retain on-task attention, performance is impaired. Yet, anxiety also has the potential to increase effort. Therefore, if the anxious individual is motivated enough to devote additional attentional resources to the task, it compensates the lack of resources and performance can be enhanced (Derakshan & Eysenck, 2009; Eysenck et al., 2007; Janelle & Naugle, 2012).

Building on PET, attentional control theory (ACT; Eysenck et al., 2007) was designed to specify which cognitive functions are affected by anxiety. Specifically, ACT stipulates that anxiety disrupts the balance between two attentional systems; the goal-directed attentional system and the stimulus-driven attentional system. The goal-directed attentional system is influenced by the individual's current goals, expectations, and knowledge whereas the stimulus-driven attentional system responds to salient stimuli. Anxious individuals preferentially attend to threat-related stimuli whether internal (e.g., worries) or external (e.g., task-irrelevant distractors). This lack of attentional control under stressful circumstances prevents performers from maintaining their attention on relevant task-stimuli (goal-directed attentional system) resulting in performance impairment (Derakshan & Eysenck, 2009; Eysenck et al., 2007). PET and ACT are similar in essence to the distraction theories (Wine, 1971) which suggest that shifting attention toward task-irrelevant cues changes what was initially a single-task performance into a dual-task challenge where the task at hand and the distractions compete for attentional resources (Beilock & Carr, 2001).

Different from distraction theories, conscious processing theories highlight the impact of self-consciousness in the anxiety–performance relationship (Beilock & Carr, 2001; Janelle & Naugle, 2012). Namely, according to the reinvestment theory (Masters, 1992; Masters & Maxwell, 2008), when anxiety rises, individuals tend to focus inward in an attempt to consciously control aspects of their movements. By reinvesting explicit knowledge about how to perform, the automaticity that usually defines high-level performance is disrupted. Accordingly, the explicit monitoring theory (Baumeister, 1984) stipulates that increased attention paid to skill processes and their step-by-step control leads to a deterioration of well-learned or proceduralized performances.

Although distraction theories and conscious processing theories may appear contradictory, they turn out to be complementary. In fact, they have different domains of applicability depending on how much the motor task/skill relies on executive function such as working memory. Anxious athletes performing a task that requires complex decision-making in action will suffer more from dual-task interferences whereas athletes executing automatized motor skills will suffer from bringing their attention to the step-by-step process (Beilock & Carr, 2001). Empirical evidence in the motor domain supports the CCM (e.g., Duncan et al., 2016), the PET (e.g., Cooke et al., 2011; M. Wilson, Smith, & Holmes, 2007), the ACT (e.g., Nibbeling, Daanen, Gerritsma, Hofland, & Oudejans, 2012; M. R. Wilson, Wood, & Vine, 2009) and the reinvestment theory (e.g., Cooke et al., 2010; Kinrade, Jackson, & Ashford, 2010). Taken together, these cognitive theories provide a rationale for how performance alteration arises as a function of the interaction between individual dispositional characteristics and the environment (Janelle & Naugle, 2012).

Emotion-performance relationship

While several theories have focused on anxiety to explain how emotions impact performance, research has also been conducted within a framework that considers other emotions (Janelle & Naugle, 2012). At the dawn of the 1990s, the assumption that individualized affective profiles might be the best way to predict optimal sport performance inspired important theoretical advancement (Janelle et al., 2018). Namely, Hanin (1989) developed the Zones of Optimal Functioning (ZOF), a sports-specific model initially articulated around athletes' optimal levels of state anxiety. The fact that this first model was mainly descriptive, and did not explain why some individuals perform better or worse than others under a certain level of anxiety, was highly criticized (Gould & Tuffey, 1996).

To go beyond pre-event anxiety, the ZOF further evolved into the Individual Zone of Optimal Functioning (IZOF; Hanin, 1995). This idiographic approach integrates functional and dysfunctional patterns of various emotions to study the subjective emotional experiences related to individual optimal and poor performances (Harmison, 2011; Ruiz, Raglin, & Hanin, 2017). According to the most recent version of the model (Hanin, 2000), to fully explore the structure and function of emotional experience, different dimensions must be considered (i.e., form, intensity, time, context, and content). Among these dimensions, emotional content is critical for the functional interpretation of one's emotional experience. Compared to the nomothetic approach used by most researchers (i.e., standardized emotion questionnaires), emotional content is an idiosyncratic method that combines hedonic tone and functionality. Hedonic tone refers to the positive or negative valence attributed to emotions. Examples of positive emotions are active, calm, excited, and brave, whereas afraid, angry, and anxious are considered negative emotions (Hanin, 2000). Functionality denotes the helpful or harmful impact of such emotion on performance.

The four global categories derived from the IZOF approach are positive helpful (P+), positive harmful (P–), negative helpful (N+), and negative harmful (N–). In addition, to be *quantifiable* (i.e., the amount of each category's experiences), these categories can be rated in terms of *intensity*. This method allows the examination of the direction of all the discrete emotions experienced by athletes during competition. It can also provide guidance on how energy can be mobilized and used during sport events. For instance, P+ are known to stimulate energy generation and help sustain effort while N+ are strong energy producers. In contrast, P– and N– are associated with decreased effort, ineffective resource recruitment, and energy misuse (Martinent et al., 2012). Extensive empirical evidence has supported this emotion-performance relationship model (see Ruiz et al., 2017 for a review).

Building on this conceptualization, Martinent et al., (2013) recently identified four multivariate affective profiles relying on various configurations of intensity and directionality of positive and negative affective states. The *high positive affect facilitators profile* represents individuals for which positive affects (e.g., active, enthusiastic, excited) are high and facilitative, whereas negative affects (i.e., afraid and upset) are low and debilitative. The *low affect debilitators profile* regrouped athletes for which positive affect is substantially low and highly debilitative, whereas negative affect is somewhat low as well as neutral to debilitative. The *facilitators profile* describes individuals for which all affects (i.e., positive, afraid, and upset) are perceived as facilitative. Finally, *high negative affect debilitators profile* refers to those for which negative affects are high and highly debilitative.

In terms of the emotion-performance relationship, it has been shown that *low affect debilitators profile* is negatively linked to competitive goal achievement. These results corroborate the IZOF's postulate that dysfunctional emotional states demobilize energy. On the other hand, facilitators profile was associated with increased likelihood of goal attainment. Similarly, athletes identified as *high negative affect debilitators profile* were less likely to reach their competitive goal than *high positive affect facilitators profile* athletes. Overall, these results highlight the performance advantages of experiencing intense positive facilitating affect compared to negative debilitating ones (Martinent et al., 2013). This trend provides a direction to the IZOF conclusion which stipulates that successful performance is predicted by emotional intensity that lies within previously established optimal zones and outside non-optimal ones.

Although the impact of emotions on performance varies from one person to another, experiencing positive functional emotions presents some advantages. Therefore, we now aim to explore whether specific genes predispose individuals to experience positive emotions over negative ones.

Variability in emotions and emotion regulation

What makes some people more prone than others to adaptive/maladaptive behaviors in response to increased stress/emotional load? Imagine an athlete experiencing a stressful event, such as losing an important competition, and, as a result, feeling frustrated. In response, various emotion regulation strategies are possible. Some may use the event as motivation to perform better. Others might accept the result and carry on. Some might worry excessively about career implications becoming increasingly agitated. This variation in emotions and emotion regulation originates from two main sources: variability in environmental factors affecting emotion and variability in genetic factors related to the biological mechanisms underlying emotions.

Twin studies provide a means of examining the source of emotion regulation by quantifying both genetic (i.e., heritable) and environmental contributions. There have been a few twin studies on emotion regulation (Canli, Ferri, & Duman, 2009; Hawn, Overstreet. Stewart, & Amstadter, 2015). First twin studies focused mainly on emotion associated traits (e.g., personality characteristics; Jang, Livesley, & Vernon, 1996) and self-report emotion regulation difficulties (Weinberg, Venables, Proudfit, & Patrick, 2015) with less emphasis on certain emotion regulation strategies (Canli et al., 2009). However, a growing number of studies exploring individual differences in emotion regulation and temperament among infants and children suggest that the processes underlying emotion regulation are moderately attributed to heritability (Goldsmith, Pollak, & Davidson, 2008). Overall, the literature consistently suggests a moderate degree of heritability to the processes associated with emotion regulation across the lifespan (0.25–0.55) (Canli et al., 2009; Coccaro, Ong, Seroczynski, & Bergeman, 2012; Hawn, Paul, Thomas, Miller, & Amstadter, 2015). For example, in a study conducted among adult twins, heritability estimates of ~0.4 were found to influence liability and intensity of emotional experiences; specifically, anger and anxiety (Coccaro et al., 2012) Furthermore, brain activity occurring during periods of time where emotion regulation is believed to be actively occurring (i.e., viewing of images) appears to be moderately heritable (0.45–0.55) (Kanakam, Krug, Raoult, Collier, & Treasure, 2013) with multiple genetic variants contributing to its interpersonal variability (Barzman, Geise, & Lin, 2015; Hawn, Overstreet, et al., 2015; Leighton, Botto, Silva, Jiménez, & Luyten, 2017). HPA-axis genes are associated with stress-related endophenotypes including cortisol response and reduced brain volumes (Gerritsen et al., 2017). The pivotal genetic variants associated with emotional regulation are located on genes which relate to the biological mechanisms such as HPA/HPG axes, oxytocin, dopamine, and serotonin. These are described in Table 4.1.

Summary

Emotion regulation refers to the mechanisms involved in modulating emotional reactions to accomplish goals. The capacity to regulate is a finite cognitive resource. Dysregulated behaviors appear when adaptive emotional regulation efforts deteriorate, and in turn, affect motor performance. This ongoing process is influenced by both genetic and environmental factors (see Figure 4.4)

Variability in emotion regulation might result from variation in genes related to the biological mechanism underlying emotion regulation. Genetic variation was studied mainly in daily life models or in pathopsychological models. Despite the importance of emotion regulation to motor performance, the link between genetic variability – emotion regulation – and motor performance has not been studied so far.

Table 4.1 Main genetic variants related to emotional regulation

Gene	Relation to emotional regulation
Serotonin *5-HTT* The serotonin transporter	5-HTTLPR polymorphism, which determines serotonin synaptic signaling (Beitchman et al., 2006) is associated with: • HPA axis reactivity to psychosocial stress (Miller, Wankerl, Stalder, Kirschbaum, & Alexander, 2013) • Frontal lobe activity during emotional regulation processes (Grossmann et al., 2011) • Levels of cortisol in response to the stressor (Manuck, Flory, Ferrell, Mann, & Muldoon, 2000) • Prolonged cortisol activity after a stressor (Gotlib, Joormann, Minor, & Hallmayer, 2008) • sensitivity to error processing in event-related potential experiments (Althaus et al., 2009) • anxiety and reduced gray matter volume in limbic regions and alterations in neural circuit activation (Weger & Sandi, 2018)
Catecholamine system *DRD2,3,4* dopamine receptors D2, D3, D4	Taq1 A polymorphism in *DRD2*, which affects receptor binding affinity (Thompson et al., 1997) is associated with greater sensitivity to negative feedback among A allele carriers (Althaus et al., 2009) Polymorphism in DRD2 (Wacker, Reuter, Hennig, & Stemmler, 2005) (Kim et al., 2013), DRD3 (Henderson et al., 2000) and DRD4 (Tochigi et al., 2006) are associated with high anxiety trait
COMT enzyme that degrades dopamine	Val156Met polymorphism affect dopamine catabolizing activity (Männistö & Kaakkola, 1999), with Val allele having higher activity Met allele is associated with severe emotion dysregulation in children and adolescents (Egan et al., 2001; Tunbridge, Harrison, & Weinberger, 2006; Waugh, Dearing, Joormann, & Gotlib, 2009), higher scores of anxiety and neuroticism and lower scores of extraversion (Eley et al., 2003; Hoth et al., 2006; Stein, Fallin, Schork, & Gelernter, 2005) Val allele carriers were more likely to become irritable when their expected rewards were delayed (Boettiger et al., 2007)
MAOA monoamine oxidase-A regulates monoamine transmitter levels in CNS	uVNTR polymorphism affects gene expression (Saito et al., 2002) Carriers of the variant associated with low gene expression have a higher propensity for aggression and impulsivity (Huang et al., 2004; Manuck et al., 2000), reduced left middle frontal gyrus activation, and left amygdala and posterior thalamic activation in response to an anger trigger (Alia-Klein et al., 2009)

BDNF Brain Derived Neurotrophic Factor	Val66Met poly morphism Met allele alters intracellular trafficking and packaging of pro-BDNF and, consequently, the regulated secretion of the mature peptide (Egan et al., 2003; U. E. Lang, Hellweg, Sander, & Gallinat, 2009) Associated with: • higher levels of anxiety and neuroticism (Hashimoto, 2007; U. E. Lang et al. 2005; Moreira et al., 2015) • higher scores of "anticipatory worry" and "fear of uncertainty" (Montag, Basten, Stelzel, Fiebach, & Reuter, 2010)
GABAergic system *GABRA6* GABA(A) α6 receptor subunit	Pro385Ser polymorphism is associated with higher neuroticism scores (Sen et al., 2004) T1521C polymorphism is associated with anticipatory worry, fear of uncertainty, shyness, and fatigability (Arias et al., 2012) T allele carriers exhibit increased levels of HPA axis hormones in response to acute stress (Uhart, McCaul, Oswald, Choi, & Wand, 2004)
HPA axis *CRHR1* Corticotrophin releasing hormone receptor 1	TAT haplotype is the key activator of the HPA axis, binding to receptors that initiate the stress response, culminating with release of cortisol from the adrenal cortex (Müller & Wurst, 2004) Associated with: • cortisol response to psychosocial stress (Mahon et al. 2013) • resilient functioning among children (Cicchetti & Rogosch 2012; Mahon et al., 2013) • moderates the effect of childhood maltreatment on cortisol responses to the Dex/CRH test (DeYoung, Cicchetti, & Rogosch, 2011; Tyrka et al., 2009)
Oxytocin *OXTR* Oxytocin receptor	rs53576 A/G polymorphism Carriers of the A allele have an increased sensitivity to stress, reduced social skills, negative mental health outcomes, and lower levels of optimism, mastery, and self-esteem (Saphire-Bernstein, Way, Kim, Sherman, & Taylor, 2011)

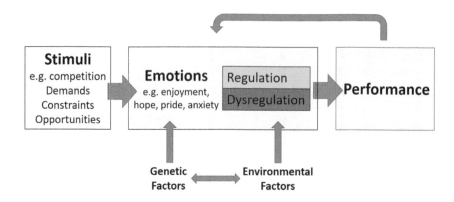

Figure 4.4 The ongoing process of emotion regulation/dysregulation and performance.

References

Alia-Klein, N., Goldstein, R. Z., Tomasi, D., Woicik, P. A., Moeller, S. J., Williams, B., ... Volkow, N. D. (2009). Neural mechanisms of anger regulation as a function of genetic risk for violence. *Emotion, 9*(3), 385–96.

Althaus, M., Groen, Y., Wijers, A. A., Mulder, L. J. M., Minderaa, R. B., Kema, I. P., ... Hoekstra, P. J. (2009). Differential effects of 5-HTTLPR and DRD2/ANKK1 polymorphisms on electrocortical measures of error and feedback processing in children. *Clinical Neurophysiology: Official Journal of the International Federation of Clinical Neurophysiology, 120*(1), 93–107. https://doi.org/10.1016/j.clinph.2008.10.012

Anderson, A. K. (2007). Feeling emotional: The amygdala links emotional perception and experience. *Social Cognitive and Affective Neuroscience, 2*(2), 71–2. https://doi.org/10.1093/scan/nsm022

APA (2000). *Diagnostic and statistical manual of mental disorders: DSM-IV-TR*. Fourth Edition. Washington, DC: American Psychiatric Association.

Arent, S. M., & Landers, D. M. (2003). Arousal, anxiety, and performance: A reexamination of the Inverted-U Hypothesis. *Research Quarterly for Exercise and Sport, 74*(4), 436–44.

Arias, B., Aguilera, M., Moya, J., Sáiz, P. A., Villa, H., Ibáñez, M. I., ... Fañanás, L. (2012). The role of genetic variability in the SLC6A4, BDNF and GABRA6 genes in anxiety-related traits. *Acta Psychiatrica Scandinavica, 125*(3), 194–202. https://doi.org/10.1111/j.1600-0447.2011.01764.x

Axelrod, J., & Reisine, T. D. (1984). Stress hormones: Their interaction and regulation. *Science, 224*(4648), 452–9.

Balk, Y. A., Adriaanse, M. A., De Ridder, D. T. D., & Evers, C. (2013). Coping under pressure: Employing emotion regulation strategies to enhance performance under pressure. *Journal of Sport and Exercise Psychology, 35*(4), 408–18.

Barrett, L. F., & Russell, J. A. E. (2015). *The psychological construction of emotion*. New York, NY: Guilford Press.

Barzman, D., Geise, C., & Lin, P.-I. (2015). Review of the genetic basis of emotion dysregulation in children and adolescents. *World Journal of Psychiatry, 5*(1), 112–7. https://doi.org/10.5498/wjp.v5.i1.112

Baumeister, R. F. (1984). Choking under pressure: Self-consciousness and paradoxical effects of incentives on skillful performance. *Journal of Personality and Social Psychology Quarterly, 46*, 610–20.

Baumeister, R. F., & Showers, C. J. (1986). A review of paradoxical performance effects: Choking under pressure in sports and mental tests. *European Journal of Social Psychology, 16*, 361–83. doi:10.1002/ejsp. 2420160405

Beilock, S. L., & Carr, T. H. (2001). On the fragility of skilled performance: What governs choking under pressure? *Journal of Experimental Psychology: General, 130*(4), 701–25. http://dx.doi.org/10.1037/0096-3445.130.4.701

Beilock, S. L., & Gray, R. (2007). Why do athletes choke under pressure? In G. Tenenbaum & R. C. Eklund (Eds.), *Handbook of sport psychology* (3rd ed., pp. 425–44). Hoboken, NJ: Wiley.

Beitchman, J. H., Baldassarra, L., Mik, H., De Luca, V., King, N., Bender, D., … Kennedy, J. L. (2006). Serotonin transporter polymorphisms and persistent, pervasive childhood aggression. *American Journal of Psychiatry, 163*(6), 1103–5. https://doi.org/10.1176/ajp. 2006.163.6.1103

Biondi, M., & Picardi, A. (1999). Psychological stress and neuroendocrine function in humans: The last two decades of research. *Psychotherapy and Psychosomatics, 68*(3), 114–50. https://doi.org/10.1159/000012323

Boettiger, C. A., Mitchell, J. M., Tavares, V. C., Robertson, M., Joslyn, G., D'Esposito, M., & Fields, H. L. (2007). Immediate reward bias in humans: Fronto-parietal networks and a role for the catechol-o-methyltransferase 158val/val genotype. *Journal of Neuroscience, 27*(52), 14383–91. https://doi.org/10.1523/JNEUROSCI.2551-07.2007

Bonnet, L., Comte, A., Tatu, L., Millot, J.-L., Moulin, T., & Medeiros de Bustos, E. (2015). The role of the amygdala in the perception of positive emotions: An "intensity detector." *Frontiers in Behavioral Neuroscience, 9*, 178. https://doi.org/10.3389/fnbeh.2015.00178

Canli, T., Ferri, J., & Duman, E. A. (2009). Genetics of emotion regulation. *Neuroscience, 164*(1), 43–54. https://doi.org/10.1016/j.neuroscience.2009.06.049

Canli, T., & Lesch, K.-P. (2007). Long story short: The serotonin transporter in emotion regulation and social cognition. *Nature Neuroscience, 10*(9), 1103–9. https://doi.org/10.1038/nn1964

Cannon, W. B. (1929). *Bodily changes in pain, hunger, fear and rage*. Oxford, England: Appleton.

Cannon, W. B. (1932). *The wisdom of the body*. New York, NY: W. W. Norton.

Chrousos, G. P., & Gold, P. W. (1992). The concepts of stress and stress system disorders: Overview of physical and behavioral homeostasis. *JAMA, 267*(9), 1244–52. doi:10.1001/jama.1992.03480090092034

Cicchetti, D., & Rogosch, F. A. (2012). Gene × environment interaction and resilience: Effects of child maltreatment and serotonin, corticotropin releasing hormone, dopamine, and oxytocin genes. *Development and Psychopathology, 24*(2), 411–27. https://doi.org/10.1017/S0954579412000077

Coccaro, E. F., Ong, A. D., Seroczynski, A. D., & Bergeman, C. S. (2012). Affective intensity and lability: Heritability in adult male twins. *Journal of Affective Disorders, 136*(3), 1011–6. https://doi.org/10.1016/j.jad.2011.06.042

Cooke, A., Kavussanu, M., McIntyre, D., Boardley, I. D., & Ring, C. (2011). Effects of competitive pressure on expert performance: Underlying psychological, physiological, and kinematic mechanisms. *Psychophysiology, 48*(8), 1146–56.

Cooke, A., Kavussanu, M., McIntyre, D., & Ring, C. (2010). Psychological, muscular and kinematic factors mediate performance under pressure. *Psychophysiology, 47*(6), 1109–18.

Cottyn, J., De Clercq, D., Pannier, J.-L., Crombez, G., & Lenoir, M. (2006). The measurement of competitive anxiety during balance beam performance in gymnasts. *Journal of Sports Sciences, 24*(2), 157–64.

de Kloet, E. R., Joëls, M., & Holsboer, F. (2005). Stress and the brain: From adaptation to disease. *Nature Reviews Neuroscience, 6*(6), 463–75. https://doi.org/10.1038/nrn1683

de Kloet, E. R., Vreugdenhil, E., Oitzl, M. S., & Joëls, M. (1998). Brain corticosteroid receptor balance in health and disease. *Endocrine Reviews, 19*(3), 269–301. https://doi.org/10.1210/edrv.19.3.0331

Derakshan, N., & Eysenck, M. W. (2009). Anxiety, processing efficiency, and cognitive performance: New developments from attentional control theory. *European Psychologist, 2*, 168. doi:10.1027/1016-9040.14.2.168

DeRijk, R. H. (2009). Single nucleotide polymorphisms related to HPA axis reactivity. *Neuroimmunomodulation, 16*(5), 340–52. https://doi.org/10.1159/000216192

DeYoung, C. G., Cicchetti, D., & Rogosch, F. A. (2011). Moderation of the association between childhood maltreatment and neuroticism by the corticotropin-releasing hormone receptor 1 gene. *Journal of Child Psychology and Psychiatry, 52*(8), 898–906. https://doi.org/10.1111/j.1469-7610.2011.02404.x

Duncan, M. J., Smith, M., Bryant, E., Eyre, E., Cook, K., Hankey, J., … Jones, M. V. (2016). Effects of increasing and decreasing physiological arousal on anticipation timing performance during competition and practice. *European Journal of Sport Science, 16*(1), 27–35.

Edmonds, W. A., Tenenbaum, G., Mann, D. T. Y., Johnson, M., & Kamata, A. (2008). The effect of biofeedback training on affective regulation and simulated car-racing performance: A multiple case study analysis. *Journal of Sports Sciences, 26*(7), 761–73.

Egan, M. F., Goldberg, T. E., Kolachana, B. S., Callicott, J. H., Mazzanti, C. M., Straub, R. E., … Weinberger, D. R. (2001). Effect of COMT Val108/158 Met genotype on frontal lobe function and risk for schizophrenia. *Proceedings of the National Academy of Sciences of the United States of America, 98*(12), 6917–22. https://doi.org/10.1073/pnas.111134598

Egan, M. F., Kojima, M., Callicott, J. H., Goldberg, T. E., Kolachana, B. S., Bertolino, A., … Weinberger, D. R. (2003). The BDNF val66met polymorphism affects activity-dependent secretion of BDNF and human memory and hippocampal function. *Cell, 112*(2), 257–69. Retrieved from www.ncbi.nlm.nih.gov/pubmed/12553913

Ekkekakis, P. (2012). Affect, mood, and emotion. In G. Tenenbaum, R. C. Eklund, & A. Kamata (Eds.), *Measurement in sport and exercise psychology* (pp. 321–32). Champaign, IL: Human Kinetics.

Eley, T. C., Tahir, E., Angleitner, A., Harriss, K., McClay, J., Plomin, R., … Craig, I. (2003). Association analysis of MAOA and COMT with neuroticism assessed by peers. *American Journal of Medical Genetics, 120B*(1), 90–6. https://doi.org/10.1002/ajmg.b.20046

Engert, V., Efanov, S. I., Duchesne, A., Vogel, S., Corbo, V., & Pruessner, J. C. (2013). Differentiating anticipatory from reactive cortisol responses to psychosocial stress. *Psychoneuroendocrinology, 38*(8), 1328–37. https://doi.org/10.1016/j.psyneuen.2012.11.018

Eysenck, M. W., & Calvo, M. G. (1992). Anxiety and performance: The processing efficiency theory. *Cognition and Emotion, 6*(6), 409–34. doi:10.1080/02699939208409696

Eysenck, M. W., Derakshan, N., Santos, R., & Calvo, M. G. (2007). Anxiety and cognitive performance: Attentional control theory. *Emotion, 7*(2), 336–53.

Frankenhaeuser, M., Lundberg, U., & Forsman, L. (1980). Dissociation between sympathetic-adrenal and pituitary-adrenal responses to an achievement situation characterized by high controllability: Comparison between type A and type B males and females. *Biological Psychology, 10*(2), 79–91. Retrieved from www.ncbi.nlm.nih.gov/pubmed/7437488

Gallagher, M., & Holland, P. C. (1994). The amygdala complex: Multiple roles in associative learning and attention. *Proceedings of the National Academy of Sciences of the United States of America, 91*(25), 11771–6. https://doi.org/10.1073/pnas.91.25.11771

Gaudreau, P., Amiot, C. E., & Vallerand, R. J. (2009). Trajectories of affective states in adolescent hockey players: Turning point and motivational antecedents. *Developmental Psychology, 45*(2), 307.

Gerritsen, L., Milaneschi, Y., Vinkers, C. H., van Hemert, A. M., van Velzen, L., Schmaal, L., & Penninx, B. W. (2017). HPA axis genes, and their interaction with childhood maltreatment, are related to cortisol levels and stress-related phenotypes. *Neuropsychopharmacology, 42*(12), 2446–55. https://doi.org/10.1038/npp.2017.118

Goldsmith, H. H., Pollak, S. D., & Davidson, R. J. (2008). Developmental neuroscience perspectives on emotion regulation. *Child Development Perspectives, 2*(3), 132–40. https://doi.org/10.1111/j.1750-8606.2008.00055.x

Gotlib, I. H., Joormann, J., Minor, K. L., & Hallmayer, J. (2008). HPA axis reactivity: A mechanism underlying the associations among 5-HTTLPR, stress, and depression. *Biological Psychiatry, 63*(9), 847–51. https://doi.org/10.1016/j.biopsych.2007.10.008

Gould, D., & Tuffey, S. (1996). Zones of optimal functioning research: A review and critique, 53. *Anxiety Stress Coping, 9*(1), 53–68.

Grossmann, T., Johnson, M. H., Vaish, A., Hughes, D. A., Quinque, D., Stoneking, M., & Friederici, A. D. (2011). Genetic and neural dissociation of individual responses to emotional expressions in human infants. *Developmental Cognitive Neuroscience, 1*(1), 57–66. https://doi.org/10.1016/J.DCN.2010.07.001

Hanin, Y. L. (1989). Interpersonal and intragroup anxiety in sports. In D. Hackfort & C. D. Spielberger (Eds.), *Anxiety in sports: An international perspective* (pp. 19–28). New York, NY: Hemisphere.

Hanin, Y. L. (1995). Individual zones of optimal functioning (IZOF) model: An idiographic approach to performance anxiety. In K. Henschen & W. Straub (Eds.), *Sport psychology: An analysis of athlete behavior* (pp. 103–19). Longmeadow, MA: Movement Publications.

Hanin, Y. L. (2000). *Emotions in sport.* Champaign, IL: Human Kinetics.

Hardy, L. (1990). A catastrophe model of anxiety and performance. In J. G. Jones & L. Hardy (Eds.), *Stress and performance in sport* (pp. 81–106). Chichester, England: Wiley.

Hardy, L. (1996). Testing the predictions of the cusp catastrophe model of anxiety and performance. *Sport Psychologist, 10*, 140–56.

Harmison, R. J. (2011). Peak performance in sport: Identifying ideal performance states and developing athletes' psychological skills. *Sport, Exercise, and Performance Psychology, 1*, 3–18. doi:10.1037/2157-3905.1.S.3

Hashimoto, K. (2007). BDNF variant linked to anxiety-related behaviors. *BioEssays, 29*(2), 116–19. https://doi.org/10.1002/bies.20534

Hawn, S. E., Overstreet, C., Stewart, K. E., & Amstadter, A. B. (2015). Recent advances in the genetics of emotion regulation: A review. *Current Opinion in Psychology, 3*, 108–16. https://doi.org/10.1016/j.copsyc.2014.12.014

Hawn, S. E., Paul, L., Thomas, S., Miller, S., & Amstadter, A. B. (2015). Stress reactivity to an electronic version of the trier social stress test: A pilot study. *Frontiers in Psychology, 6*, 724. doi:10.3389/fpsyg.2015.00724

Henderson, A. S., Korten, A. E., Jorm, A. F., Jacomb, P. A., Christensen, H., Rodgers, B., … Easteal, S. (2000). COMT and DRD3 polymorphisms, environmental exposures, and personality traits related to common mental disorders. *American Journal of Medical Genetics, 96*(1), 102–7. https://doi.org/10.1002/(SICI)1096-8628(20000207)96: 1102::AID-AJMG203.0.CO;2-3

Henry, J. P. (1992). Biological basis of the stress response. *Integrative Physiological and Behavioral Science: The Official Journal of the Pavlovian Society, 27*(1), 66–83. Retrieved from www.ncbi.nlm.nih.gov/pubmed/1576090

Herman, J. P. (2012). Neural pathways of stress integration: Relevance to alcohol abuse. *Alcohol Research: Current Reviews, 34*(4), 441–7. Retrieved from www.ncbi.nlm.nih. gov/pubmed/23584110

Herman, J. P., McKlveen, J. M., Ghosal, S., Kopp, B., Wulsin, A., Makinson, R., … Myers, B. (2016). Regulation of the hypothalamic-pituitary-adrenocortical stress response. *Comprehensive Physiology, 6*(2), 603–21. https://doi.org/10.1002/cphy.c150015

Het, S., Ramlow, G., & Wolf, O. T. (2005). A meta-analytic review of the effects of acute cortisol administration on human memory. *Psychoneuroendocrinology, 30*(8), 771–84. https://doi.org/10.1016/j.psyneuen.2005.03.005

Hirai, T., Korogi, Y., Yoshizumi, K., Shigematsu, Y., Sugahara, T., & Takahashi, M. (2000). Limbic lobe of the human brain: Evaluation with turbo fluid-attenuated inversion-recovery MR imaging. *Radiology, 215*(2), 470–5. https://doi.org/10.1148/ radiology.215.2.r00ma06470

Hjemdahl, P. (2000). Cardiovascular system and stress. In G. Fink (Ed.), *Encyclopedia of stress* (Vol. 1, pp. 389–403). San Diego, CA: Academic Press.

Hoth, K. F., Paul, R. H., Williams, L. M., Dobson-Stone, C., Todd, E., Schofield, P. R., … Gordon, E. (2006). Associations between the *COMT Val/Met* polymorphism, early life stress, and personality among healthy adults. *Neuropsychiatric Disease and Treatment, 2*(2), 219–25. https://doi.org/10.2147/nedt.2006.2.2.219

Huang, J., Zhu, H., Haggarty, S. J., Spring, D. R., Hwang, H., Jin, F., … Schreiber, S. L. (2004). Finding new components of the target of rapamycin (TOR) signaling network through chemical genetics and proteome chips. *Proceedings of the National Academy of Sciences of the United States of America, 101*(47), 16594–9.

Jacks, D. E., Sowash, J., Anning, J., McGloughlin, T., & Andres, F. (2002). Effect of exercise at three exercise intensities on salivary cortisol. *Journal of Strength and Conditioning Research, 16*(2), 286–9. Retrieved from www.ncbi.nlm.nih.gov/pubmed/ 11991783

Janelle, C. M., Fawver, B., & Beatty, G. F. (2018). Emotions and sport performance. In G. Tenenbaum & B. Eklund (Eds.), *Handbook of sport psychology* (4th ed.). New York, NY: Wiley.

Janelle, C. M., & Naugle, K. M. (2012). Emotional reactivity. In G. Tenenbaum, R. C. Eklund, & A. Kamata (Eds.), *Measurement in sport and exercise psychology* (pp. 333–48). Champaign, IL: Human Kinetics.

Jang, K. L., Livesley, W. J., & Vernon, P. A. (1996). Heritability of the big five personality dimensions and their facets: A twin study. *Journal of Personality, 64*(3), 577–91. Retrieved from www.ncbi.nlm.nih.gov/pubmed/8776880

Kamata, A., Tenenbaum, G., & Hanin, Y. L. (2002). Individual Zone of Optimal Functioning (IZOF): A probabilistic estimation. *Journal of Sport and Exercise Psychology, 24*(2), 189–208.

Kanakam, N., Krug, I., Raoult, C., Collier, D., & Treasure, J. (2013). Social and emotional processing as a behavioural endophenotype in eating disorders: A pilot investigation in twins. *European Eating Disorders Review: The Journal of the Eating Disorders Association, 21*(4), 294–307. https://doi.org/10.1002/erv.2232

Kim, H.-N., Roh, S.-J., Sung, Y. A., Chung, H. W., Lee, J.-Y., Cho, J., … Kim, H.-L. (2013). Genome-wide association study of the five-factor model of personality in young Korean women. *Journal of Human Genetics, 58*(10), 667–74. https://doi.org/10.1038/jhg.2013.75

Kinrade, N. P., Jackson, R. C., & Ashford, K. J. (2010). Dispositional reinvestment and skill failure in cognitive and motor tasks. *Psychology of Sport and Exercise, 11*, 312–19. doi:10.1016/j.psychsport.2010.02.005

Krugers, H. J., Karst, H., & Joëls, M. (2012). Interactions between noradrenaline and corticosteroids in the brain: From electrical activity to cognitive performance. *Frontiers in Cellular Neuroscience, 6*, 15. https://doi.org/10.3389/fncel.2012.00015

Kudielka, B. M., & Kirschbaum, C. (2007). Biological bases of the stress response. In M. al Absi (Ed.), *Stress and addiction: Biological and psychological mechanism* (pp. 3–19). Amsterdam, the Netherlands: Elsevier. https://doi.org/10.1016/B978-012370632-4/50004-8

Kupfermann, I. (1991). Hypothalamus and limbic system: Peptidergic neurons, homeostasis, and emotional behaviour. In E. R. Kandel, J. H. Schwartz, & T. M. Jessell (Eds.), *Principles of neural science* (pp. 735–49). Norwalk, CT: Appleton and Lange.

Lang, P. J. (1995). The emotion probe: Studies of motivation and attention. *The American Psychologist, 50*, 372–85.

Lang, P. J., & Bradley, M. M. (2010). Emotion and the motivational brain. *Biological Psychology, 84*(3), 437–50.

Lang, P. J., & Bradley, M. M. (2013). Appetitive and defensive motivation: Goal-directed or goal-determined? *Emotion Review: Journal of the International Society for Research on Emotion, 5*(3), 230–4. https://doi.org/10.1177/1754073913477511

Lang, U. E., Hellweg, R., Kalus, P., Bajbouj, M., Lenzen, K. P., Sander, T., … Gallinat, J. (2005). Association of a functional BDNF polymorphism and anxiety-related personality traits. *Psychopharmacology, 180*(1), 95–9. https://doi.org/10.1007/s00213-004-2137-7

Lang, U. E., Hellweg, R., Sander, T., & Gallinat, J. (2009). The Met allele of the BDNF Val66Met polymorphism is associated with increased BDNF serum concentrations. *Molecular Psychiatry, 14*(2), 120–2. https://doi.org/10.1038/mp.2008.80

Lazarus, R. S. (2000). How emotions influence performance in competitive sports. *Sport Psychologist, 14*, 229–52.

Leighton, C., Botto, A., Silva, J. R., Jiménez, J. P., & Luyten, P. (2017). Vulnerability or sensitivity to the environment? Methodological issues, trends, and recommendations in gene-environment interactions research in human behavior. *Frontiers in Psychiatry, 8*(106). https://doi.org/10.3389/fpsyt.2017.00106

Levi, L. (1971). *Society, stress and disease. Vol. 1. The psyehosocial environment and psychosomatic diseases*. Proceedings of an International Interdisciplinary Symposium held in Stockholm, April 1970. Retrieved from www.cabdirect.org/cabdirect/abstract/19722700465

Linares, O. A., Jacquez, J. A., Zech, L. A., Smith, M. J., Sanfield, J. A., Morrow, L. A., … Halter, J. B. (1987). Norepinephrine metabolism in humans. Kinetic analysis and model. *The Journal of Clinical Investigation, 80*(5), 1332–41. https://doi.org/10.1172/JCI113210

Lovallo, W. R. (2016). *Stress and health: Biological and psychological interactions* (3rd ed.). Los Angeles, CA: SAGE Publications.

Lundberg, U. (1983). Sex differences in behaviour pattern and catecholamine and cortisol excretion in 3-6-year-old day-care children. *Biological Psychology, 16*(1–2), 109–17. Retrieved from www.ncbi.nlm.nih.gov/pubmed/6850021

Lundqvist, C., & Kenttä, G. (2010). Positive emotions are not simply the absence of the negative ones: Development and validation of the Emotional Recovery Questionnaire (EmRecQ). *The Sport Psychologist, 24*(4), 468–88. doi:10.1123/tsp. 24.4.468

Mahon, P. B., Zandi, P. P., Potash, J. B., Nestadt, G., & Wand, G. S. (2012). Genetic association of FKBP5 and CRHR1 with cortisol response to acute psychosocial stress in healthy adults. *Psychopharmacology, 227*(2), 231–41.

Männistö, P. T., & Kaakkola, S. (1999). Catechol-O-methyltransferase (COMT): Biochemistry, molecular biology, pharmacology, and clinical efficacy of the new selective COMT inhibitors. *Pharmacological Reviews, 51*(4), 593–628. Retrieved from www.ncbi.nlm.nih.gov/pubmed/10581325

Manuck, S. B., Flory, J. D., Ferrell, R. E., Mann, J. J., & Muldoon, M. F. (2000). A regulatory polymorphism of the monoamine oxidase-A gene may be associated with variability in aggression, impulsivity, and central nervous system serotonergic responsivity. *Psychiatry Research, 95*(1), 9–23. Retrieved from www.ncbi.nlm.nih. gov/pubmed/10904119

Martens, R., Vealey, R. S., & Burton, D. (1990). *Competitive anxiety in sport* Champaign, IL: Human Kinetics.

Martinent, G., Campo, M., & Ferrand, C. (2012). A descriptive study of emotional process during competition: Nature, frequency, direction, duration and co-occurrence of discrete emotions. *Psychology of Sport and Exercise, 13*, 142–51. doi:10.1016/j. psychsport.2011.10.006

Martinent, G., Gareau, A., Lienhart, N., Nicaise, V., & Guillet-Descas, E. (2018). Emotion profiles and their motivational antecedents among adolescent athletes in intensive training settings. *Psychology of Sport and Exercise, 35*, 198–206. doi:10.1016/j. psychsport.2018.01.001

Martinent, G., Guillet-Descas, E., & Moiret, S. (2015). Reliability and validity evidence for the French Psychological Need Thwarting Scale scores: Significance of a distinction between thwarting and satisfaction of basic psychological needs. *Psychology of Sport and Exercise, 20*, 29–39. doi:10.1016/j.psychsport.2015.04.005

Martinent, G., Nicolas, M., Gaudreau, P., & Campo, M. (2013). A cluster analysis of affective states before and during competition. *Journal of Sport and Exercise Psychology, 35*(6), 600–11.

Mason, J. W. (1968a). A review of psychoendocrine research on the pituitary-adrenal cortical system. *Psychosomatic Medicine, 30*(Suppl. 5), S576–607. Retrieved from www.ncbi.nlm.nih.gov/pubmed/4303377

Mason, J. W. (1968b). A review of psychoendocrine research on the sympathetic-adrenal medullary system. *Psychosomatic Medicine, 30*(Suppl. 5), S631–53. Retrieved from www.ncbi.nlm.nih.gov/pubmed/4974233

Mason, J. W. (1971). A re-evaluation of the concept of "non-specificity" in stress theory. *Journal of Psychiatric Research, 8*(3), 323–33. Retrieved from www.ncbi.nlm.nih.gov/ pubmed/4331538

Masters, R. (1992). Knowledge, knerves and know-how: The role of explicit versus implicit knowledge in the breakdown of a complex motor skill under pressure. *British Journal of Psychology, 83*, 343–58. doi:10.1111/j.2044-8295.1992.tb02446.x

Masters, R., & Maxwell, J. (2008). The theory of reinvestment. *International Review of Sport and Exercise Psychology, 1*(2), 160–83.

McCorry, L. K. (2007). Physiology of the autonomic nervous system. *American Journal of Pharmaceutical Education, 71*(4), 78. Retrieved from www.ncbi.nlm.nih.gov/pubmed/17786266

McEwen, B. S. (1991). Non-genomic and genomic effects of steroids on neural activity. *Trends in Pharmacological Sciences, 12*(4), 141–7. Retrieved from www.ncbi.nlm.nih.gov/pubmed/2063480

McEwen, B. S. (1994). Steroid hormone actions on the brain: When is the genome involved? *Hormones and Behavior, 28*(4), 396–405. https://doi.org/10.1006/hbeh.1994.1036

McEwen, B. S. (2003). Early life influences on life-long patterns of behavior and health. *Mental Retardation and Developmental Disabilities Research Review, 9*(3), 149–54.

McGaugh, J. L. (2004). The amygdala modulates the consolidation of memories of emotionally arousing experiences. *Annual Review of Neuroscience, 27*(1), 1–28. https://doi.org/10.1146/annurev.neuro.27.070203.144157

Mesagno, C., & Marchant, D. (2013). Characteristics of polar opposites: An exploratory investigation of choking-resistant and choking-susceptible athletes. *Journal of Applied Sport Psychology, 25*(1), 72–91.

Millan, M. J. (2003). The neurobiology and control of anxious states. *Progress in Neurobiology, 70*(2), 83–244. Retrieved from www.ncbi.nlm.nih.gov/pubmed/12927745

Miller, R., Wankerl, M., Stalder, T., Kirschbaum, C., & Alexander, N. (2013). The serotonin transporter gene-linked polymorphic region (5-HTTLPR) and cortisol stress reactivity: A meta-analysis. *Molecular Psychiatry, 18*(9), 1018–24. https://doi.org/10.1038/mp.2012.124

Montag, C., Basten, U., Stelzel, C., Fiebach, C. J., & Reuter, M. (2010). The BDNF Val66Met polymorphism and anxiety: Support for animal knock-in studies from a genetic association study in humans. *Psychiatry Research, 179*(1), 86–90. https://doi.org/10.1016/j.psychres.2008.08.005

Moreira, F. P., Fabião, J. D., Bittencourt, G., Wiener, C. D., Jansen, K., Oses, J. P., … Ghisleni, G. (2015). The Met allele of BDNF Val66Met polymorphism is associated with increased BDNF levels in generalized anxiety disorder. *Psychiatric Genetics, 25*(5), 201–7. https://doi.org/10.1097/YPG.0000000000000097

Müller, M. B., & Wurst, W. (2004). Getting closer to affective disorders: The role of CRH receptor systems. *Trends in Molecular Medicine, 10*(8), 409–15. https://doi.org/10.1016/j.molmed.2004.06.007

Murray, E. A. (2007). The amygdala, reward and emotion. *Trends in Cognitive Sciences, 11*(11), 489–97. https://doi.org/10.1016/J.TICS.2007.08.013

Nibbeling, N., Daanen, H. A. M., Gerritsma, R. M., Hofland, R. M., & Oudejans, R. R. D. (2012). Effects of anxiety on running with and without an aiming task. *Journal of Sports Sciences, 30*(1), 11–19.

Pacak, K., & McCarty, R. (2000). Acute stress response: Experimental. In G. Fink (Ed.), *Encyclopedia of stress* (pp. 8–17). San Diego, CA: Academic Press.

Papez, J. W. (1937). A proposed mechanism of emotion. *Archives of Neurology and Psychiatry, 38*(4), 725. https://doi.org/10.1001/archneurpsyc.1937.02260220069003

Parfitt, G., Hardy, L., & Pates, L. (1995). Somatic anxiety, physiological arousal and performance: Differential effects upon a high anaerobic, low memory demand task. *International Journal of Sport Psychology, 26*, 196–213.

Parfitt, G., Jones, J. G., & Hardy, L. (1990). Multidimensional anxiety and performance. In L. G. Jones & L. Hardy (Eds.), *Stress and performance in sport* (pp. 43–80). Chichester, England: Wiley.

Paz, R., & Pare, D. (2013). Physiological basis for emotional modulation of memory circuits by the amygdala. *Current Opinion in Neurobiology, 23*(3), 381–6. https://doi.org/10.1016/j.conb.2013.01.008

Perkins, D., Wilson, G. V., & Kerr, J. H. (2001). The effects of elevated arousal and mood on maximal strength performance in athletes. *Journal of Applied Sport Psychology, 13*(3), 239–59.

Rajmohan, V., & Mohandas, E. (2007). The limbic system. *Indian Journal of Psychiatry, 49*(2), 132–9. https://doi.org/10.4103/0019-5545.33264

Ritz, T., George, C., & Dahme, B. (2000). Respiratory resistance during emotional stimulation: Evidence for a nonspecific effect of experienced arousal? *Biological Psychology, 52*(2), 143–60.

Ruiz, M. C., Raglin, J. S., & Hanin, Y. L. (2017). The individual zones of optimal functioning (IZOF) model (1978–2014): Historical overview of its development and use. *International Journal of Sport and Exercise Psychology, 15*(1), 41–63.

Sabatinelli, D., Fortune, E. E., Li, Q., Siddiqui, A., Krafft, C., Oliver, W. T., … Jeffries, J. (2011). Emotional perception: Meta-analyses of face and natural scene processing. *NeuroImage, 54*(3), 2524–33. https://doi.org/10.1016/j.neuroimage.2010.10.011

Saito, T., Lachman, H. M., Diaz, L., Hallikainen, T., Kauhanen, J., Salonen, J. T., … Tiihonen, J. (2002). Analysis of monoamine oxidase A (MAOA) promoter polymorphism in Finnish male alcoholics. *Psychiatry Research, 109*(2), 113–9. Retrieved from www.ncbi.nlm.nih.gov/pubmed/11927135

Saphire-Bernstein, S., Way, B. M., Kim, H. S., Sherman, D. K., & Taylor, S. E. (2011). Oxytocin receptor gene (OXTR) is related to psychological resources. *Proceedings of the National Academy of Sciences of the United States of America, 108*(37), 15118–22. https://doi.org/10.1073/pnas.1113137108

Savage, J. E., Sawyers, C., Roberson-Nay, R., & Hettema, J. M. (2017). The genetics of anxiety-related negative valence system traits. *American Journal of Medical Genetics Part B: Neuropsychiatric Genetics, 174*(2), 156–77. https://doi.org/10.1002/ajmg.b.32459

Schommer, N. C., Hellhammer, D. H., & Kirschbaum, C. (2003). Dissociation between reactivity of the hypothalamus-pituitary-adrenal axis and the sympathetic-adrenal-medullary system to repeated psychosocial stress. *Psychosomatic Medicine, 65*(3), 450–60.

Selye, H. (1936). A syndrome produced by diverse nocuous agents. *Nature, 138*(3479), 32. https://doi.org/10.1038/138032a0

Selye, H. (1956). *The stress of life.* New York, NY: McGraw-Hill Book Co.

Selye, H. (1976). Forty years of stress research: Principal remaining problems and misconceptions. *Canadian Medical Association Journal, 115*(1), 53–6. Retrieved from www.ncbi.nlm.nih.gov/pubmed/1277062

Sen, S., Villafuerte, S., Nesse, R., Stoltenberg, S. F., Hopcian, J., Gleiberman, L., … Burmeister, M. (2004). Serotonin transporter and GABA(A) alpha 6 receptor variants are associated with neuroticism. *Biological Psychiatry, 55*(3), 244–9. https://doi.org/10.1016/j.biopsych.2003.08.006

Sonstroem, R. J., & Bernardo, P. (1982). Intraindividual pregame state anxiety and basketball performance: A re-examination of the Inverted-U Curve. *Journal of Sport Psychology, 4*(3), 235–45.

Spielberger, C. D. (1972). Anxiety as an emotional state. In C. D. Spielberger (Ed.), *Anxiety: Current trends and theory and research* (Vol. 1). New York, NY: Academic Press.

Steimer, T. (2002). The biology of fear- and anxiety-related behaviors. *Dialogues in Clinical Neuroscience, 4*(3), 231–49. Retrieved from www.ncbi.nlm.nih.gov/pubmed/22033741

Stein, M. B., Fallin, M. D., Schork, N. J., & Gelernter, J. (2005). COMT polymorphisms and anxiety-related personality traits. *Neuropsychopharmacology, 30*(11), 2092–102. https://doi.org/10.1038/sj.npp. 1300787

Thompson, J., Thomas, N., Singleton, A., Piggott, M., Lloyd, S., Perry, E. K., … Court, J. A. (1997). D2 dopamine receptor gene (DRD2) Taq1 A polymorphism: Reduced dopamine D2 receptor binding in the human striatum associated with the A1 allele. *Pharmacogenetics, 7*(6), 479–84. Retrieved from www.ncbi.nlm.nih.gov/pubmed/9429233

Tochigi, M., Hibino, H., Otowa, T., Kato, C., Marui, T., Ohtani, T., … Sasaki, T. (2006). Association between dopamine D4 receptor (DRD4) exon III polymorphism and neuroticism in the Japanese population. *Neuroscience Letters, 398*(3), 333–6. https://doi.org/10.1016/J.NEULET.2006.01.020

Tunbridge, E. M., Harrison, P. J., & Weinberger, D. R. (2006). Catechol-o-methyltransferase, cognition, and psychosis: Val158Met and beyond. *Biological Psychiatry, 60*(2), 141–51. https://doi.org/10.1016/j.biopsych.2005.10.024

Tyng, C. M., Amin, H. U., Saad, M. N. M., & Malik, A. S. (2017). The influences of emotion on learning and memory. *Frontiers in Psychology, 8*, 1454. https://doi.org/10.3389/fpsyg.2017.01454

Tyrka, A. R., Price, L. H., Gelernter, J., Schepker, C., Anderson, G. M., & Carpenter, L. L. (2009). Interaction of childhood maltreatment with the corticotropin-releasing hormone receptor gene: Effects on hypothalamic-pituitary-adrenal axis reactivity. *Biological Psychiatry, 66*(7), 681–5. https://doi.org/10.1016/j.biopsych.2009.05.012

Uhart, M., McCaul, M. E., Oswald, L. M., Choi, L., & Wand, G. S. (2004). GABRA6 gene polymorphism and an attenuated stress response. *Molecular Psychiatry, 9*(11), 998–1006. https://doi.org/10.1038/sj.mp. 4001535

Ulrich-Lai, Y. M., & Herman, J. P. (2009). Neural regulation of endocrine and autonomic stress responses. *Nature Reviews. Neuroscience, 10*(6), 397–409. https://doi.org/10.1038/nrn2647

Valentino, R. J., & Van Bockstaele, E. (2008). Convergent regulation of locus coeruleus activity as an adaptive response to stress. *European Journal of Pharmacology, 583*(2–3), 194–203. https://doi.org/10.1016/j.ejphar.2007.11.062

Vallerand, R. J., & Blanchard, C. M. (2000). The study of emotion in sport and exercise: Historical, definitional, and conceptual perspectives. In Y. L. Hanin (Ed.), *Emotions in sport* (pp. 3–37). Champaign, IL: Human Kinetics.

van der Lei, H., Tenenbaum, G., & Land, W. M. (2016). Individual arousal-related performance zones effect on temporal and behavioral patterns in golf routines. *Psychology of Sport and Exercise, 26*, 52–60. http://dx.doi.org/10.1016/j.psychsport.2016.06.005

van Paridon, K. N., Timmis, M. A., Nevison, C. M., & Bristow, M. (2017). The anticipatory stress response to sport competition: A systematic review with meta-analysis of cortisol reactivity. *BMJ Open Sport and Exercise Medicine, 3*(1), e000261. https://doi.org/10.1136/bmjsem-2017-000261

Wacker, J., Reuter, M., Hennig, J., & Stemmler, G. (2005). Sexually dimorphic link between dopamine D2 receptor gene and neuroticism-anxiety. *Neuroreport, 16*(6),

611–14. Retrieved from https://insights.ovid.com/crossref?an=00001756-200504250-0 0019

Waugh, C. E., Dearing, K. F., Joormann, J., & Gotlib, I. H. (2009). Association between the catechol-O-methyltransferase Val158Met polymorphism and self-perceived social acceptance in adolescent girls. *Journal of Child and Adolescent Psychopharmacology, 19*(4), 395–401. https://doi.org/10.1089/cap. 2008.0141

Weger, M., & Sandi, C. (2018). High anxiety trait: A vulnerable phenotype for stress-induced depression. *Neuroscience and Biobehavioral Reviews, 87*, 27–37. https://doi.org/10.1016/J.NEUBIOREV.2018.01.012

Weinberg, A., Venables, N. C., Proudfit, G. H., & Patrick, C. J. (2015). Heritability of the neural response to emotional pictures: Evidence from ERPs in an adult twin sample. *Social Cognitive and Affective Neuroscience, 10*(3), 424–34. https://doi.org/10.1093/scan/nsu059

Weymar, M., & Schwabe, L. (2016). Amygdala and emotion: The bright side of it. *Frontiers in Neuroscience, 10*, 224. https://doi.org/10.3389/fnins.2016.00224

Wilson, M. R., Smith, N. C., & Holmes, P. S. (2007). The role of effort in influencing the effect of anxiety on performance: Testing the conflicting predictions of processing efficiency theory and the conscious processing hypothesis. *British Journal of Psychology, 3*, 411. doi:10.1348/000712606X133047

Wilson, M. R., Wood, G., & Vine, S. J. (2009). Anxiety, attentional control, and performance impairment in penalty kicks. *Journal of Sport and Exercise Psychology, 31*(6), 761–75.

Wine, J. (1971). Test anxiety and direction of attention. *Psychological Bulletin, 76*, 92–104.

Yerkes, R. M., & Dodson, J. D. (1908). The relation of strength of stimulus to rapidity of habit-formation. *Journal of Comparative Neurology and Psychology, 18*, 459–82. doi:10.1002/cne.920180503

5 Genetics, self-regulation, coping skills, and adaptation

Coping and self-regulation are essential constructs and foundations of the psychological adaptation process required by the performer to achieve success. When facing challenges, the use of coping skills and resources allows the performer to deploy cognitive and behavioral efforts to manage external and internal demands. Similarly, self-regulation skills enable the individual to adjust goal and behavior to maintain the balance, manifesting in optimal performance. While both environmental and genetic factors have direct, long-lasting influences on an individual's ability to self-regulate, these factors also interact with each other in critical ways. On one hand, environmental factors such as parental attachment can shape the epigenetics and the expression of the individual genotype; on the other hand, gene variations may increase vulnerability to certain environmental pathogens.

The pathway toward excellence in the motor domain is complex and winding. Thus, the development of expertise requires athletes to navigate through a myriad of challenges in their career to accomplish their goal (Collins & MacNamara, 2012; Jordet, 2015). The ability of the athlete to cope, self-regulate, and, finally, to adapt is crucial for talent development and realization (Schinke et al., 2010). Although interrelated, coping, self-regulation, and adaptation processes play a different role in the achievement of an optimal performance. Adaptation is the end objective of a process that reflects the athlete's capacity to act and react functionally in his/her environment (Schinke et al., 2010; Tenenbaum, Lane, Razon, Lidor, & Schinke, 2015). To achieve psychological adaptation, the use of effective coping skills and self-regulation strategies is imperative. As briefly outlined in Chapter 3, different personality traits may account for variation in individuals' capacity to cope with adversity.

It is well accepted that there is remarkable interpersonal variation in self-regulation, coping skills, and resilience. A set of processes and mechanisms underlie these traits making it a complex multidimensional construct, influenced by genes, environment, and gene-environment interactions. The aim of the current chapter is thus to explore more in-depth the theoretical models explaining the links between adaptation and motor performance, and to identify the role of genetics in this relationship.

Appraisal, coping, and performance

In Chapter 4 we highlighted the impact of emotions on motor performance. Namely, depending on individual factors, athletes' performance may improve or decline when experiencing specific emotions. In the event of a debilitative emotional experience, possessing efficient coping skills becomes a pivotal asset to maintain a high level of performance. To better capture the role of the coping mechanism in the adaptation process, it is first essential to understand how emotions are elicited and how the mechanism influences subsequent actions and reactions (Lazarus, 2000).

At the dawn of the twenty-first century, Lazarus (2000) presented the cognitive-motivational-relational theory of emotions. According to this theory, the emotions involved in an adaptational encounter depend on how individuals appraise the meaning of an event for their well-being. Emotional experience also relies on the implementation of the coping process (Lazarus, 2000). Specifically, after appraising whether the environment has the potential to endanger personal goals *(primary appraisal)*, the athlete can deploy, if needed, appropriate coping skills to deal with aspects of the problem or with the emotions associated with it *(secondary appraisal)* (Lazarus, 1999, 2000). If the environment is assessed as a threat, or perceived as potentially harmful, and the athlete possesses few effective coping skills, the likelihood of experiencing debilitative emotion increases. On the other hand, perception of challenge or benefit along with high ability to cope with the challenging situation may result in pleasant emotional experience. A reciprocal process exists between appraisal and coping. In other words, if perceived threat is successfully alleviated through coping, future appraisal of similar situations may be interpreted positively (Nicholls et al., 2014). This ongoing process can lead to optimal adaptation to challenging sport situations (Tenenbaum et al., 2009).

Appraisal

From a cognitive perspective, the appraisal of stimuli in the environment is the first cognitive process leading to action organization (Tenenbaum et al., 2009). Primary appraisal refers to a judgment of the person-environment relationship that is influenced by personal goals, values, beliefs, and intentions. In line with this concept, Ntoumanis, Edmunds, and Duda (2009), demonstrated that appraisals are shaped by the goal at sake. Namely, performers adopting *self-determined goals* tended to appraise situations as a challenge whereas those setting *controlled goals* assessed situations as a threat. Theories underlying self-determined goals are discussed in more details in Chapter 6. Nevertheless, the notion that different goal motives are influencing appraisals has been supported empirically in sport (Adie, Duda, & Ntoumanis, 2010; Kavussanu et al., 2014; Nicholls et al., 2014). Accordingly, the achievement goal perspectives provide a perceptual-cognitive foundation in which to form cognitive appraisals (McGregor and Elliot, 2002). Unfortunately, research examining the relationship between appraisal and objective performance is scarce. Yet, some findings revealed that challenge appraisal is positively associated with pleasant emotions, which are subsequently linked to performance satisfaction. On the other hand, when a situation is assessed as a threat, unpleasant emotions are elicited impacting negatively on performance satisfaction (Nicholls et al., 2012).

Appraisal outcomes are stored in memory thereby potentially influencing the assessment of future similar situations (Tenenbaum et al., 2009). Because appraisal is triggered by environmental stimuli, this cognitive function appears to rely more heavily on environmental conditions than on genetic predisposition. Yet, is it possible that we were born with an inclination toward one or the other types of appraisal? In the next section we elaborate on this issue.

Appraisal is triggered by environmental stimuli, which evoke cognitive process, and therefore situated in neural circuits. The target brain region of appraisal is commonly believed to be the amygdala, a key structure that supports the elaboration of external and internal emotional stimuli (Cunningham, Arbuckle, Jahn, Mowrer, & Abduljalil, 2011; Cunningham, Van Bavel, & Johnsen, 2008) and facilitates the formation of emotional memories (Paz & Pare, 2013). Other structures include the ventral striatum, dorsolateral prefrontal cortex, superior temporal sulcus, somatosensory-related cortices, orbitofrontal cortex, medial prefrontal cortex, fusiform gyrus, cerebellum, and anterior cingulate (Petta, Pelachaud, & Cowie, 2011). Genetic variability associated with amygdala and neural processes related to appraisal contribute to the remarkable interpersonal variability in stimuli appraisal.

Though large-scale twin studies have shown that the amygdala volume is highly heritable (Hulshoff Pol et al., 2006; Kremen et al., 2010) its molecular genetic architecture remains to be determined. Several variants in genes expressed in the amygdala, such as serotonin transporter (*SLC6A4*), oxytocin receptor (*OXTR*), stathmin protein (*STMN1*), and anandamide (AEA) catabolic enzyme (*FAAH*) were studied in relation to interpersonal variability in amygdala structure and function. The main genetic variants related to the amygdala structure and function are described in Table 5.1.

Coping skills

Secondary appraisals involve the evaluation of the available coping skill. Coping skills enable the athlete to invest cognitive and behavioral efforts directed to manage specific external and internal demands (Lazarus & Folkman, 1984). Nicholls and Polman (2007) conducted a systematic review of coping in sport revealing several models and approaches. First, Lazarus and Folkman's (1984) model refers to *problem-focused coping* as strategies used to alter the stressful situation, whereas *emotion-focused coping* entails strategies which aimed to manage the emotional distress associated with the situation. In sport, the *approach-avoidance model* (Roth & Cohen, 1986) is often used to categorize athletes' coping responses. *Approach coping strategies* are those in which the athlete confronts the problem to actively address, remove, or change the stressor, while *avoidance coping* includes attempts to disengage from that stressor. In line

Table 5.1 Genetic variants related to the amygdala structure and function

Genetic variants	Relation to amygdala
Serotonin transporter (*SLC6A4*) 5-HTTLPR (rs22531) s allele showing a 43-bp reduction (Kraft, Slager, McGrath, & Hamilton, 2005; Wendland, Martin, Kruse, Lesch, & Murphy, 2006) and reduced mRNA transcription levels (Heils et al., 1996)	s allele associated with: • increased amygdala function at rest (Rao et al., 2007) • amygdala response to emotional stimuli (Hariri et al., 2002; Lemogne et al., 2011; Munafò, Brown, & Hariri, 2008; Serretti, Kato, De Ronchi, & Kinoshita, 2007) • amygdala volume (Scherk et al., 2009; Stjepanović, Lorenzetti, Yücel, Hawi, & Bellgrove, 2013)
Tandem repeat (STin2) Alleles: 10-/12-repeats 12-repeat allele has been reported to be a transcriptional enhancer (MacKenzie & Quinn, 1999)	12-repeat homozygotes displayed lower serotonin transporter availability in the brain (Bah et al., 2008)
Oxytocin receptor (*OXTR*) rs53576	Response of the amygdala during facial emotion processing as well as a reported effect on amygdala volume in male participants (Tost et al., 2010)
Stathmin 1 (*STMN1*) rs182455	Amygdala volume (Stjepanović et al., 2013)
Fatty acid amide hydrolase (*FAAH*) C385A (rs324420) A allele – FAAH vulnerability to proteolytic degradation, and therefore elevated AEA levels (Chiang, Gerber, Sipe, & Cravatt, 2004)	Variation in reactivity to threat (Hariri et al., 2009) enhances fronto-amygdala connectivity (Dincheva et al., 2015)

with the two previous frameworks, Gaudreau and Blondin (2002) introduced a model of coping grounded in sport, which includes three dimensions of coping: *task-oriented coping, distraction-oriented coping*, and *disengagement-oriented coping*. Task-oriented coping involves directly addressing the source of stress and deliberately attempting to reduce or remove the stressors. Distraction-oriented coping corresponds to strategies that can be used to direct one's attention momentarily on things that are unrelated to sport competition; whereas disengagement-oriented coping represents strategies that are used to disengage oneself from processes that generally lead to goal attainment.

In the sport psychology literature, there has been a tendency to consider approach strategies as adaptive and avoidance strategies as maladaptive. Some evidence supports this assumption by showing that approaching a problem and dealing with emotions are strategies that benefit goal attainment (Gaudreau & Blondin, 2004) and performance (Hill & Hemmings, 2015; Levy, Nicholls, & Polman, 2011; Nicholls et al., 2012). For instance, findings revealed that strategies such as rushing and denial are associated with choking episodes, while cognitive restructuring is associated with increased performances (Hill & Hemmings, 2015). Yet, some evidence points toward the negative effect of approach strategies on performance. For instance, Mesagno and Marchant (2013) explored the strategies used by athletes labeled as chocking susceptible and chocking resistant during a low- and high-pressure netball task. Findings revealed that choking susceptible possesses few coping strategies, and those were mostly approach ones, which contributes to performance deterioration under pressure. Trying to deal with the situation at hand could have created an additional distraction, thereby negatively influencing performance (Eysenck & Calvo, 1992; Eysenck, Derakshan, Santos, & Calvo, 2007; Wine, 1971). These studies highlight the lack of consensus about the link between coping dimensions and performance.

To circumvent this confusion, some researchers examined perceived coping effectiveness. In sport, an emotional-focused strategy such as venting negative emotions may be effective and adaptative although in other social situations such a strategy is considered inappropriate. Furthermore, a coping response may be beneficial in a specific moment, but totally inefficient in another sport context. Therefore, when examining the link between coping and performance, perceived efficacy and context must be considered (Pensgaard & Duda, 2003). More specifically, coping effectiveness is dependent upon individual differences in appraisal, the type of threat, the stage of stressful encounter, and the outcome modality (Lazarus, 1999). A study examining the effects of emotions and coping effectiveness on athletes' performances at the Sydney 2000 Olympic Games showed that perceived coping effectiveness was the only significant predictor of objective performance (Pensgaard and Duda, 2003). *Controllability* of the situation is another important factor influencing the effectiveness of coping strategies. According to the goodness-of-fit model (Folkman, 1992), when a situation is under the athlete's control, problem-focused coping should be favored, whereas emotion-focused strategies should be used when facing an uncontrollable challenge. This framework was supported by empirical evidence (see Nicholls & Polman, 2007 for a review).

Coping-related genes

Both environmental conditions and individual differences influence coping. It is well accepted that coping strategies are important for relieving stress, but different individuals may prefer different coping strategies. The mechanisms underlying an individual preference of coping strategy are unclear, but specific genetic factors may play a key role in determining the coping strategy preferred in a given situation (Aizawa et al., 2015). In a systematic review of genetic influences on coping, Dunn and Conley (2015) identified 19 studies that measured coping style or a specific coping domain. Nine of them estimated coping heritability, and ten were candidate gene association studies. The high heritability estimates (0.68–0.72) support a nonadditive genetic component to coping. The main genetic variants associated with coping that were identified in candidate gene case–control association are summarized in Table 5.2.

Table 5.2 Genetic variants related to coping

Gene (genetic variants)	Coping domain/style (coping measure)	Relation to coping
SLC64A (5-HTTLPR)	Drinking to cope/enhance (MAUS)	L/L carriers more likely to drink to cope than S/S carriers (Armeli, Conner, Covault, Tennen, & Kranzler, 2008)
	Emotional appraisal of fear, sadness, and joy (SAQ)	s-carriers significantly associated with coping ability for fear and sadness compared to noncarriers (Szily, Bowen, Unoka, Simon, & Kéri, 2008)
	Coping with stress (ABM, CUS)	SLC64A 5-HTTLPR promoter polymorphism was associated with using fewer problem-solving strategies (Wilhelm et al., 2007)
ADRB2 (+491 G/A) (Haplotype Gly16/Glu27)	Active coping, emotional coping (SVF) Anger-in/anger-out coping strategies (SASS)	Association between the ADRB2 gene and the active coping style (Busjahn et al. 2002) Haplotype Gly16/Glu27, race, and anger-in interaction indicated higher anger-in carriers had higher resting SBP. Interactions with anger-in were present in Black men only (Poole, Snieder, Davis, & Treiber, 2006)
BDNF (Val66Met rs6265)	Emotion-focused coping, problem-focused coping (SCOPE)	Emotion-focused coping varied as a function of BDNF genotype, such that individuals with at least one Met allele endorsed more emotion-focused coping than those with a Val/Val genotype (Caldwell et al., 2013)
	Emotion-focused strategies, seeking social support, self-control, and distancing (STAI, BDI)	Associations between BDNF and emotion-focused strategies, seeking social support, self-control, and distancing critical attitudes (Aizawa et al., 2015)
NTRK2 (rs11140800, rs1187286, rs1867283, rs1147198, rs10868235)	Emotion-focused strategies, seeking social support, self-control, and distancing (STAI, BDI)	Significant associations between NTRK2 and cognitive strategies, problem-solving, confrontive-coping, seeking social support, distancing and positive reappraisal, and all seven ego-related factors. In the SASS, the minor allele rs1867283 of NTRK2 had a significantly higher score than the heterozygote
MAOA	Self-coping, seeking others, avoidance (ACOPE)	In high-MAOA-activity genotype groups, significant association between self-coping and fewer depressive symptoms (Cicchetti, Rogosch, & Sturge-Apple, 2007)
ACE (rs8066276)	Coping styles (SVF)	ACE intronic SNP (rs8066276) was significantly associated with positive coping style distraction (Heck et al., 2009)
OXTR (G/A rs53576)	Emotional support seeking (ND)	AA genotype carriers reported more emotional support–seeking than GG/AG genotype carriers (Kim et al., 2010)
DRD2 (Taq1A, rs1800497)	Drinking to cope, coping motives (DMQ-R)	The link between coping motives and alcohol outcomes was stronger among those A1 allele carriers

Source: partially adapted from Dunn and Conley (2015).

Notes
ABM = Anti-Depressive Behavior Measure; ACOPE = Adolescent-Coping Orientation for Problem Experiences; CUS = Coping under Stress; DMQ-R = Drinking Motive Questionnaire–Revised; MAUS = Motivations for Alcohol Use Scale; ND = no data; SAES = Spielberger's Anger Expression Scale; SAQ = Scherer's Appraisal Questionnaire; SCOPE = Survey of Coping Profile Endorsement; SNP = single-nucleotide polymorphism; SVF = Stress verarbeitungs fragebogen; SBP = Systolic Blood Pressure; STAI = State-Trait Anxiety Inventory; BDI = Beck Depression Inventory; and SASS = Social Adaptation Self-Evaluation Scale.

Self-regulation

Slightly different from coping, self-regulation refers to the organizational framework that enables the athlete to adjust his or her behaviors and goals to perform (Zeidner, Boekaerts, & Pintrich, 2000). Thoughts, emotions, and behaviors are the motivational components that must be regulated by the athlete to achieve desired outcomes (Schinke, Tenenbaum, Lidor, & Battochio, 2010). The capacity to self-regulate initial psychological state has been reported by elite athletes as an essential psychological process leading to positive performance outcome (Anderson, Hanrahan, & Mallett, 2014). Self-regulation strategies (e.g., self-talk, goal setting, mental imagery) are often combined in a pre-performance routine (PPR) allowing athletes to gain control over the motivational components underlying performance.

A PPR is a repeatable series of motor and mental activities performed prior to undertaking a task (Lidor & Singer, 2003). Increasing evidence in various sports, such as gymnastics (Gröpel & Beckmann, 2017), tennis (Lautenbach, Laborde, Klämpfl, & Achtzehn, 2015), bowling (Mesagno et al., 2008), Australian rules football (Mesagno & Mullane-Grant, 2010), cricket (Cotterill, 2011), volleyball (Lidor & Mayan, 2005), and soccer (Hazell, Cotterill, & Hill, 2014) indicates that a PPR is an effective mental technique which optimizes the athlete's performance of a closed skill task. Interestingly, when under various pressure conditions, the quality of the PPR is affected. For instance, findings revealed that professional soccer players from the most merited European nations rush their preparation leading to less successful penalty shots in major competitions compared to their lower public status countries counterparts (Jordet, 2009). Although Jordet attributed these results to the fact that players from renowned countries perceived a shootout as a treat (i.e., they must score to maintain their reputation), and the outcome as uncontrollable (i.e., attributed to luck), it may also have something to do with their self-control capacity in such a context. The next section explores the influence of self-control in the athlete's capacity to regulate emotion, thoughts, and behaviors.

Self-control

To enable athletes to effectively regulate thoughts, emotions, and actions, self-control must be solicited. According to the strength-energy model (Baumeister, Bratslavsky, Muraven, & Tice, 1998), self-control is a limited resource. Specifically, self-control refers to the ability to voluntary control behaviors or the capacity to resist immediate temptations to achieve long-term goals. When encountering challenges, athletes may experience self-regulatory failure if they possess limited individual capacity (trait approach) or if the demand of the situation consumes all their resources (state approach) leaving them in a state of ego-depletion. Self-control has implications in adherence to exercise, commitment to training, and competition performance (Englert, 2017).

First, because individuals need to resist the temptation to stay comfortable on their couch to invest themselves in an exhausting workout, findings revealed that higher trait self-control individuals are more physically active than their less resourceful counterparts (Stork, Graham, Bray, & Martin Ginis, 2017). In this vein, ego-depleted athletes (i.e., lack of self-control resources) performed a significantly lower number of press-ups and sit-ups than those in a state with temporarily available self-control strength (Dorris, Power, & Kenefick, 2012). Self-control also allowed athletes to commit to different types of practice requirement and go through challenges during arduous training conditions (Tedesqui & Young, 2015). Accordingly, a higher level of trait self-control was associated with more hours of soccer-specific practice in professional soccer players (Toering & Jordet, 2015). Similarly, Tedesqui and Young (2017) demonstrated that self-control was associated with engagement in mandatory and voluntary practice for senior athletes, but not for junior ones. This can be explained by a lower involvement of external support such as parents and coaches at the senior level requiring more self-control from the athlete directly at that level. Furthermore, self-control has been found to help athletes stay involved in the developmental path of their main sport.

Finally, evidence is pointing toward the mediating role of self-control in the anxiety–performance relationship. Specifically, whereas ego-depleted participants performed significantly worse in both a basketball free throw task and a darts task as anxiety increased, those with fully available self-control maintained their level of performance under the same conditions. The role of self-control on attention regulation can provide an explanation to these results. As described by distraction theories (Eysenck & Calvo, 1992; Eysenck et al., 2007), anxiety can disrupt attention processes by switching the focus from relevant task-cues to irrelevant ones (see Chapter 4). To be able to discount irrelevant cues and keep the focus on what matters to perform optimally, selective attention must be solicited. Interestingly, selective attention is thought to be influenced by self-control (Schmeichel & Baumeister, 2010). To test this assumption, eye-tracking technology was used to assess gaze behavior – a relevant indicator of efficient attention regulation (Wilson, Smith, & Holmes, 2007). Findings revealed that in a state of high anxiety, ego-depleted participants showed less-efficient gaze behaviors and performed worse than non-depleted participants supporting the relationship between self-control and selective attention (Englert, Zwemmer, Bertrams, & Oudejans, 2015). In this vein, Englert, Bertrams, Furley, and Oudejans (2015) showed that sufficient levels of self-control allow participants to block external distraction efficiently thereby leading to a higher level of performance.

The ability to regulate emotions, thoughts, and behaviors is imperative for athletic performance since self-control is required for proficient execution of plans. To elucidate what influences self-regulation and self-control we outline the role of genetics in both processes. Individual differences in executive attention, working memory, emotion, and their interaction within the self-regulation concept are described in Figure 5.1.

Twin and adoption studies have shown moderate to substantial heritability for attention and effortful control, working memory, and negative emotionality (Lemery & Goldsmith, 2002). Molecular genetic studies identified several genetic variants related to self-control. Most of them related to the dopaminergic system (Faraone et al., 2005). These genetic variants and others are introduced in Chapter 6.

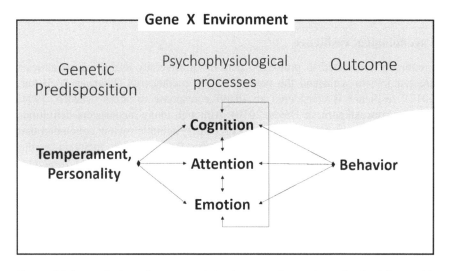

Figure 5.1 Dynamic interplay among behavior, genetics, and psychophysiology with respect to self-regulation (Bell & Deater-Deckard, 2007).

Adaptation

The outcome of positive appraisal and efficient use of coping skills and self-regulation strategies is *adaptation*. In line with this idea, Tenenbaum et al. (2015) developed the Two Perception Probabilistic Concept of Adaptation (TPPCA). This framework suggests that the degree of adaptation is a function of the difference between how one perceives the environment/task (e.g., challenging, threatening, etc.), and how one perceives his/her own ability/ capacity (i.e., self-efficacy) to interact and cope with the environmental/task demands. Therefore, in the pursuit of a given goal, if one perceives the environment/task as challenging and feels he/she possesses the appropriate set of skills to deal with the presented challenge, the probability of adequate adaptation increases resulting in above-expected performance, positive affects (e.g., happiness) and optimal behavioral response (e.g., approach behaviors). On the other hand, the probability of poor adaptation is augmented when one perceives the environment/task as threatening and feels he/she lacks the skills to deal with the environmental demands. Poor adaptation may lead to under-expected performance, negative affect (e.g., frustration), and suboptimal behavioral response (e.g., avoidance behaviors). The TPPCA also encompass slow and fast adaptation processes. *Fast adaptation* processes require immediate responses, such as the self-regulatory responses that an individual must make just before, during, or shortly after a performance when another performance is scheduled. *Slow adaptation* processes involve ongoing adaptation to long-term life and athletic career demands. If these demands represent significant adversity, such as catastrophic injuries or prolonged performance slumps, psychological resilience may be required to reach adaptation.

Psychological resilience

Frequently associated to prolonged periods of adversity during which athletes are required to withstand the pressures they encountered (Fletcher & Sarkar, 2012), resilience is considered an adaptive response to stress (Masten, 1994; Zautra, Arewasikporn, & Davis, 2010). Although many inconsistent definitions of resilience appear in the literature, a recent systematic review concluded that resilience is "a dynamic process encompassing the capacity to maintain regular functioning through diverse challenges or to rebound through the use of facilitative resources" (Bryan, O'Shea, & MacIntyre, 2017, p. 8).

In Chapter 3, resilience is presented as a trait-like characteristic. Yet, most recent research considers resilience as a state-like construct (Bryan et al., 2017). In fact, Richardson (2002) presented a model describing the three waves of resilience. The first wave, *resilient qualities*, describes the internal and external characteristics required to cope with or bounce back from setbacks (trait-like). The second wave focuses on how those qualities are acquired (state-like). This wave describes the dynamic process involving the disruption of body and mind homeostasis and its reintegration into one of the four forms: resilient reintegration, reintegration back to homeostasis, reintegration with loss, and dysfunctional reintegration (see Figure 5.2). Resilient reintegration is the optimal form because it involves insight and growth through disruption. This assumption is supported by Zautra et al. (2010) in their conceptualization which stipulates that resilience is evidenced by rapid and effective emotional recovery from adversity, while sustaining an approach motivation and potentially gaining new learning from the experience. Finally, the third wave pertains to what and where is the motivation to reintegrate resiliently. Some resilience theories claim that there is a force within everyone that drives them to seek self-actualization.

To systematically examine the relationship between psychological resilience and optimal sport performance, Fletcher and Sarkar (2012) developed a grounded theory of psychological resilience (see Figure 5.3). Twelve Olympic champions were asked about the way they withstood episodes of high stress throughout their athletic careers. Results revealed that *challenge appraisal* and *meta-cognition of stressors* are central components to the model. Champions confirmed that perceiving stressors as an opportunity to grow and learn was imperative for success; especially at the peak of their sporting journey. Furthermore, athletes became skilled at evaluating their own thoughts (i.e., meta-cognition), and using mental strategies to restructure their feelings and thoughts when necessary. This cognitive control process also contributed positively to their capacity to handle pressure. To support the two central aspects of the model, five main psychological factors were identified by athletes; *positive personality, motivation, confidence, focus*, and *perceived social support*. Optimizing these characteristics allowed athletes to improve their capacity to face

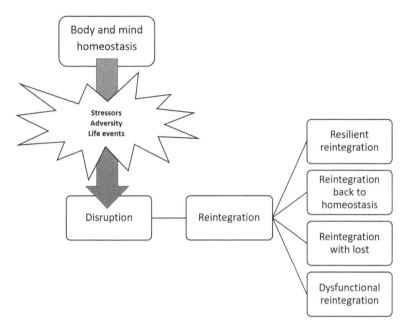

Figure 5.2 The resilience model
Source: based on Richardson (2002).

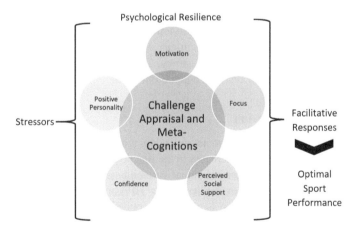

Figure 5.3 A grounded theory of psychological resilience and optimal sport performance
(Fletcher & Sarkar, 2012).

adversity. To summarize, taking responsibility for one's thoughts, feelings, and actions facilitate responses to stressful situations which thereafter result in optimal performance.

Several researchers have used the grounded theory of psychological resilience to explore the impact of this adaptative psychological construct in the motor domain. For instance, findings revealed that athletes who are high in resilience and benefit from informational and tangible social support from coaches are less prone to negative stress-induced outcomes such as burnout (Lu et al., 2016). Resilience also influences the type of coping strategies used by athletes. Empirical evidence has shown that athletes exhibiting elevated levels of resilient qualities favored task-oriented coping rather than distraction or disengagement coping when stress increases during a season (Secades et al., 2016). Finally, resilience was positively associated to competitive swimming performance. Specifically, a significant interaction between resilience and cortisol secretion (i.e., a hormone associated with physiological arousal) was revealed suggesting a moderating role of resilience in the cortisol-performance relationship. Resilience was also directly associated with athletic performance through positive appraisal of the situation (Meggs, Golby, Mallett, Gucciardi, & Polman, 2016).

To succinctly summarize the impact of resilience in sport, Fletcher and Sarkar (2016) recently suggested two conceptualizations of resilience. First, *robust resilience* refers to the protective qualities that allow performers to sustain their well-being and performance under pressure. On the other hand, *rebound resilience* reflects the capacity of an athlete to bounce back when minor or temporary disruptions happen to rapidly return to an optimal level of well-being or performance. Although resilience is profoundly influenced by a wide range of environmental factors (Fletcher & Sarkar, 2016), the complex interaction between these environmental conditions and individuals' genetic make-up determines the degree of adaptability of neurochemical stress response systems to new adverse exposures (Feder, Nestler, & Charney, 2009). We expand on the impact of genes in the expression of resilient adaptations next.

Genes, resilience, and adaptation

Numerous hormones, neurotransmitters, and neuropeptides are involved in the acute psychobiological responses to stress. Differences in the function, balance, and interaction of these factors underlie the inter-individual variability in stress resilience. The main biological systems related to resilience are: HPA axis, noradrenergic systems, and dopaminergic, serotonergic systems, neuropeptide Y, and BDNF.

The HPA axis was described in Chapter 4. Briefly, corticotropin-releasing hormone (CRH) is released by the hypothalamus in response to stress, leading to activation of the HPA axis and the release of cortisol. Early life stress has been linked to chronically high levels of CRH (Heim & Nemeroff, 2001). Although the short-term actions of cortisol are protective and promote adaptation, sustained exposure to abnormally high levels of cortisol can challenge health (Karlamangla, Singer, McEwen, Rowe, & Seeman, 2002). Excessive cortisol in the brain is associated with complex structural effects in the hippocampus and amygdala (Brown, Woolston, & Frol, 2008; McEwen & Milner, 2007). Resilience is associated with the capacity to constrain stress-induced increases in CRH and cortisol through an elaborate negative feedback system, involving optimal function and balance of glucocorticoid and mineralocorticoid receptors (Charney, 2004; de Kloet, DeRijk, & Meijer, 2007; de Kloet, Joëls, & Holsboer, 2005). Dehydroepi-androsterone (DHEA), which is also released in response to stress, has antigluco-corticoid effects in the brain. Higher DHEA sulfate/cortisol ratios in individuals undergoing rigorous military survival training indicates higher resilience to stress (Morgan et al., 2004). DHEA also affects the GABA (γ-aminobutyric acid)-ergic system, which plays a part in resilience (Dubrovsky, 2005).

Polymorphisms of the CRH type 1 receptor gene (*CRHR1*) are associated with cortisol response to psychosocial stress (Mahon, Zandi, Potash, Nestadt, & Wand, 2013), Post Traumatic Stress Disorder (PTSD) (both lifetime and early onset) (Boscarino, Erlich, Hoffman, & Zhang, 2012), and self-reported resilience and quality of life (Sleijpen, Heitland, Mooren, & Kleber, 2017).

Polymorphisms in CRHR1 also showed Gene X Environment interaction for resilient functioning (Cicchetti & Rogosch, 2012) and depressive symptoms (Bradley et al., 2008; Ressler et al., 2009). Functional variants of the brain miner-alocorticoid and glucocorticoid receptor (GR) genes have been identified in humans (de Kloet et al., 2007). For example, carriers of the N363S variant of the GR gene were shown to exhibit higher cortisol responses to the Trier Social Stress Test (DeRijk & de Kloet, 2008). Polymorphisms in *FKBP5* (the gene that codes for a "chaperone" protein that regulates GR sensitivity) were found to interact with the severity of childhood abuse in the prediction of PTSD symptoms in adults (E. B. Binder et al., 2008; Tamman et al., 2017; Watkins et al., 2016; Zimmermann et al., 2011). Genetic variations in FKBP5 modulated recovery from psychosocial stress (Ising et al., 2008) and cortisol response to psychosocial stress (Mahon et al., 2013).

Serotonergic systems. Serotonin neurons project widely in the brain. Acute stress is associated with increased serotonin turnover in several brain regions, including the amygdala, the nucleus accumbens, and the PFC. Serotonin modu-lates neural responses to stress, with both anxiogenic and anxiolytic effects (depending on the brain region and receptor subtype involved) (Charney, 2004). Serotonin function is also closely linked to mood regulation. A naturally occurring variation in the promoter of the human serotonin transporter gene (5-HTTLPR; also known as SLC6A4) was described in Chapter 4. The s allele is associated with elevated risk for depression on exposure to stressful life events in some but not all studies (Munafò, Durrant, Lewis, & Flint, 2009); and with increased sus-ceptibility to stress (Munafò et al., 2008; Pezawas et al., 2005). A recent study found an association between the long allele of 5-HTTLPR l allele is associated with emotional resilience (Stein, Campbell-Sills, & Gelernter, 2009).

Noradrenergic and dopaminergic systems. Stress leads to the release of noradrenaline from brainstem nuclei, most importantly the locus coeruleus. The result is increased noradrenergic stimulation of numerous forebrain areas implicated in emotional behavior, such as the amygdala, the nucleus accumbens, the prefrontal cortex (PFC), and the hippocampus (Charney, 2003; McGaugh, 2004). Dopamine neurons are activated in response to reward or the expectation of reward and generally are inhibited by aversive stimuli, as detailed below. Recently it was found that resilience to stress is associated with gene expression alterations in dopaminergic and serotonergic pathways (Azadmarzabadi, Haghighatfard, & Mohammadi, 2018).

COMT is an enzyme that metabolizes catecholamines including norepinephrine, epinephrine, and dopamine. The most common variation of the *COMT* gene is the Val158Met polymorphism (rs4680) in which a single G/A base-pair substitution leads to a valine (val) to methionine (met) substitution at codon 158 (Lachman et al., 1996). This met substitution reduces the activity of COMT enzyme to one-quarter of what was originally encoded by the val allele (Lachman et al., 1996). A significant effect of the COMT polymorphism on resilience and a gene-gene interaction effect between the COMT and BDNF on resilience were observed for healthy males (Gerritsen et al., 2017). Met-carriers were found to have higher extracellular DA levels in the prefrontal cortex (J. Chen et al., 2004), higher circulating levels of neurotransmitters (Heinz & Smolka, 2006), lower resilience to negative mood states, and increased limbic reactivity to unpleasant stimuli (Heinz & Smolka, 2006; Schmack et al., 2008).

Children carrying the met allele showed a higher cortisol response to stress (Armbruster et al., 2012). The *COMT* Val158Met polymorphism has been linked to deficits in stress response and emotional resilience, and was found to influence the risk of development of post trauma stress disorder (PTSD) (Heinz & Smolka, 2006; Kolassa, Kolassa, Ertl, Papassotiropoulos, & De Quervain, 2010; Skelton, Ressler, Norrholm, Jovanovic, & Bradley-Davino, 2012). *COMT* Val158Met polymorphism's effect on resilience can be modulated by *BDNF* Val66Met polymorphism in males. Polymorphisms in the dopamine receptor genes, including *DRD2* and *DRD4*, and in the dopamine transporter gene *DAT1* have also been implicated in stress responsivity, emotion processing, and susceptibility to PTSD and depression (Wu et al., 2013)

Neuropeptide Y (NPY). NPY, a neuropeptide that is widely distributed in the brain, has anxiolytic-like effects and promotes protective responses in the face of stress (Wu et al., 2011). NPY also counteracts the anxiogenic effects of CRH in the amygdala, the hippocampus, the hypothalamus, and the locus coeruleus, and resilience might involve maintaining a balance between NPY and CRH levels during stress (Sajdyk, Shekhar, & Gehlert, 2004). NPY levels during rigorous military training were associated with better performance (Morgan et al., 2000). NPY is also associated with resilience to PTSD in animal (Cohen et al., 2012) and human (Kautz, Charney, & Murrough, 2017). Genetic variations of *NPY* contributed to individual susceptibility to stress (Wu et al., 2013). Two *NPY* haplotypes represented by three SNPs correlated with increased susceptibility to anxiety disorders (Donner et al., 2012). Genetic variants in the premotor region are associated with NPY release, and lower haplotype-driven NPY expression predicted weakened resilient response to stress (Zhang et al., 2012; Zhou et al., 2008).

BDNF. BDNF, an important nerve growth factor that is found at high levels in the brain, is known to be essential for the development and maintenance of the neurons (D. K. Binder & Scharfman, 2004). BDNF function is modulated by physical activity (Phillips, 2017). Though stress produces distinct effects on *BDNF* in the amygdala and the PFC, BDNF in these regions has not yet been studied in resilience models. A common SNP of rs6265 in the *BDNF* gene causes a substitution of valine (Val) to methionine (Met) at codon 66 in the prodomain (Val66Met), which influences activity-dependent release of the BDNF protein (Kuczewski, Porcher, & Gaiarsa, 2010). The BDNF Val66Met polymorphism has been reported to be associated with cognitive (Egan et al., 2003; Hariri et al., 2003) and emotional dysfunctions (Z.-Y. Chen et al., 2006; Soliman et al., 2010). The *BDNF* Val66Met polymorphism was found to moderate the relation between physical activity and depressive symptoms (Mata, Thompson, & Gotlib, 2010).

Summary

Identifying the genetic components of self-regulation, coping skills, adaptation, and resilience, as well as emotion regulation is an intricate task. Not only due to the inconsistency in these traits' definition and measuring tools, but also because these traits are interrelated and interconnected, and therefore situated on overlapping biological mechanisms. Thus, genetic variance related to the dopaminergic system may affect adaptation, coping, and self-regulation-related traits. Moreover, each genetic polymorphism makes a small contribution to the more complex trait. In this respect some "oligo" genes such as serotonin receptor gene were identified as imperative to these psychological states, traits, and processes.

References

Adie, J. W., Duda, J. L., & Ntoumanis, N. (2010). Achievement goals, competition appraisals, and the well- and ill-being of elite youth soccer players over two competitive seasons. *Journal of Sport and Exercise Psychology, 32*(4), 555–79.

Aizawa, S., Ishitobi, Y., Masuda, K., Inoue, A., Oshita, H., Hirakawa, H., … Akiyoshi, J. (2015). Genetic association of the transcription of neuroplasticity-related genes and variation in stress-coping style. *Brain and Behavior, 5*(9), e00360. https://doi.org/10.1002/brb3.360

Anderson, R., Hanrahan, S. J., & Mallett, C. J. (2014). Investigating the optimal psychological state for peak performance in Australian elite athletes. *Journal of Applied Sport Psychology, 26*(3), 318–33.

Armbruster, D., Mueller, A., Strobel, A., Lesch, K.-P., Brocke, B., & Kirschbaum, C. (2012). Children under stress – COMT genotype and stressful life events predict cortisol increase in an acute social stress paradigm. *The International Journal of Neuropsychopharmacology, 15*(9), 1229–39. https://doi.org/10.1017/S1461145711001763

Armeli, S., Conner, T. S., Covault, J., Tennen, H., & Kranzler, H. R. (2008). A serotonin transporter gene polymorphism (5-HTTLPR), drinking-to-cope motivation, and negative life events among college students. *Journal of Studies on Alcohol and Drugs, 69*(6), 814–23. Retrieved from www.ncbi.nlm.nih.gov/pubmed/18925339

Azadmarzabadi, E., Haghighatfard, A., & Mohammadi, A. (2018). Low resilience to stress is associated with candidate gene expression alterations in the dopaminergic signalling pathway. *Psychogeriatrics, 18*(3), 190–201. https://doi.org/10.1111/psyg.12312

Bah, J., Lindström, M., Westberg, L., Manneräs, L., Ryding, E., Henningsson, S., … Eriksson, E. (2008). Serotonin transporter gene polymorphisms: Effect on serotonin transporter availability in the brain of suicide attempters. *Psychiatry Research: Neuro-imaging, 162*(3), 221–9. https://doi.org/10.1016/j.pscychresns.2007.07.004

Baumeister, R. F., Bratslavsky, E., Muraven, M., & Tice, D. M. (1998). Ego depletion: Is the active self a limited resource? *Journal of Personality and Social Psychology, 74*(5), 1252–65.

Bell, M. A., & Deater-Deckard, K. (2007). Biological systems and the development of self-regulation: Integrating behavior, genetics, and psychophysiology. *Journal of Developmental and Behavioral Pediatrics, 28*(5), 409–20. https://doi.org/10.1097/DBP.0b013e3181131fc7

Binder, D. K., & Scharfman, H. E. (2004). Brain-derived neurotrophic factor. *Growth Factors, 22*(3), 123–31. Retrieved from www.ncbi.nlm.nih.gov/pubmed/15518235

Binder, E. B., Bradley, R. G., Liu, W., Epstein, M. P., Deveau, T. C., Mercer, K. B., … Ressler, K. J. (2008). Association of FKBP5 polymorphisms and childhood abuse with risk of posttraumatic stress disorder symptoms in adults. *JAMA, 299*(11), 1291. https://doi.org/10.1001/jama.299.11.1291

Boscarino, J. A., Erlich, P. M., Hoffman, S. N., & Zhang, X. (2012). Higher FKBP5, COMT, CHRNA5, and CRHR1 allele burdens are associated with PTSD and interact with trauma exposure: Implications for neuropsychiatric research and treatment. *Neuropsychiatric Disease and Treatment, 8*, 131–9. https://doi.org/10.2147/NDT.S29508

Bradley, R. G., Binder, E. B., Epstein, M. P., Tang, Y., Nair, H. P., Liu, W., … Ressler, K. J. (2008). Influence of child abuse on adult depression. *Archives of General Psychiatry, 65*(2), 190. https://doi.org/10.1001/archgenpsychiatry.2007.26

Bryan, C., O'Shea, D., & MacIntyre, T. (2017). Stressing the relevance of resilience: A systematic review of resilience across the domains of sport and work. *International Review of Sport and Exercise Psychology.* doi:10.1080/1750984X.2017.1381140

Brown, E. S., Woolston, D. J., & Frol, A. B. (2008). Amygdala volume in patients receiving chronic corticosteroid therapy. *Biological Psychiatry, 63*(7), 705–9. https://doi.org/10.1016/j.biopsych.2007.09.014

Busjahn, A., Freier, K., Faulhaber, H.-D., Li, G. H., Rosenthal, M., Jordan, J., … Luft, F. C. (2002). Beta-2 adrenergic receptor gene variations and coping styles in twins. *Biological Psychology, 61*(1–2), 97–109. Retrieved from www.ncbi.nlm.nih.gov/pubmed/12385671

Caldwell, W., McInnis, O. A., McQuaid, R. J., Liu, G., Stead, J. D., Anisman, H., & Hayley, S. (2013). The role of the Val66Met polymorphism of the brain derived neurotrophic factor gene in coping strategies relevant to depressive symptoms. *PloS One, 8*(6), e65547. https://doi.org/10.1371/journal.pone.0065547

Charney, D. S. (2003). Neuroanatomical circuits modulating fear and anxiety behaviors. *Acta Psychiatrica Scandinavica. Supplementum, 417*, 38–50. Retrieved from www.ncbi.nlm.nih.gov/pubmed/12950435

Charney, D. S. (2004). Psychobiological mechanisms of resilience and vulnerability: Implications for successful adaptation to extreme stress. *American Journal of Psychiatry, 161*(2), 195–216. https://doi.org/10.1176/appi.ajp.161.2.195

Chen, J., Lipska, B. K., Halim, N., Ma, Q. D., Matsumoto, M., Melhem, S., … Weinberger, D. R. (2004). Functional analysis of genetic variation in Catechol-O-Methyltransferase (COMT): Effects on mRNA, protein, and enzyme activity in postmortem human brain. *The American Journal of Human Genetics, 75*(5), 807–21. https://doi.org/10.1086/425589

Chen, Z.-Y., Jing, D., Bath, K. G., Ieraci, A., Khan, T., Siao, C.-J., … Lee, F. S. (2006). Genetic variant BDNF (Val66Met) polymorphism alters anxiety-related behavior. *Science, 314*(5796), 140–3. https://doi.org/10.1126/science.1129663

Chiang, K. P., Gerber, A. L., Sipe, J. C., & Cravatt, B. F. (2004). Reduced cellular expression and activity of the P129T mutant of human fatty acid amide hydrolase: Evidence for a link between defects in the endocannabinoid system and problem drug use. *Human Molecular Genetics, 13*(18), 2113–9. https://doi.org/10.1093/hmg/ddh216

Cicchetti, D., & Rogosch, F. A. (2012). Gene × environment interaction and resilience: Effects of child maltreatment and serotonin, corticotropin releasing hormone, dopamine, and oxytocin genes. *Development and Psychopathology, 24*(2), 411–27. https://doi.org/10.1017/S0954579412000077

Cicchetti, D., Rogosch, F. A., & Sturge-Apple, M. L. (2007). Interactions of child maltreatment and serotonin transporter and monoamine oxidase A polymorphisms: Depressive symptomatology among adolescents from low socioeconomic status backgrounds. *Development and Psychopathology, 19*(4), 1161–80. https://doi.org/10.1017/S0954579407000600

Cohen, H., Kozlovsky, N., Alona, C., Matar, M. A., & Joseph, Z. (2012). Animal model for PTSD: From clinical concept to translational research. *Neuropharmacology, 62*(2), 715–24.

Cohen, H., Liu, T., Kozlovsky, N., Kaplan, Z., Zohar, J., & Mathé, A. A. (2012). The Neuropeptide Y (NPY)-ergic system is associated with behavioral resilience to stress exposure in an animal model of post-traumatic stress disorder. *Neuropsychopharmacology, 37*(2), 350–63. https://doi.org/10.1038/npp.2011.230

Collins, D., & MacNamara, A. (2012). The rocky road to the top: Why talent needs trauma. *Sports Medicine, 42*(11), 907–14.

Cotterill, S. T. (2011). Experiences of developing pre-performance routines with elite cricket players. *Journal of Sport Psychology in Action, 2*, 81–9.

Cunningham, W. A., Arbuckle, N. L., Jahn, A., Mowrer, S. M., & Abduljalil, A. M. (2011). Reprint of: Aspects of neuroticism and the amygdala: Chronic tuning from motivational styles. *Neuropsychologia, 49*(4), 657–62. https://doi.org/10.1016/j.neuropsychologia.2011.02.027

Cunningham, W. A., Van Bavel, J. J., & Johnsen, I. R. (2008). Affective flexibility. *Psychological Science, 19*(2), 152–60. https://doi.org/10.1111/j.1467-9280.2008.02061.x

de Kloet, E. R., DeRijk, R. H., & Meijer, O. C. (2007). Therapy insight: Is there an imbalanced response of mineralocorticoid and glucocorticoid receptors in depression? *Nature Clinical Practice Endocrinology and Metabolism, 3*(2), 168–79. https://doi.org/10.1038/ncpendmet0403

de Kloet, E. R., Joëls, M., & Holsboer, F. (2005). Stress and the brain: From adaptation to disease. *Nature Reviews Neuroscience, 6*(6), 463–75. https://doi.org/10.1038/nrn1683

DeRijk, R. H., & de Kloet, E. R. (2008). Corticosteroid receptor polymorphisms: Determinants of vulnerability and resilience. *European Journal of Pharmacology, 583*(2–3), 303–11. https://doi.org/10.1016/j.ejphar.2007.11.072

Dincheva, I., Drysdale, A. T., Hartley, C. A., Johnson, D. C., Jing, D., King, E. C., … Lee, F. S. (2015). FAAH genetic variation enhances fronto-amygdala function in mouse and human. *Nature Communications, 6*(1), 6395. https://doi.org/10.1038/ncomms7395

Donner, J., Sipilä, T., Ripatti, S., Kananen, L., Chen, X., Kendler, K. S., … Hovatta, I. (2012). Support for involvement of glutamate decarboxylase 1 and neuropeptide y in anxiety susceptibility. *American Journal of Medical Genetics Part B: Neuropsychiatric Genetics, 159B*(3), 316–27. https://doi.org/10.1002/ajmg.b.32029

Dorris, D. C., Power, D. A., & Kenefick, E. (2012). Investigating the effects of ego depletion on physical exercise routines of athletes. *Psychology of Sport and Exercise, 13*(2), 118–25.

Dubrovsky, B. O. (2005). Steroids, neuroactive steroids and neurosteroids in psychopathology. *Progress in Neuro-Psychopharmacology and Biological Psychiatry, 29*(2), 169–92. https://doi.org/10.1016/j.pnpbp.2004.11.001

Dunn, S. H., & Conley, Y. P. (2015). A systematic review of genetic influences on coping. *Biological Research for Nursing, 17*(1), 87–93. https://doi.org/10.1177/1099800414527340

Egan, M. F., Kojima, M., Callicott, J. H., Goldberg, T. E., Kolachana, B. S., Bertolino, A., … Weinberger, D. R. (2003). The BDNF val66met polymorphism affects activity-dependent secretion of BDNF and human memory and hippocampal function. *Cell, 112*(2), 257–69. Retrieved from www.ncbi.nlm.nih.gov/pubmed/12553913

Englert, C. (2017). Ego depletion in sports: Highlighting the importance of self-control strength for high-level sport performance. *Current Opinion in Psychology, 16*, 1–5.

Englert, C., Bertrams, A., Furley, P., & Oudejans, R. R. D. (2015). Is ego depletion associated with increased distractibility? Results from a basketball free throw task. *Psychology of Sport and Exercise, 18*, 26–31.

Englert, C., Zwemmer, K., Bertrams, A., & Oudejans, R. R. (2015). Ego depletion and attention regulation under pressure: Is a temporary loss of self-control strength indeed related to impaired attention regulation? *Journal of Sport amd Exercise Psychology, 37*(2), 127–37.

Eysenck, M. W., & Calvo, M. G. (1992). Anxiety and performance: The processing efficiency theory. *Cognition and Emotion, 6*(6), 409–34.

Eysenck, M. W., Derakshan, N., Santos, R., & Calvo, M. G. (2007). Anxiety and cognitive performance: Attentional control theory. *Emotion, 7*(2), 336–53.

Faraone, S. V., Perlis, R. H., Doyle, A. E., Smoller, J. W., Goralnick, J. J., Holmgren, M. A., & Sklar, P. (2005). Molecular genetics of attention-deficit/hyperactivity disorder. *Biological Psychiatry, 57*(11), 1313–23. https://doi.org/10.1016/j.biopsych.2004.11.024

Feder, A., Nestler, E. J., & Charney, D. S. (2009). Psychobiology and molecular genetics of resilience. *Nature Reviews Neuroscience, 10*(6), 446–57.

Folkman, S. (1992). Making the case for coping. In B. N. Carpenter (Ed.), *Personal coping: Theory, research and application* (pp. 31–46). Westport, CT: Praeger.

Fletcher, D., & Sarkar, M. (2012). A grounded theory of psychological resilience in olympic champions. *Psychology of Sport and Exercise, 13*, 669–78. http://dx.doi.org/10.1016/j.psychsport.2012.04.007

Fletcher, D., & Sarkar, M. (2016). Mental fortitude training: An evidence-based approach to developing psychological resilience for sustained success. *Journal of Sport Psychology in Action, 7*(3), 135–57, doi:10.1080/21520704.2016.1255496

Gaudreau, P., & Blondin, J.-P. (2002). Development of a questionnaire for the assessment of coping strategies employed by athletes in competitive sports settings. *Psychology of Sport and Exercise, 3*, 1–34.

Gaudreau, P., & Blondin, J.-P. (2004). Different athletes cope differently during a sport competition: A cluster analysis of coping. *Personality and Individual Differences, 36*(8), 1865–77.

Gerritsen, L., Milaneschi, Y., Vinkers, C. H., van Hemert, A. M., van Velzen, L., Schmaal, L., & Penninx, B. W. (2017). HPA axis genes, and their interaction with childhood maltreatment, are related to cortisol levels and stress-related phenotypes. *Neuropsychopharmacology, 42*(12), 2446–55. https://doi.org/10.1038/npp.2017.118

Gröpel, P., & Beckmann, J. (2017). A pre-performance routine to optimize competition performance in artistic gymnastics. *The Sport Psychologist, 31*, 199–207.

Hariri, A. R., Goldberg, T. E., Mattay, V. S., Kolachana, B. S., Callicott, J. H., Egan, M. F., & Weinberger, D. R. (2003). Brain-derived neurotrophic factor val66met polymorphism affects human memory-related hippocampal activity and predicts memory performance. *The Journal of Neuroscience: The Official Journal of the Society for Neuroscience, 23*(17), 6690–4. Retrieved from www.ncbi.nlm.nih.gov/pubmed/12890761

Hariri, A. R., Gorka, A., Hyde, L. W., Kimak, M., Halder, I., Ducci, F., … Manuck, S. B. (2009). Divergent effects of genetic variation in endocannabinoid signaling on human threat- and reward-related brain function. *Biological Psychiatry, 66*(1), 9–16. https://doi.org/10.1016/j.biopsych.2008.10.047

Hariri, A. R., Mattay, V. S., Tessitore, A., Kolachana, B., Fera, F., Goldman, D., … Weinberger, D. R. (2002). Serotonin transporter genetic variation and the response of the human amygdala. *Science, 297*(5580), 400–3. https://doi.org/10.1126/science.1071829

Hazell, J., Cotterill, S. T., & Hill, D. M. (2014). An exploration of pre-performance routines, self-efficacy, anxiety and performance in semi-professional soccer. *European Journal of Sport Science, 14*(6), 603–10.

Heck, A., Lieb, R., Ellgas, A., Pfister, H., Lucae, S., Erhardt, A., … Ising, M. (2009). Polymorphisms in the angiotensin-converting enzyme gene region predict coping styles in healthy adults and depressed patients. *American Journal of Medical Genetics Part B: Neuropsychiatric Genetics, 150B*(1), 104–14. https://doi.org/10.1002/ajmg.b.30784

Heils, A., Teufel, A., Petri, S., Stöber, G., Riederer, P., Bengel, D., & Lesch, K. P. (1996). Allelic variation of human serotonin transporter gene expression. *Journal of Neurochemistry, 66*(6), 2621–4. Retrieved from www.ncbi.nlm.nih.gov/pubmed/8632190

Heim, C., & Nemeroff, C. B. (2001). The role of childhood trauma in the neurobiology of mood and anxiety disorders: Preclinical and clinical studies. *Biological Psychiatry, 49*(12), 1023–39. Retrieved from www.ncbi.nlm.nih.gov/pubmed/11430844

Heinz, A., & Smolka, M. N. (2006). The effects of catechol O-methyltransferase genotype on brain activation elicited by affective stimuli and cognitive tasks. *Reviews in the Neurosciences, 17*(3), 359–67. Retrieved from www.ncbi.nlm.nih.gov/pubmed/16878403

Hill, D. M., & Hemmings, B. (2015). A phenomenological exploration of coping responses associated with choking in sport. *Qualitative Research in Sport, Exercise and Health, 7*(4), 521–38.

Hulshoff Pol, H. E., Schnack, H. G., Posthuma, D., Mandl, R. C. W., Baare, W. F., van Oel, C., … Kahn, R. S. (2006). Genetic contributions to human brain morphology and intelligence. *Journal of Neuroscience, 26*(40), 10235–42. https://doi.org/10.1523/JNEUROSCI.1312-06.2006

Ising, M., Depping, A.-M., Siebertz, A., Lucae, S., Unschuld, P. G., Kloiber, S., … Holsboer, F. (2008). Polymorphisms in the FKBP5 gene region modulate recovery from psychosocial stress in healthy controls. *European Journal of Neuroscience, 28*(2), 389–98. https://doi.org/10.1111/j.1460-9568.2008.06332.x

Jordet, G. (2015). Psychological characteristics of expert performers. In J. Baker & D. Farrow (Eds.), *Routledge handbook of sport expertise* (pp. 106–20). London: Routledge.

Karlamangla, A. S., Singer, B. H., McEwen, B. S., Rowe, J. W., & Seeman, T. E. (2002). Allostatic load as a predictor of functional decline. MacArthur studies of successful aging. *Journal of Clinical Epidemiology, 55*(7), 696–710. Retrieved from www.ncbi.nlm.nih.gov/pubmed/12160918

Kautz, M., Charney, D. S., & Murrough, J. W. (2017). Neuropeptide Y, resilience, and PTSD therapeutics. *Neuroscience Letters, 649*, 164–9. https://doi.org/10.1016/j.neulet.2016.11.061

Kavussanu, M., Dewar, A. J., & Boardley, I. D. (2014). Achievement goals and emotions in athletes: The mediating role of challenge and threat appraisals. *Motiv Emot, 38*(4), 589–99.

Kim, H. S., Sherman, D. K., Sasaki, J. Y., Xu, J., Chu, T. Q., Ryu, C., … Taylor, S. E. (2010). Culture, distress, and oxytocin receptor polymorphism (OXTR) interact to influence emotional support seeking. *Proceedings of the National Academy of Sciences, 107*(36), 15717–21. https://doi.org/10.1073/pnas.1010830107

Kolassa, I.-T., Kolassa, S., Ertl, V., Papassotiropoulos, A., & De Quervain, D. J.-F. (2010). The risk of posttraumatic stress disorder after trauma depends on traumatic load and the Catechol-O-Methyltransferase Val158Met polymorphism. *Biological Psychiatry, 67*(4), 304–8. https://doi.org/10.1016/j.biopsych.2009.10.009

Kraft, J. B., Slager, S. L., McGrath, P. J., & Hamilton, S. P. (2005). Sequence analysis of the serotonin transporter and associations with antidepressant response. *Biological Psychiatry, 58*(5), 374–81. https://doi.org/10.1016/j.biopsych.2005.04.048

Kremen, W. S., Prom-Wormley, E., Panizzon, M. S., Eyler, L. T., Fischl, B., Neale, M. C., … Fennema-Notestine, C. (2010). Genetic and environmental influences on the size of specific brain regions in midlife: The VETSA MRI study. *NeuroImage, 49*(2), 1213–23. https://doi.org/10.1016/j.neuroimage.2009.09.043

Kuczewski, N., Porcher, C., & Gaiarsa, J.-L. (2010). Activity-dependent dendritic secretion of brain-derived neurotrophic factor modulates synaptic plasticity. *European Journal of Neuroscience, 32*(8), 1239–44. https://doi.org/10.1111/j.1460-9568.2010.07378.x

Lachman, H. M., Papolos, D. F., Saito, T., Yu, Y. M., Szumlanski, C. L., & Weinshilboum, R. M. (1996). Human catechol-O-methyltransferase pharmacogenetics: Description of a functional polymorphism and its potential application to neuropsychiatric disorders. *Pharmacogenetics, 6*(3), 243–50. Retrieved from www.ncbi.nlm.nih.gov/pubmed/8807664

Lautenbach, F., Laborde, S., Klämpfl, M., & Achtzehn, S. (2015). A link between cortisol and performance: An exploratory case study of a tennis match. *International Journal of Psychophysiology, 98*(2, Pt. 1), 167–73.

Lazarus, R. S. (1999). *Stress and emotion: A new synthesis*. New York, NY: Springer Publishing Co.

Lazarus, R. S. (2000). How emotions influence performance in competitive sports. *Sport Psychologist, 14*(3), 229–52.

Lazarus, R. S., & Folkman, S. (1984). *Stress, appraisal, and coping*. New York, NY: Springer.

Lemery, K. S., & Goldsmith, H. H. (2002). Genetic and environmental influences on preschool sibling cooperation and conflict: Associations with difficult temperament and parenting style. *Marriage and Family Review, 33*(1), 77–99.

Lemogne, C., Gorwood, P., Boni, C., Pessiglione, M., Lehéricy, S., & Fossati, P. (2011). Cognitive appraisal and life stress moderate the effects of the 5-HTTLPR polymorphism on amygdala reactivity. *Human Brain Mapping, 32*(11), 1856–67. https://doi.org/10.1002/hbm.21150

Levy, A. R., Nicholls, A. R., & Polman, R. C. (2011). Pre-competitive confidence, coping, and subjective performance in sport. *Scandanavian Journal of Medicine & Science in Sports, 21*(5), 721–9.

Lidor, R., & Mayan, Z. (2005). Can beginning learners benefit from preperformance routines when serving in volleyball? *The Sport Psychologist, 19*(4), 343–63.

Lidor, R., & Singer, R. N. (2003). Preperformance routines in self-paced tasks: Developmental and educational consideration. In R. Lidor & K. P. Hennschen (Eds.), *The psychology of team sport* (pp. 69–98). Morgantown, WV: Fitness Information Technology.

Lu, F. J. H., Lee, W. P., Chang, Y. K., Chou, C. C., Hsu, Y. W., Ju-Han Lin, J. H., & Gill, D. L. (2016). Interaction of athletes' resilience and coaches' social support on the stress-burnout relationship: A conjunctive moderation perspective. *Psychology of Sport and Exercise, 22*, 202–9.

MacKenzie, A., & Quinn, J. (1999). A serotonin transporter gene intron 2 polymorphic region, correlated with affective disorders, has allele-dependent differential enhancer-like properties in the mouse embryo. *Proceedings of the National Academy of Sciences of the United States of America, 96*(26), 15251–5. Retrieved from www.ncbi.nlm.nih.gov/pubmed/10611371

Mahon, P. B., Zandi, P. P., Potash, J. B., Nestadt, G., & Wand, G. S. (2013). Genetic association of FKBP5 and CRHR1 with cortisol response to acute psychosocial stress in healthy adults. *Psychopharmacology, 227*(2), 231–41. https://doi.org/10.1007/s00213-012-2956-x

Masten, A. S. (1994). Resilience in individual development: Successful adaptation despite risk and adversity. In M. C. Wang & E. W. Gordon (Eds.), *Educational resilience in inner-city America: Challenges and prospects* (pp. 3–25). Hillsdale, NJ: Lawrence Erlbaum Associates, Inc.

Mata, J., Thompson, R. J., & Gotlib, I. H. (2010). BDNF genotype moderates the relation between physical activity and depressive symptoms. *Health Psychology, 29*(2), 130–3. https://doi.org/10.1037/a0017261

McEwen, B. S., & Milner, T. A. (2007). Hippocampal formation: Shedding light on the influence of sex and stress on the brain. *Brain Research Reviews, 55*(2), 343–55. https://doi.org/10.1016/j.brainresrev.2007.02.006

McGaugh, J. L. (2004). The amygdala modulates the consolidation of memories of emotionally arousing experiences. *Annual Review of Neuroscience, 27*(1), 1–28. https://doi.org/10.1146/annurev.neuro.27.070203.144157

McGregor, H. A., & Elliot, A. J. (2002). Achievement goals as predictors of achievement-relevant processes prior to task engagement. *Journal of Educational Psychology, 94*(2), 381–395.

Meggs, J., Golby, J., Mallett, C. J., Gucciardi, D. F., & Polman, R. C. (2016). The cortisol awakening response and resilience in elite swimmers. *International Journal of Sports Medicine, 37*(2), 169–74.

Mesagno, C., & Marchant, D. (2013). Characteristics of polar opposites: An exploratory investigation of choking-resistant and choking-susceptible athletes. *Journal of Applied Sport Psychology, 25*(1), 72–91.

Mesagno, C., Marchant, D., & Morris, T. (2008). A pre-performance routine to alleviate choking in "choking-susceptible" athletes. *The Sport Psychologist, 22*(4), 439–57.

Mesagno, C., & Mullane-Grant, T. (2010). A comparison of different pre-performance routines as possible choking interventions. *Journal of Applied Sport Psychology, 22*(3), 343–60.

Morgan, C. A., Southwick, S., Hazlett, G., Rasmusson, A., Hoyt, G., Zimolo, Z., & Charney, D. (2004). Relationships among plasma dehydroepiandrosterone sulfate and cortisollevels, symptoms of dissociation, and objective performance in humans exposedto acute stress. *Archives of General Psychiatry, 61*(8), 819. https://doi.org/10.1001/archpsyc.61.8.819

Morgan, C. A., Wang, S., Southwick, S. M., Rasmusson, A., Hazlett, G., Hauger, R. L., & Charney, D. S. (2000). Plasma neuropeptide-Y concentrations in humans exposed to military survival training. *Biological Psychiatry, 47*(10), 902–9. Retrieved from www.ncbi.nlm.nih.gov/pubmed/10807963

Munafò, M. R., Brown, S. M., & Hariri, A. R. (2008). Serotonin transporter (5-HTTLPR) genotype and amygdala activation: A meta-analysis. *Biological Psychiatry, 63*(9), 852–7. https://doi.org/10.1016/j.biopsych.2007.08.016

Munafò, M. R., Durrant, C., Lewis, G., & Flint, J. (2009). Gene × environment interactions at the serotonin transporter locus. *Biological Psychiatry, 65*(3), 211–19. https://doi.org/10.1016/j.biopsych.2008.06.009

Nicholls, A. R., Perry, J. L., & Calmeiro, L. (2014). Precompetitive achievement goals, stress appraisals, emotions, and coping among athletes. *Journal of Sport and Exercise Psychology, 36*(5), 433–45.

Nicholls, A. R., & Polman, R. C. (2007). Coping in sport: A systematic review. *Journal of Sports Sciences, 25*(1), 11–31.

Nicholls, A. R., Polman, R. C., & Levy, A. R. (2012). A path analysis of stress appraisals, emotions, coping, and performance satisfaction among athletes. *Psychology of Sport and Exercise, 13*, 263–70.

Ntoumanis, N., Edmunds, J., & Duda, J. L. (2009). Understanding the coping process from a self-determination theory perspective. *British Journal of Health Psychology, 14*(2), 249–60.

Paz, R., & Pare, D. (2013). Physiological basis for emotional modulation of memory circuits by the amygdala. *Current Opinion in Neurobiology, 23*(3), 381–6. https://doi.org/10.1016/j.conb.2013.01.008

Pensgaard, A. M., & Duda, J. L. (2003). Sydney 2000: The interplay between emotions, coping, and the performance of Olympic-level athletes. *Sport Psychologist, 17*(3), 253–67.

Petta, P., Pelachaud, C., & Cowie, R. (2011). *Emotion-oriented systems: The humaine handbook*. Berlin, Germany: Springer.

Pezawas, L., Meyer-Lindenberg, A., Drabant, E. M., Verchinski, B. A., Munoz, K. E., Kolachana, B. S., ... Weinberger, D. R. (2005). 5-HTTLPR polymorphism impacts human cingulate-amygdala interactions: A genetic susceptibility mechanism for depression. *Nature Neuroscience, 8*(6), 828–34. https://doi.org/10.1038/nn1463

Phillips, C. (2017). Brain-derived neurotrophic factor, depression, and physical activity: Making the neuroplastic connection. *Neural Plasticity, 2017*, 1–17. https://doi.org/10.1155/2017/7260130

Poole, J. C., Snieder, H., Davis, H. C., & Treiber, F. A. (2006). Anger suppression and adiposity modulate association between ADRB2 haplotype and cardiovascular stress reactivity. *Psychosomatic Medicine, 68*(2), 207–12. https://doi.org/10.1097/01.psy.0000204925.18143.4f

Rao, H., Gillihan, S. J., Wang, J., Korczykowski, M., Sankoorikal, G. M. V., Kaercher, K. A., ... Farah, M. J. (2007). Genetic variation in serotonin transporter alters resting brain function in healthy individuals. *Biological Psychiatry, 62*(6), 600–6. https://doi.org/10.1016/j.biopsych.2006.11.028

Ressler, K. J., Bradley, B., Mercer, K. B., Deveau, T. C., Smith, A. K., Gillespie, C. F., ... Binder, E. B. (2009). Polymorphisms in CRHR1 and the serotonin transporter loci: Gene × gene × environment interactions on depressive symptoms. *American Journal of Medical Genetics Part B: Neuropsychiatric Genetics, 9999B*(3), 812–24. https://doi.org/10.1002/ajmg.b.31052

Richardson, G. E. (2002). The metatheory of resilience and resiliency. *Journal of Clinical Psychology, 58*(3), 307–21.

Roth, S., & Cohen, L. J. (1986). Approach, avoidance, and coping with stress. *American Psychologist, 41*(7), 813–19.

Sajdyk, T. J., Shekhar, A., & Gehlert, D. R. (2004). Interactions between NPY and CRF in the amygdala to regulate emotionality. *Neuropeptides, 38*(4), 225–34. https://doi.org/10.1016/j.npep. 2004.05.006

Secades, X. G., Molinero, O., Salguero, A., Barquín, R. R., la Vega, R. de, & Márquez, S. (2016). Relationship between resilience and coping strategies in competitive sport. *Perceptual and Motor Skills, 122*(1), 336–49. https://doi.org/10.1177/ 0031512516631056

Scherk, H., Gruber, O., Menzel, P., Schneider-Axmann, T., Kemmer, C., Usher, J., ... Falkai, P. (2009). 5-HTTLPR genotype influences amygdala volume. *European Archives of Psychiatry and Clinical Neuroscience, 259*(4), 212–17. https://doi.org/10.1007/s00406-008-0853-4

Schinke, R., Tenenbaum, G., Lidor, R., & Battochio, R. (2012). Adaptation processes affecting performance in elite sport. *Journal of Clinical Sport Psychology, 6*, 180–95.

Schinke, R., Yungblut, H., Blodgett, A., Eys, M., Peltier, D., Ritchie, S., & Recollet-Saikkonen, D. (2010). The role of families in youth sport programming in a canadian aboriginal reserve. *Journal of Physical Activity and Health, 7*, 156–66.

Schmack, K., Schlagenhauf, F., Sterzer, P., Wrase, J., Beck, A., Dembler, T., ... Gallinat, J. (2008). Catechol-O-methyltransferase val158met genotype influences neural processing of reward anticipation. *NeuroImage, 42*(4), 1631–8. https://doi.org/10.1016/j.neuroimage.2008.06.019

Schmeichel, B. J., & Baumeister, R. F. (2010). Effortful attention control. In B. Bruya (Ed.), *Effortless attention: A new perspective in the cognitive science of attention and action* (pp. 29–49). Cambridge, MA: MIT Press.

Serretti, A., Kato, M., De Ronchi, D., & Kinoshita, T. (2007). Meta-analysis of serotonin transporter gene promoter polymorphism (5-HTTLPR) association with selective serotonin reuptake inhibitor efficacy in depressed patients. *Molecular Psychiatry, 12*(3), 247–57. https://doi.org/10.1038/sj.mp. 4001926

Skelton, K., Ressler, K. J., Norrholm, S. D., Jovanovic, T., & Bradley-Davino, B. (2012). PTSD and gene variants: New pathways and new thinking. *Neuropharmacology, 62*(2), 628–37. https://doi.org/10.1016/j.neuropharm.2011.02.013

Sleijpen, M., Heitland, I., Mooren, T., & Kleber, R. (2017). Resilience in refugee and Dutch adolescents: Genetic variability in the corticotropin releasing hormone receptor 1. *Personality and Individual Differences, 111*, 211–14.

Soliman, F., Glatt, C. E., Bath, K. G., Levita, L., Jones, R. M., Pattwell, S. S., … Casey, B. J. (2010). A genetic variant BDNF polymorphism alters extinction learning in both mouse and human. *Science, 327*(5967), 863–6. https://doi.org/10.1126/science. 1181886

Stein, M. B., Campbell-Sills, L., & Gelernter, J. (2009). Genetic variation in 5HTTLPR is associated with emotional resilience. *American Journal of Medical Genetics Part B: Neuropsychiatric Genetics, 150B*(7), 900–6. https://doi.org/10.1002/ajmg.b.30916

Stjepanović, D., Lorenzetti, V., Yücel, M., Hawi, Z., & Bellgrove, M. A. (2013). Human amygdala volume is predicted by common DNA variation in the stathmin and serotonin transporter genes. *Translational Psychiatry, 3*(7), e283. https://doi.org/10.1038/tp. 2013.41

Stork, M. J., Graham, J. D., Bray, S. R., & Martin Ginis, K. A. (2017). Using self-reported and objective measures of self-control to predict exercise and academic behaviors among first-year university students. *Journal of Health Psychology, 22*(8), 1056–66.

Szily, E., Bowen, J., Unoka, Z., Simon, L., & Kéri, S. (2008). Emotion appraisal is modulated by the genetic polymorphism of the serotonin transporter. *Journal of Neural Transmission, 115*(6), 819–22. https://doi.org/10.1007/s00702-008-0029-4

Tamman, A. J. F., Sippel, L. M., Han, S., Neria, Y., Krystal, J. H., Southwick, S. M., … Pietrzak, R. H. (2017). Attachment style moderates effects of *FKBP5* polymorphisms and childhood abuse on post-traumatic stress symptoms: Results from the national health and resilience in veterans study. *The World Journal of Biological Psychiatry*, 1–12. https://doi.org/10.1080/15622975.2017.1376114

Tedesqui, R. A. B., & Young, B. W. (2015). Perspectives on active and inhibitive self-regulation relating to the deliberate practice activities of sport experts. *Talent Development and Excellence, 7*(1), 29–39.

Tedesqui, R. A. B., & Young, B. W. (2017). Associations between self-control, practice and skill level in sport expertise development. *Research Quarterly for Exercise and Sport, 88*(1), 108–13.

Tenenbaum, G., Hatfield, B. D., Eklund, R. C., Land, W. M., Calmeiro, L., Razon, S., & Schack, T. (2009). A conceptual framework for studying emotions-cognitions-performance linkage under conditions that vary in perceived pressure. *Progress in Brain Research, 174*, 159–78.

Tenenbaum, G., Lane, A., Razon, S., Lidor, R., & Schinke, R. (2015). Adaptation: A two-perception probabilistic conceptual framework. *Journal of Clinical Sport Psychology, 9*(1), 1–23.

Toering, T., & Jordet, G. (2015). Self-control in professional soccer players. *Journal of Applied Sport Psychology, 27*(3), 335–50.

Tost, H., Kolachana, B., Hakimi, S., Lemaitre, H., Verchinski, B. A., Mattay, V. S., … Meyer-Lindenberg, A. (2010). A common allele in the oxytocin receptor gene (OXTR) impacts prosocial temperament and human hypothalamic-limbic structure and function. *Proceedings of the National Academy of Sciences, 107*(31), 13936–41. https://doi. org/10.1073/pnas.1003296107

Watkins, L. E., Han, S., Harpaz-Rotem, I., Mota, N. P., Southwick, S. M., Krystal, J. H., … Pietrzak, R. H. (2016). FKBP5 polymorphisms, childhood abuse, and PTSD symptoms: Results from the national health and resilience in veterans study. *Psychoneuroendocrinology, 69*, 98–105. https://doi.org/10.1016/j.psyneuen.2016.04.001

Wendland, J. R., Martin, B. J., Kruse, M. R., Lesch, K.-P., & Murphy, D. L. (2006). Simultaneous genotyping of four functional loci of human SLC6A4, with a reappraisal of 5-HTTLPR and rs25531. *Molecular Psychiatry, 11*(3), 224–6. https://doi.org/10.1038/sj.mp. 4001789

Wilhelm, K., Siegel, J. E., Finch, A. W., Hadzi-Pavlovic, D., Mitchell, P. B., Parker, G., & Schofield, P. R. (2007). The long and the short of it: Associations between 5-HTT genotypes and coping with stress. *Psychosomatic Medicine, 69*(7), 614–20. https://doi.org/10.1097/PSY.0b013e31814cec64

Wilson, M., Smith, N. C., & Holmes, P. S. (2007). The role of effort in influencing the effect of anxiety on performance: Testing the conflicting predictions of processing efficiency theory and the conscious processing hypothesis. *British Journal of Psychology, 98*(3), 411–28.

Wine, J. (1971). Test anxiety and direction of attention. *Psychological Bulletin, 76*(2), 92–104. http://dx.doi.org/10.1037/h0031332

Wu, G., Feder, A., Cohen, H., Kim, J. J., Calderon, S., Charney, D. S., & Mathé, A. A. (2013). Understanding resilience. *Frontiers in Behavioral Neuroscience, 7*(10). https://doi.org/10.3389/fnbeh.2013.00010

Wu, G., Feder, A., Wegener, G., Bailey, C., Saxena, S., Charney, D., & Mathé, A. A. (2011). Central functions of neuropeptide Y in mood and anxiety disorders. *Expert Opinion on Therapeutic Targets, 15*(11), 1317–31. https://doi.org/10.1517/14728222.2011.628314

Zautra, A. J., Arewasikporn, A., & Davis, M. C. (2010). Resilience: Promoting well-being through recovery, sustainability, and growth. *Research in Human Development, 7*(3), 221–38. https://doi.org/10.1080/15427609.2010.504431

Zeidner, M., Boekaerts, M., & Pintrich, P. R. (2000). Self-regulation: Directions and challenges for future research. In M. Boekaerts, P. R. Pintrich, & M. Zeidner (Eds.), *Handbook of self-regulation* (pp. 749–68). San Diego, CA: Academic Press.

Zhang, K., Rao, F., Pablo Miramontes-Gonzalez, J., Hightower, C. M., Vaught, B., Chen, Y., … O'Connor, D. T. (2012). Neuropeptide Y (NPY). *Journal of the American College of Cardiology, 60*(17), 1678–89. https://doi.org/10.1016/j.jacc.2012.06.042

Zhou, Z., Zhu, G., Hariri, A. R., Enoch, M.-A., Scott, D., Sinha, R., … Goldman, D. (2008). Genetic variation in human NPY expression affects stress response and emotion. *Nature, 452*(7190), 997–1001. https://doi.org/10.1038/nature06858

Zimmermann, P., Brückl, T., Nocon, A., Pfister, H., Binder, E. B., Uhr, M., … Ising, M. (2011). Interaction of FKBP5 gene variants and adverse life events in predicting depression onset: Results from a 10-year prospective community study. *The American Journal of Psychiatry, 168*(10), 1107–16. https://doi.org/10.1176/appi.ajp.2011.10111577

6   Genetics and environmental determinants of motivation

Motivation is conceptualized as the "internal and/or external forces that produce the initiation, intensity, and persistence of behavior." Intrinsic motivation involves performing an activity for one's own pleasure and drive whereas extrinsic motivation involves engaging in an activity as a means to an end. Both types of motivation strongly impact motor performance. New concepts introduce more dimensions to this psychological construct. The identification of the capability to take part in activity is a challenging task, determined by intrinsic and extrinsic factors as well as by the interaction between them. While it is well established that genetics have a large influence on "body-related" phenotypes (e.g., strength, muscle size, endurance capacity, etc), less is known about genetic variants related to motivation, self-efficacy, and self-determination, which interactively may influence the tendency to practice in physical activities, though genetic markers determine to some extent both (a) motivation for certain types of physical activities, and (b) the quality of performance in these activities

According to Ryan and Deci (2017), motivation concerns the *energizing, direction, regulation,* and *persistence* of behavior. Therefore, sport and exercise contexts represent an appropriate environment to study motivation (Standage & Ryan, 2012). Whether it is to sustain intense periods of training regimen or to maintain consistent exercise behaviors, self-determined motivation appears to be a key factor (Standage & Ryan, 2018). To thoroughly capture the role of self-determined behaviors in the achievement of sport success, researchers have mainly focused on athletes' phenomenological experiences and the nature of the social environment in which they evolve. Adding to this empirical knowledge, the current chapter aims to explore the biological factors underlying self-determined behaviors.

Definitions and theories

SDT is a multidimensional and empirically based meta-theory of human motivation. It assumes that humans are proactive, self-motivated organisms, who naturally engage in optimal challenges and seek novel experiences to grow psychologically and integrate into a coherent sense of self. These natural developmental tendencies interplay with the social environment which forms the foundation of SDT meta-theory. Most recent formulations of SDT have divided the meta-theory into various sub-theories, each of which is designed to explain a set of motivationally based phenomena (Martin-Krumm & Tarquinio, 2011). The five SDT sub-theories are cognitive evaluation theory (CET), organismic integration theory (OIT), basic psychological needs theory (BPNT), causality orientation theory (COT), and goal contents theory (GCT). Before digging into the genetic aspect of motivation, the research associated with these environmental sub-theories is reviewed.

Cognitive evaluation theory

Intrinsic motivation refers to doing an activity for the inherent satisfaction of the activity itself as opposed to doing it to reach or avoid separable consequences. Intrinsically motivated individuals are curious, seek learning opportunities, and are devoted to the mastery of a variety of skills. Although humans are naturally inclined toward intrinsic motivational tendencies, maintaining and fostering this propensity requires supportive conditions (Ryan & Deci, 2000). The CET serves as a theoretical foundation to examines specific social and environmental factors that facilitate or thwart an individual's intrinsically motivated behaviors.

CET maintains that social-contextual events such as rewards, competition, feedback, choice, punishment, and surveillance can alter an individual's intrinsic motivation (Ryan & Deci, 2000). For instance, in a comprehensive meta-analysis aimed at exploring the effect of extrinsic rewards on intrinsic motivation, Deci, Koestner, and Ryan (1999) showed that all tangible and expected rewards undermine free choice motivation. Accordingly, because elite sport environments focus on winning and large financial incentives (e.g., professional sport), it promotes a lower level of intrinsic motivation (Vallerand, Deci, & Ryan, 1987; Vallerand, Gauvin, & Halliwell, 1986). Yet, a distinction exists between rewards that provide information and those aiming at controlling the individuals. Specifically, CET stipulates that informational events satisfy the psychological needs for *competence* and *autonomy* leading to increased intrinsic motivation, whereas controlling events undermine autonomy impacting negatively on intrinsic behaviors. Therefore, if external rewards are perceived by athletes as providing information about competence rather than recognized as controlling, it can enhance their perception of competence, which in turn will affect positively their intrinsic motivation (Mageau & Vallerand, 2003; Mallett & Harrahan, 2004; Readdy, Raabe, & Harding, 2014).

Readdy et al. (2014) tested this assumption on collegiate football players by implementing an off-season extrinsic reward system. To enhance the effectiveness of the program, the researcher used the three factors that were shown to be especially important in determining how an athlete perceives a reward: namely, *reward contingent* (i.e., task- or performance-oriented), the degree to which the environment is controlling or non-controlling, and the cue value (Deci et al., 1999). This reward program was successful in increasing athletes' intrinsic motivation, but not basic psychological needs. Being in opposition to the theory of SDT, the authors argued that the program may not have created meaningful competition or success feedback for the players.

Indeed, it has been shown that specific types of competition, and the presence of success or failure feedback, are important social factors that influence needs satisfaction (Vallerand & Losier, 1999). Specifically, it has been argued that successful performance impacts positively intrinsic motivation through need satisfaction and positive affect, whereas failure triggers negative affect thereby undermining motivation (Blanchard, Mask, Vallerand, de la Sablonnière, & Provencher, 2007; Gillet, Berjot, & Gobance, 2009; Standage, Duda, & Pensgaard, 2005). This evidence supports one of the postulates of the *hierarchical model of intrinsic and extrinsic motivation* (HMIEM) (Vallerand, 1997, 2007). Based on SDT assumptions, HMIEM is concerned with the antecedents and consequences linked to various forms of motivation. Accordingly, to fully capture motivational processes, this framework highlights the necessity to consider the three constructs of motivation; namely, intrinsic motivation, extrinsic motivation, and amotivation. The next section defines thoroughly the construct of extrinsic motivation.

Organismic integration theory

Whereas CET focuses on intrinsic motivation, OIT is concerned with the various levels of extrinsically regulated behaviors. Compared to amotivation, which is defined as a state of lacking the intention to act, extrinsic motivation refers to the performance of an activity in order to attain some separable outcomes (Ryan & Deci, 2000). Depending on the degree to which behaviors are autonomous or controlled, OIT illustrates motivation on a continuum ranging from the less internalized to the more internalized motivated behaviors (see Figure 6.1). Here, the term *internalization* refers to a process whereby people adapt external values, beliefs, and behavioral regulations from social contexts to themselves (Standage & Ryan, 2018, p. X). The four levels of internalization are *external regulation, introjection, identification*, and *integration* (Deci & Ryan, 1985; Ryan & Deci, 2000).

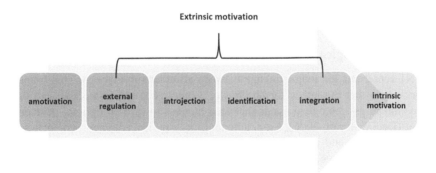

Figure 6.1 Organismic integration theory. Types of motivation are aligned on a continuum ranging from amotivation to intrinsic motivations through extrinsic motivation.

External regulation represents behaviors that are adopted to satisfy external pressure. Under externally regulated conditions, people usually act to obtain external reward, gain social recognition, or avoid negative consequences. Although efficient to achieve short-term goals, externally regulated behaviors are rarely maintained over time (Deci & Ryan, 1985). The next three internalization levels are characterized by an internal rather than an external source of control or pressure. First, *introjection* refers to a partially internalized controlled behavior. Under this type of regulation, people force themselves into an activity to avoid shame and guilt or gain ego and pride (Standage & Ryan, 2018). The following level, *identification*, is more autonomous since it represents behaviors that are valued because of their contribution to the achievement of one's personal goal (Ryan & Deci, 2000). Although more internalized, these behaviors are still instrumental because usefulness guides participation in the activity rather than enjoyment (Deci & Ryan, 2000). Finally, the fullest form of internalization of extrinsic motivation is *integration*. At this stage, behaviors become in harmony with other aspects of an individual's values and identity resulting in self-determined extrinsic motivation (Deci & Ryan, 2000). Despite sharing many attributes with intrinsic motivation, integrated behaviors are still considered to be extrinsically regulated as they are performed to achieve a separable outcome (Ryan & Deci, 2002).

Behavioral regulations have been examined as a predictor of several outcomes within sport and exercise settings (Standage & Ryan, 2018). Namely, empirical evidence highlights the significant contribution of both intrinsic motivation and identified regulation to enhance bouts of moderate intensity exercise (Standage, Sebire, & Loney, 2008). In the sport setting, intrinsic motivation as well as identified regulation were positively associated with persistent behaviors whereas external regulation was significantly predicting dropout over time (Pelletier, Fortier, Vallerand, & Brière, 2001). Self-determined motivation has also been positively associated with objective performance during two seasons among youth elite tennis players. Performance was thereafter positively linked to the satisfaction of the three basic psychological needs which are introduced next (Gillet, Vallerand, & Rosnet, 2009).

Basic psychological needs theory

BPNT represents the major linkage between all other sub-theories. This framework posits that the needs for *autonomy*, *competence*, and *relatedness* are the three innate psychological needs that feed humans toward an optimal development (Deci & Ryan, 2000). First, autonomy is experienced when people feel a sense of choice and perceive their actions are congruent with their integrated sense of self. The need for competence, on the other hand, is satisfied when individuals feel they have the capacities to achieve their goal. Finally, the relatedness need is met when humans feel a sense of belongingness to and by others in a particular context. When the social environment provides the resources to fulfill these needs, the likelihood of optimal development increases. Yet, if these needs are thwarted, people may experience physical and mental ill-being leading to developmental decline (Deci & Ryan, 2012; Ryan & Deci, 2017).

Taking an environmental perspective, sport psychology research points toward the essential role of the coach in nurturing the satisfaction of the three psychological needs (Mallett, 2005). For instance, findings revealed that coaches' autonomy facilitates athletes' self-determined motivation toward their sport activity. Autonomy-supportive environment increases contextual motivation which in turn leads to optimal situational self-determined behaviors and performance (Gillet, Vallerand, Amoura, & Baldes, 2010; Mallett, 2005). Coaching behaviors that encourage the athletes' perspective, build trust in their abilities, and acknowledge their choices and decision-making are not only positively associated with athletes' perception of autonomy, but also with an increased sense of competence and relatedness (Adie, Duda, & Ntoumanis, 2012). Indeed, meaningful coach-athlete relationship has been shown to be an essential factor underlying athletes' intrinsic motivation (Mageau & Vallerand, 2003; N. Williams, Whipp, Jackson, & Dimmock, 2013).

Sharing some conceptual similarities with SDT basic needs theory, the *dispositional motive approach* (McClelland, 1985) must be considered when studying the genetic basis of motivation. According to this framework, individuals respond differently to environmental incentives depending on implicit motive dispositions. Namely, three implicit motive dispositions are crucial to describe and explain human behavior. First, *implicit achievement motive* refers to the desire to surpass standards of excellence. Second, striving for positive and stable interpersonal relationships is defined as *implicit affiliation motive*. Lastly, *implicit power motive* is concerned with influencing and controlling other people (McClelland, 1985). People thus vary in their capacities to experience the attainment of certain types of incentives as rewarding. For instance, it has been demonstrated that athletes with a stronger *implicit affiliation motive* reach flow experience more frequently when their need for relatedness is satisfied (Brandstätter & Schüler, 2013). Similarly, athletes higher in implicit achievement motive benefit greatly from an environment that supports their need for competence (Schüler, Sheldon, & Fröhlich, 2010). Recently, researchers have tested the influence of a fourth implicit achievement motive – the *implicit autonomy disposition* – on flow experience and well-being. Findings revealed that, in an autonomy-supportive environment, athletes higher in implicit autonomy disposition derived more flow – an intrinsically motivating experience (Csikszentmihalyi, 1996) – and report greater well-being (Schüler, Sheldon, Prentice, & Halusic, 2016).

Causality orientations theory

Parallel to OIT conceptualization, COT is concerned with individual's consistent and stable pattern of thinking stemming from repeated interactions with their social environment. The three orientations are labeled the *autonomy orientation*, the *controlled orientation*, and the *impersonal orientation* (Ryan & Deci, 2017). These orientations are influenced by the frequency to which individuals have been exposed to autonomy-supportive, controlling, or amotivating environments respectively. First, autonomy orientation is characterized by a high interest in self-selected goals as well as integrated regulated or intrinsically motivated behaviors. On the other hand, people adopting a controlled orientation are less attuned with their interests and values making them more prone to adopt external and introjected regulation behaviors. Finally, impersonal orientation refers to individual's perception of incompetence resulting in behaviors that lack intentionality (Standage & Ryan, 2018).

Research investigating the effect of causality orientations on performance in the sport and exercise setting is quite scarce. Yet, Rose, Parfitt, and Williams (2005) showed that high levels of autonomy orientation significantly influenced the adoption and maintenance of regular exercise behaviors. Furthermore, because, to a certain extent, all people have the three causality orientations (Weinstein, Deci, & Ryan, 2011), some researchers use priming to trigger automatic and unconscious causality orientations. For instance, a scrambled sentence task was used to prime autonomous or neutral motivational orientation in recreationally active undergraduate students. Results revealed that autonomous motivational priming stimulates enjoyment, perceived competence and positive attitude toward high-intensity interval training (Brown, Teseo, & Bray, 2016). This empirical evidence supports COT theoretical proposition.

Goal content theory

The GCT is concerned with the goals people pursue (Standage & Ryan, 2018). According to Kasser and Ryan (1993, 1996), when individuals pursue personal growth, affiliation, community contribution, and/or maintenance of physical health, their goals are considered *intrinsic*. On the other hand, seeking financial success, social recognition, and/or attractiveness represents *extrinsic* goals.

Somewhat tied to GCT, *achievement goal theory* (Maehr & Nicholls, 1980) has attracted a substantial level of interest in sport and exercise psychology (Roberts, Treasure, & Conroy, 2007). According to this framework, motivation can be understood through the function and meaning an individual gives to his or her achievement behavior. Achievement goals influence achievement beliefs which thereafter guide decision-making and behavior in achievement contexts. J. G. Nicholls (1984) argues that achievement goals and behavior are dependent on two conceptions of ability. On one hand, an undifferentiated conception of ability reflects a perception that effort and ability are directly linked. On the other hand, when adopting a differentiated conception of ability and effort, people tend to dissociate their ability from the level of effort they invest while performing a task. These two conceptualizations form the criteria used by individuals to not only set goals, but also determine their success and failure. Accordingly, *personal theory of achievement* (J. G. Nicholls, 1989) stipulates that when adopting an undifferentiated conception, the goal of action is to develop mastery, self-improvement, or learning (i.e., *mastery-oriented goals*) which stimulates a *task involvement* motivational state. On the other hand, a differentiated conception of ability leads to the establishment of *ego-oriented goals*, which implies outperforming others with equal effort, or performing equal to others using less effort. This other-referenced type of goal triggers an ego involvement motivational state.

Building on the *personal theory of achievement*, Elliot and McGregor (2001) designed the *2 × 2 achievement goal framework*. In addition to the *mastery vs. ego-oriented goal dimensions*, the *approach vs avoidance dimensions* were added. Therefore, athletes can be inclined toward four types of goals:

(A) Mastery Approach (MAp; mastering self-referenced skills).
(B) Mastery Avoidance (MAv; avoiding the demonstration of self-referenced incompetence).
(C) Performance Approach (PAp; attaining normatively referenced competence).
(D) Performance avoidance (PAv; avoiding the demonstration of norma-tively referenced incompetence).

Of these four types of goal, Mastery Approach goal has shown to result in the most positive effects. Namely, it has been linked to athletes' well-being (Adie, Duda, & Ntoumanis, 2010), pleasant emotions (A. R. Nicholls, Perry, & Calmeiro, 2014), precompetitive state-anxiety (C.-H. Li, 2013), and performance (Lochbaum & Smith, 2015).

The reasons people articulate to explain the achievement or failure of their goal is also known to influence motivational state in subsequent situations (Rees, Ingledew, & Hardy, 2005). Popular in the 1980s, *attribution theories* are concerned with the explanations people assign to specific events (Allen, 2012). A central premise within attribution research is that there is a dimensional structure underlying the explana-tions people give for events. The initial model designed by Weiner (1971), stipulates that two dimensions are defining attributions: *locus of causality* and *stability*. Locus of causality is concerned with the internal or external explanation a person is assign-ing to a situation. The stability dimension, on the other hand, refers to whether the cause of an event is interpreted as stable or unstable over time. A further version of the model adds a third dimension (Weiner, 1979), *controllability*, which refers to the perception that a situation is controllable or uncontrollable by the person. The learned helplessness hypothesis (Maier & Seligman, 1976) also enriched the attribu-tion framework by adding the *globality* and *universality* dimensions (Abramson, Seligman, & Teasdale, 1978). Specifically, when a person is experiencing an uncon-trollable event, he/she can generalize the uncontrollability of the situation to all other situations he/she might experience or consider the cause as specific to the current event (i.e., global vs. specific). An individual can also establish the cause of an event as being unique to himself or common to all people (i.e., personal vs. universal). A limited amount of research has explored the impact of attribution on elite athletes' future performance. Yet, results of research investigating the influence of attribution on 80 athletes indicated that when failure is perceived as controllable and unstable the likelihood of future success is increased (Coffee, Rees, & Haslam, 2009).

Taking into consideration the theories and research findings, most sport psy-chologists are studying the impact of fostering the three psychological needs on motor performance. An important view of SDT is that these needs are known to be universal, i.e., they are not acquired or promoted through a value system but rather have a similar effect on human development independently of culture, gender, developmental stage and context (Standage & Ryan, 2018). Yet, although these three needs must be fulfilled to stimulate self-determined behaviors, the degree to which each need must be satisfied may differ among people. Individual differences indeed interact with the influence of each need satisfaction on intrinsic motivation (Schüler et al., 2016). From a genetic standpoint, these postulates have important implications since they underlie the role of nature in the process of enhancing human intrinsic motivation.

Genetic lookout on motivation

Theoretically, studies on genetics of motivation in sport evolved from two distinguished domains: *sport participation* and *sport performance.* However, this discrimination is fallacious. While *sport participation* can be linked directly to the multifactorial trait of motivation, *sport performance* is the outcome of many traits interacting together in a specific context. Therefore, when trying to figure out the genetic basis of motivation, it is actually the genetic basis of motivation toward sport participation/physical activity/exercise, rather than to sport performance. In other words, everybody is motivated to perform well, but not everybody is motivated to practice, train, exercise, and put in an effort in order to perform well.

In line with this idea, a study investigating the impact of intrinsic motivation on student performance showed that the relationship between students' intrinsic motivation at the start of the semester and performance over time was fully mediated by mastery goals. In other words, intrinsically motivated students set themselves goals that are oriented toward the mastery of a task which increases their engagement with proactive study (Cerasoli & Ford, 2014). Similar observations have been made in sport. For instance, the study of harmonious passion, which refers to an autonomous internalization of the activity into the person's identity (Vallerand et al., 2003), has revealed a positive link with performance (Vallerand et al., 2008). Yet, the relationship between this highly intrinsic motivational state and performance was mediated by deliberate practice – a structured form of activity aimed at improving performance. A subsequent study in the same direction added goal orientation to the model explaining performance (Vallerand et al., 2008). Findings revealed that passionate athletes pursue mastery goals which predict greater engagement in deliberate practice. The amount of deliberate practice an athlete is involved in is then directly linked to performance. This evidence supports the assumption that motivation is a fuel to engage in relevant training behaviors and it is these behaviors that influence performance subsequently.

The genetic basis of motivation to sport participation

Voluntary physical activity essentially has two relevant components, which interact with each other: *motor movement* component and *motivational/rewarding* component; both act upon (sometimes overlapping) biological mechanisms, and are therefore influenced by genetic factors. The hypothesis that physical activity level is influenced by biological mechanisms was first suggested by Richter (Richter, 1927; Richter & Wislocki, 1928) and reviewed by Rowland (1998) and Lightfoot et al. (2018). Rundquist (1933) selectively bred rats for 12 generations on the basis of daily activity, and found that heritability influenced physical activity levels. Since then, dozens of studies with both humans and animals confirmed Rundquist's conclusions that variation in physical activity is influenced by genetic variation (Lightfoot et al., 2018), with heritability estimated to range from 0.20 (Pérusse, Tremblay, Leblanc, & Bouchard, 1989) to 0.90 (Joosen, Gielen, Vlietinck, & Westerterp, 2005) – depending on the model, methods, population, age, and sex.

Lightfoot et al. (2018) introduced a conceptual model of the biological determinants of physical activity, and clustered them into three main components: *brain, cardiorespiratory system*, and *muscle* – all of which can interact and comprise a substantial genetic basis but are also influenced by various factors in the external environment. According the model (see Figure 6.2), the brain holds the "activity-stat," and serves as activity-level controller, also receiving signals from other factors that may be partly genetically regulated. The parts of the brain which are most important for motor motivation are (a) the striatum/nucleus accumbens, particularly in reward and motor movement; and (b) the ventral pallidum, which is involved in integrating dopaminergic signals from both motivational/reward centers and motor movement centers in the brain (Smith, Tindell, Aldridge, & Berridge, 2009). The activity-stat is part of the motivational regulatory system that integrates reward and punishment cues and afferent somato-visceral feedback. The motivational states are further modulated by trait-dependent individual differences in personality and

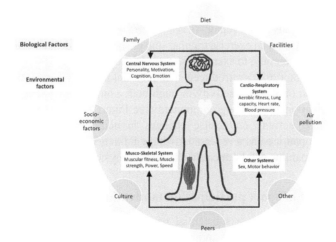

Figure 6.2 Conceptual model for the main physiological systems involved in physical activity and its regulation (Lightfoot et al., 2018).

behavior, and are influenced by complex multifactorial and redundant genetic, epigenetic, and other biological systems, with each component characterized by small effect sizes (Lightfoot et al., 2018).

The dopaminergic basis of sport participation motivation

The role of the dopaminergic system (described in Chapter 2) in monitoring and controlling the motor movement was studied through various paradigms, such as Parkinson's Disease, ADHD, addiction, and animal models (see Knab & Lightfoot, 2010 for review). The results from these studies imply that the dopaminergic system may play a role in the pleasurable/rewarding feelings associated with voluntary physical activity in humans, and thus might contribute to the observed variation in animals and humans in motivation for physical activity (Knab & Lightfoot, 2010). Moreover, dopamine and exercise show interconnected interactions, in which exercise induces changes in the dopaminergic system, and the dopaminergic system induces changes in exercise behavior. The support for these interactions comes from anatomical studies, animal models, and the use of exercise in the treatment of depression. From the anatomical perspective, dopamine functions in both the *striatum*, which is involved in motor activity (Salamone, Keller, Zigmond, & Stricker, 1989), and the *nucleus accumbens*, which is involved in anticipatory behavior (Blackburn, Phillips, Jakubovic, & Fibiger, 1989; Pfaus et al., 1990; Salamone, Cousins, McCullough, Carriero, & Berkowitz, 1994). However, these areas are integrated by neural connections.

Animal models show that dopamine depleted animals lack the motivation for doing more effortful tasks (Cousins, Atherton, Turner, & Salamone, 1996; Salamone, Cousins, & Bucher, 1994). Complementary to these finding, it was found that exercise alleviates symptoms of depression (Duman, Schlesinger, Russell, & Duman, 2008), and that trained animals showed increased D2 (MacRae, Spirduso, Walters, Farrar, & Wilcox, 1987) and D1 receptors (Liste, Guerra, Caruncho, & Labandeira-Garcia, 1997). Similarly, human exercise training studies show dependent changes in the dopamine system in response to exercise (Knab & Lightfoot, 2010).

Knab and Lightfoot (2010) introduced a model linking the dopaminergic system and regulation of physical activity through both a motor movement component and a motivational/rewarding component (see Figure 6.3). According to this model, physical activity can cause changes in neuronal signaling and dopamine levels. Dopamine has a reversed U-shape influence on dopamine: too much or too little dopamine can both cause changes in physical activity levels.

Genetic variability in sport participation motivation

Twin studies have shown that a substantial part of the variation in exercise behavior (Stubbe & de Geus, 2009) and motivational dimensions such as self-efficacy (Waaktaar & Torgersen, 2013), decision-making (Tuvblad et al., 2013), and internal motivation (Aaltonen, Kujala, & Kaprio, 2014) can be accounted for by genetic factors. However, data from molecular genetic perspective is scare.

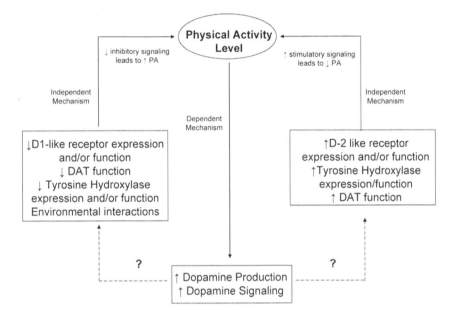

Figure 6.3 Dopamine system and regulation of physical activity (Knab & Lightfoot, 2010).

The natural candidate genetic variants related to sport performance motivation are the genetic variants in genes related to the dopaminergic (see Figure 2.4 in Chapter 2) and are natural candidates for affecting physical activity motivation.

Dopamine receptor D2, also known as *DRD2*, is a protein that, in humans, is encoded by the *DRD2* gene. The *DRD2* TaqIA polymorphism is a single nucleotide transition which creates a restriction fragment polymorphism (Velasco et al., 2002). The A1 allele has been associated with a 30–40 percent reduction in D2 dopamine receptor density compared to individuals homozygous for the A2 allele (Grandy et al., 1989; Jönsson et al., 1999; Pohjalainen et al., 1998; Thompson et al., 1997). Both polymorphisms have been associated with measures of behavioral motivation, including Cloninger's harm avoidance and novelty seeking (NS) scales (J. Chen et al., 2004).

5-Hydroxytryptamine (5-HT, serotonin) (described in Chapter 5) has long been implicated in a wide variety of emotional, cognitive, and behavioral control processes. However, its precise contribution is still not well understood. There are a growing catalog of genetic polymorphisms in the human population that modulate the functioning of particular neurotransmitters that may influence the regulation of the 5-HT system, which can be exploited to make inferences about how the system functions to produce behavior and cognition. A prominent example is a polymorphism 5-HTTLPR linked to the 5-HT transporter and involving a variable repeat sequence in the promoter region of the gene that encodes short (s) and long (l) allelic variants. The 5-HTTLPR regulates the efficacy of the 5-HT transporter

(5HTT), and the s and l alleles are associated with its reduced and increased expression, respectively, as evidenced by the analyses of postmortem tissue (Hariri & Holmes, 2006). Although one might expect that reduced expression of the 5-HTT would lead to exaggerated 5-HT transmission, in fact, the s allele has been associated with reduced 5-HT function, possibly as a result of lifelong differences in 5-HTT gene transcription leading to long-term neurochemical adaptations (Bethea et al., 2004). s-carriers exhibit a greater incidence of depression (Caspi et al., 2003). Other genetic polymorphisms of interest include those affecting the expression of tryptophan hydroxylase (the synthetic enzyme for 5-HT) and the 5-HT2A receptor.

The highly conserved factor S100B belongs to the S100 family of Ca2+– binding proteins and the *S100B* gene located on chromosome 21 at 21q22.3. It is a low molecular mass protein (21kDa) that is abundant in the central nervous system. The effects of S100B involve regulation of transcription factors, cell growth and differentiation, protein phosphorylation, and the inflammatory response (Donato et al., 2009). S100B is secreted by astrocytes and released into the extracellular space where its actions depend on the concentration at which it is released. At nanomolar concentrations, S100B has been shown to have neurotrophic effects while at micromolar concentrations it is believed to produce toxicity due to apoptosis and necrosis as well as stimulating secretion of proinflammatory mediators (Y. Li, Barger, Liu, Mrak, & Griffin, 2000). Two SNPs within the *S100B* gene, 2757C>G and 5748C>T, were found to be associated with the personality trait of self-directedness (Suchankova et al., 2011). Self-directedness is an overall estimate of adaptive strategies to adjust behavior to conceptual goals as well as coping strategies and is strongly correlated to general mental health and absence of personality disorder.

The val66met SNP is a common, functional polymorphism found in humans that results in a valine (val) to methionine (met) amino acid substitution at codon66. Individuals with at least one copy of the met allele have been shown to have a lower neuronal expression of BDNF (Z. Chen et al., 2008), smaller hippocampal volume (Pezawas et al., 2004), and impaired memory and hippocampal activation (Egan et al., 2003). Another study's findings revealed that individuals with one copy of the met allele had a more positive mood response to a bout of moderate intensity exercise (65 percent of VO$_2$max) relative to those with a val/val genotype (A. D. Bryan, Hutchinson, Seals, & Allen, 2007). *BDNF* genotype has also been shown to moderate response to an exercise intervention (A. Bryan et al., 2013), since subjects with the met allele in the intervention condition increased their aerobic exercise the most, while those with the met allele in the control condition exercised the least. The affective response to exercise influences future exercise motivation and participation (Kwan & Bryan, 2010a, 2010b; D. M. Williams et al., 2008; D. M. Williams, Dunsiger, Jennings, & Marcus, 2012). Lately it was found that regular exercisers with at least one copy of the met allele reported greater increases in intrinsic motivation during exercise and were more likely to continue exercising when given the option to stop (Caldwell Hooper, Bryan, & Hagger, 2014).

The dopamine D4 receptor (*DRD4*) gene is highly polymorphic, with two variants, tandem repeats (VNTR) and C-521T that have been reported to be associated with human approach-related traits such as NS and extraversion. Research evaluating behavioral and psychiatric phenotypes has focused largely on a variable number of tandem repeats (VNTR) polymorphism in exon III and mainly the presence or absence of the 7-repeat ("long") allele. This variant has been reported to be associated with decreased ligand binding (Asghari et al., 1994), decreased gene expression in vitro, and attenuation of cyclic adenosine monophosphate (cAMP) formation when dopamine is bound to the receptor (Asghari et al., 1995), compared with 6-repeat or fewer ("short") alleles, although there is some disagreement regarding the optimal grouping of variants. The SNP C-521T in the promoter region is associated with variation in expression of the D4 receptor, with the T allele associated with a reduction in transcription levels of up to 40 percent compared with the C allele (Okuyama, Ishiguro, Toru, & Arinami, 1999). In a meta-analysis of the association between the *DRD4* gene VNTR and C-521T polymorphisms and human approach-related personality traits, including NS, extraversion, and impulsivity it was found that the -521T polymorphism may be associated with measures of NS and impulsivity but not extraversion.

Summary

Evidence accumulated from heritability studies with twins and families, and insights from biological systems associated with behavior, indicates that motivation for exercise carries a significant genetic component. The studies consist of the correlation between motivation and participation and between participation and performance, and thus the links cannot imply a direct link between motivation and performance (see Figure 6.4). Therefore, the study of the genetic basis of motivation and sport performance centers on the genetic

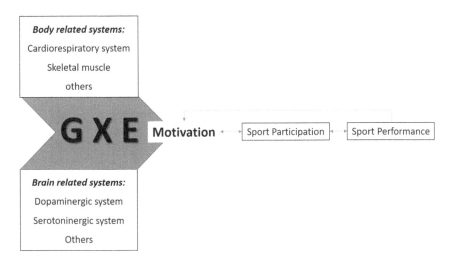

Figure 6.4 Gene-environment interaction motivation and sport performance.

basis of motivation to sport participation and on the genetic basis of motivation-related traits. Due to the complicated nature of the biological and psychological systems related to motivation, their connection with other psychological constructs (e.g., cognition, personality, emotion, etc.), and their interactions with the environment, the isolation of the genetic factors related to motivation is considered a mission impossible. The study on the genetic foundation of motivation in sports must take into consideration these complexities and establish itself accordingly.

References

Aaltonen, S., Kujala, U. M., & Kaprio, J. (2014). Factors behind leisure-time physical activity behavior based on Finnish twin studies: The role of genetic and environmental influences and the role of motives. *BioMed Research International, 2014*, 931820. https://doi.org/10.1155/2014/931820

Abramson, L. Y., Seligman, M. E., & Teasdale, J. D. (1978). Learned helplessness in humans: Critique and reformulation. *Journal of Abnormal Psychology, 87*(1), 49–74. http://dx.doi.org/10.1037/0021-843X.87.1.49

Adie, J. W., Duda, J. L., & Ntoumanis, N. (2010). Achievement goals, competition appraisals, and the well- and ill-being of elite youth soccer players over two competitive seasons. *Journal of Sport and Exercise Psychology, 32*(4), 555–79.

Adie, J. W., Duda, J. L., & Ntoumanis, N. (2012). Perceived coach-autonomy support, basic need satisfaction and the well- and ill-being of elite youth soccer players: A longitudinal investigation. *Psychology of Sport and Exercise, 13*(1), 51–9. http://dx.doi.org/10.1016/j.psychsport.2011.07.008

Allen, M. S. (2012). A systematic review of content themes in sport attribution research: 1954–2011. *International Journal of Sport and Exercise Psychology, 10*(1), 1–8. doi:10.1080/1612197X.2012.645130

Asghari, V., Sanyal, S., Buchwaldt, S., Paterson, A., Jovanovic, V., & Van Tol, H. H. (1995). Modulation of intracellular cyclic AMP levels by different human dopamine D4 receptor variants. *Journal of Neurochemistry, 65*(3), 1157–65. Retrieved from www.ncbi.nlm.nih.gov/pubmed/7643093

Asghari, V., Schoots, O., van Kats, S., Ohara, K., Jovanovic, V., Guan, H. C., ... Van Tol, H. H. (1994). Dopamine D4 receptor repeat: Analysis of different native and mutant forms of the human and rat genes. *Molecular Pharmacology, 46*(2), 364–73. Retrieved from www.ncbi.nlm.nih.gov/pubmed/8078498

Bethea, C. L., Streicher, J. M., Coleman, K., Pau, F. K.-Y., Moessner, R., & Cameron, J. L. (2004). Anxious behavior and fenfluramine-induced prolactin secretion in young rhesus macaques with different alleles of the serotonin reuptake transporter polymorphism (5HTTLPR). *Behavior Genetics, 34*(3), 295–307. https://doi.org/10.1023/B:BEGE.0000017873.61607.be

Blackburn, J. R., Phillips, A. G., Jakubovic, A., & Fibiger, H. C. (1989). Dopamine and preparatory behavior: II. A neurochemical analysis. *Behavioral Neuroscience, 103*(1), 15–23. Retrieved from www.ncbi.nlm.nih.gov/pubmed/2923667

Blanchard, C. M., Mask, L., Vallerand, R. J., de la Sablonnière, R., & Provencher, P. (2007). Reciprocal relationships between contextual and situational motivation in a sport setting. *Psychology of Sport and Exercise, 8*(5), 854–73. http://dx.doi.org/10.1016/j.psychsport.2007.03.004

Brandstätter, V., & Schüler, J. (2013). Action crisis and cost–benefit thinking: A cognitive analysis of a goal-disengagement phase. *Journal of Experimental Social Psychology, 49*(3), 543–53.

Brown, D. M., Teseo, A. J., & Bray, S. R. (2016). Effects of autonomous motivational priming on motivation and affective responses towards high-intensity interval training. *Journal of Sports Sciences, 34*(16), 1491–9.

Bryan, A. D., Hutchison, K. E., Seals, D. R., & Allen, D. L. (2007). A transdisciplinary model integrating genetic, physiological, and psychological correlates of voluntary exercise. *Health Psychology: Official Journal of the Division of Health Psychology, American Psychological Association, 26*(1), 30–9. https://doi.org/10.1037/0278-6133.26.1.30

Bryan, A., Magnan, R. E., Hooper, A. E. C., Ciccolo, J. T., Marcus, B., & Hutchison, K. E. (2013). Colorado stride (COSTRIDE): Testing genetic and physiological moderators of response to an intervention to increase physical activity. *The International Journal of Behavioral Nutrition and Physical Activity, 10*, 139. https://doi.org/10.1186/1479-5868-10-139

Caldwell Hooper, A. E., Bryan, A. D., & Hagger, M. S. (2014). What keeps a body moving? The brain-derived neurotrophic factor val66met polymorphism and intrinsic motivation to exercise in humans. *Journal of Behavioral Medicine, 37*(6), 1180–91. https://doi.org/10.1007/s10865-014-9567-4

Caspi, A., Sugden, K., Moffitt, T. E., Taylor, A., Craig, I. W., Harrington, H., … Poulton, R. (2003). Influence of life stress on depression: Moderation by a polymorphism in the 5-HTT gene. *Science, 301*(5631), 386–9. https://doi.org/10.1126/science.1083968

Cerasoli, C. P., & Ford, M. T. (2014). Intrinsic motivation, performance, and the mediating role of mastery goal orientation: A test of self-determination theory. *Journal of Psychology, 148*(3), 267–86.

Chen, J., Lipska, B. K., Halim, N., Ma, Q. D., Matsumoto, M., Melhem, S., … Weinberger, D. R. (2004). Functional analysis of genetic variation in catechol-O-methyltransferase (COMT): Effects on mRNA, protein, and enzyme activity in postmortem human brain. *American Journal of Human Genetics, 75*(5), 807–21. https://doi.org/10.1086/425589

Chen, Z., Simmons, M. S., Perry, R. T., Wiener, H. W., Harrell, L. E., & Go, R. C. P. (2008). Genetic association of neurotrophic tyrosine kinase receptor type 2 (NTRK2) with Alzheimer's disease. *American Journal of Medical Genetics. Part B, Neuropsychiatric Genetics: The Official Publication of the International Society of Psychiatric Genetics, 147*(3), 363–9. https://doi.org/10.1002/ajmg.b.30607

Coffee, P., Rees, T., & Haslam, S. A. (2009). Bouncing back from failure: The interactive impact of perceived controllability and stability on self-efficacy beliefs and future task performance. *Journal of Sports Sciences, 27*(11), 1117–24.

Cousins, M. S., Atherton, A., Turner, L., & Salamone, J. D. (1996). Nucleus accumbens dopamine depletions alter relative response allocation in a T-maze cost/benefit task. *Behavioural Brain Research, 74*(1–2), 189–97. Retrieved from www.ncbi.nlm.nih.gov/pubmed/8851929

Csikszentmihalyi, M. (1996). *Where is creativity? In creativity: Flow and the psychology of discovery and invention* (1st ed., pp. 23–50). New York, NY: HarperCollins.

Deci, E. L., Koestner, R., & Ryan, R. M. (1999). The undermining effect is a reality after all – Extrinsic rewards, task interest, and self-determination: Reply to Eisenberger, Pierce, and Cameron (1999) and Lepper, Henderlong, and Gingras (1999). *Psychological Bulletin, 125*(6), 692–700. http://dx.doi.org/10.1037/0033-2909.125.6.692

Deci, E. L., & Ryan, R. M. (1985). *Intrinsic motivation and self-determination in human behavior.* New York, NY: Springer.

Deci, E. L., & Ryan, R. M. (2000). The "what" and "why" of goal pursuits: Human needs and the self-determination of behavior. *Psychological Inquiry, 11,* 227–68.

Deci, E. L., & Ryan, R. M. (2012). Motivation, personality, and development within embedded social contexts: An overview of self-determination theory. In R. M. Ryan (Ed.), *Oxford handbook of human motivation* (pp. 85–107). Oxford, England: Oxford University Press.

Donato, R., Sorci, G., Riuzzi, F., Arcuri, C., Bianchi, R., Brozzi, F., … Giambanco, I. (2009). S100B's double life: Intracellular regulator and extracellular signal. *Biochimica et Biophysica Acta, 1793*(6), 1008–22. https://doi.org/10.1016/j.bbamcr.2008.11.009

Duman, C. H., Schlesinger, L., Russell, D. S., & Duman, R. S. (2008). Voluntary exercise produces antidepressant and anxiolytic behavioral effects in mice. *Brain Research, 1199,* 148–58. https://doi.org/10.1016/j.brainres.2007.12.047

Egan, M. F., Kojima, M., Callicott, J. H., Goldberg, T. E., Kolachana, B. S., Bertolino, A., … Weinberger, D. R. (2003). The BDNF val66met polymorphism affects activity-dependent secretion of BDNF and human memory and hippocampal function. *Cell, 112*(2), 257–69. Retrieved from www.ncbi.nlm.nih.gov/pubmed/12553913

Elliot, A. J., & McGregor, H. A. (2001). A 2×2 achievement goal framework. *Journal of Personality and Social Psychology, 80*(3), 501–19. http://dx.doi.org/10.1037/0022-3514.80.3.501

Gillet, N., Berjot, S., & Gobance, L. (2009). A motivational model of performance in the sport domain. *European Journal of Sport Science, 9*(3), 151–8.

Gillet, N., Vallerand, R. J., Amoura, S., & Baldes, B. (2010). Influence of coaches' autonomy support on athletes' motivation and sport performance: A test of the hierarchical model of intrinsic and extrinsic motivation. *Psychology of Sport and Exercise, 11,* 155–61.

Gillet, N., Vallerand, R. J., & Rosnet, E. (2009). Motivational clusters and performance in a real-life setting. *Motivation and Emotion, 33*(1), 49–62. http://dx.doi.org/10.1007/s11031-008-9115-z

Grandy, D. K., Litt, M., Allen, L., Bunzow, J. R., Marchionni, M., Makam, H., … Civelli, O. (1989). The human dopamine D2 receptor gene is located on chromosome 11 at q22-q23 and identifies a TaqI RFLP. *American Journal of Human Genetics, 45*(5), 778–85. Retrieved from www.pubmedcentral.nih.gov/articlerender.fcgi?artid=1683432&tool=pmcentrez&rendertype=abstract

Hariri, A. R., & Holmes, A. (2006). Genetics of emotional regulation: The role of the serotonin transporter in neural function. *Trends in Cognitive Sciences, 10*(4), 182–91. https://doi.org/10.1016/j.tics.2006.02.011

Jönsson, E. G., Nöthen, M. M., Grünhage, F., Farde, L., Nakashima, Y., Propping, P., & Sedvall, G. C. (1999). Polymorphisms in the dopamine D2 receptor gene and their relationships to striatal dopamine receptor density of healthy volunteers. *Molecular Psychiatry, 4*(3), 290–6. Retrieved from www.ncbi.nlm.nih.gov/pubmed/10395223

Joosen, A. M. C. P., Gielen, M., Vlietinck, R., & Westerterp, K. R. (2005). Genetic analysis of physical activity in twins. *The American Journal of Clinical Nutrition, 82*(6), 1253–9. https://doi.org/10.1093/ajcn/82.6.1253

Kasser, T., & Ryan, R. M. (1993). A dark side of the American dream: Correlates of financial success as a central life aspiration. *Journal of Personality and Social Psychology, 65*(2), 410–22.

Kasser, T., & Ryan, R. M. (1996). Further examining the American dream: Differential correlates of intrinsic and extrinsic goals. *Personality and Social Psychology Bulletin, 22*(3), 280–7. https://doi.org/10.1177/0146167296223006

Knab, A. M., & Lightfoot, J. T. (2010). Does the difference between physically active and couch potato lie in the dopamine system? *International Journal of Biological Sciences, 6*(2), 133–50. Retrieved from www.ncbi.nlm.nih.gov/pubmed/20224735

Kwan, B. M., & Bryan, A. (2010a). In-task and post-task affective response to exercise: Translating exercise intentions into behaviour. *British Journal of Health Psychology, 15*(Pt. 1), 115–31. https://doi.org/10.1348/135910709X433267

Kwan, B. M., & Bryan, A. D. (2010b). Affective response to exercise as a component of exercise motivation: Attitudes, norms, self-efficacy, and temporal stability of intentions. *Psychology of Sport and Exercise, 11*(1), 71–9. https://doi.org/10.1016/j.psychsport.2009.05.010

Li, C.-H. (2013). Predicting precompetitive state anxiety: Using the 2×2 achievement goal framework. *Perceptual and Motor Skills, 117*(2), 339–52. https://doi.org/10.2466/06.30.PMS.117x18z5

Li, Y., Barger, S. W., Liu, L., Mrak, R. E., & Griffin, W. S. (2000). S100beta induction of the proinflammatory cytokine interleukin-6 in neurons. *Journal of Neurochemistry, 74*(1), 143–50. Retrieved from www.pubmedcentral.nih.gov/articlerender.fcgi?artid=3836592&tool=pmcentrez&rendertype=abstract

Lightfoot, J. T., De Geus, E. J., Booth, F., Bray, M., Den Hoed, M., Kaprio, J., … Bouchard, C. (2018). Biological/genetic regulation of physical activity level: Consensus from GenBioPAC. *Medicine and Science in Sports and Exercise, 50*(4), 863–73. https://doi.org/10.1249/MSS.0000000000001499

Liste, I., Guerra, M. J., Caruncho, H. J., & Labandeira-Garcia, J. L. (1997). Treadmill running induces striatal Fos expression via NMDA glutamate and dopamine receptors. *Experimental Brain Research, 115*(3), 458–68. Retrieved from www.ncbi.nlm.nih.gov/pubmed/9262200

Lochbaum, M., & Smith, C., (2015). Making the cut and winning a golf putting championship: The role of approach-avoidance achievement goals. *International Journal of Golf Sciences, 4*, 50–66.

MacRae, P. G., Spirduso, W. W., Walters, T. J., Farrar, R. P., & Wilcox, R. E. (1987). Endurance training effects on striatal D2 dopamine receptor binding and striatal dopamine metabolites in presenescent older rats. *Psychopharmacology, 92*(2), 236–40. Retrieved from www.ncbi.nlm.nih.gov/pubmed/3110847

Maehr, M. L., & Nicholls, J. G. (1980). Culture and achievement motivation: A second look. In N. Warren (Ed.), *Studies in cross-cultural psychology* (Vol. 2, pp. 221–67). New York, NY: Academic Press.

Mageau, G. A., & Vallerand, R. J. (2003). The coach-athlete relationship: A motivational model. *Journal of Sports Sciences, 21*, 883–904. http://dx.doi.org/10.1080/0264041031000140374

Maier, S. F., & Seligman, M. E. (1976). Learned helplessness: Theory and evidence. *Journal of Experimental Psychology: General, 105*(1), 3–46. http://dx.doi.org/10.1037/0096-3445.105.1.3

Mallett, C. J. (2005). Self-determination theory: A case study of evidence-based coaching. *The Sport Psychologist, 19*(4), 417–29.

Mallett, C. J., & Harahan, S. J. (2004). Elite athletes; Why does the fire burn so brightly? *Psychology of Sport and Exercise, 5*, 183–200. https://doi.org/10.1016/S1469-0292(02)00043-2

Martin-Krumm, C., & Tarquinio, C. (2011). *Traité de psychologie positive*. Brussels, Belguim: C. de Boeck.

McClelland, D. C. (1985). How motives, skills, and values determine what people do. *American Psychologist, 40*(7), 812–25. http://dx.doi.org/10.1037/0003-066X. 40.7.812

Nicholls, A. R., Perry, J. L., & Calmeiro, L. (2014). Precompetitive achievement goals, stress appraisals, emotions, and coping among athletes. *Journal of Sport and Exercise Psychology, 36*(5), 433–45.

Nicholls, J. G. (1984). Achievement motivation: Conceptions of ability, subjective experience, task choice, and performance. *Psychological Review, 91*, 328–46. https:// doi.org/10.1037/0033-295X.91.3.328

Nicholls, J. G. (1989). *The competitive ethos and democratic education*. Cambridge, MA: Harvard University Press.

Okuyama, Y., Ishiguro, H., Toru, M., & Arinami, T. (1999). A genetic polymorphism in the promoter region of DRD4 associated with expression and schizophrenia. *Biochemical and Biophysical Research Communications, 258*(2), 292–5. https://doi.org/10.1006/ bbrc.1999.0630

Pelletier, L. G., Fortier, M. S., Vallerand, R. J., & Brière, N. M. (2001). Associations among perceived autonomy support, forms of self-regulation, and persistence: A prospective study. *Motivation and Emotion, 25*, 279–306. doi:10.1023/A:1014 805132406

Pérusse, L., Tremblay, A., Leblanc, C., & Bouchard, C. (1989). Genetic and environmental influences on level of habitual physical activity and exercise participation. *American Journal of Epidemiology, 129*(5), 1012–22. Retrieved from www.ncbi.nlm. nih.gov/pubmed/2705422

Pezawas, L., Verchinski, B. A., Mattay, V. S., Callicott, J. H., Kolachana, B. S., Straub, R. E., ... Weinberger, D. R. (2004). The brain-derived neurotrophic factor val66met polymorphism and variation in human cortical morphology. *The Journal of Neuroscience: The Official Journal of the Society for Neuroscience, 24*(45), 10099–102. https://doi.org/10.1523/JNEUROSCI.2680-04.2004

Pfaus, J. G., Damsma, G., Nomikos, G. G., Wenkstern, D. G., Blaha, C. D., Phillips, A. G., & Fibiger, H. C. (1990). Sexual behavior enhances central dopamine transmission in the male rat. *Brain Research, 530*(2), 345–8. Retrieved from www.ncbi.nlm.nih.gov/ pubmed/2176121

Pohjalainen, T., Rinne, J. O., Någren, K., Lehikoinen, P., Anttila, K., Syvälahti, E. K., & Hietala, J. (1998). The A1 allele of the human D2 dopamine receptor gene predicts low D2 receptor availability in healthy volunteers. *Molecular Psychiatry, 3*(3), 256–60. Retrieved from www.ncbi.nlm.nih.gov/pubmed/9672901

Readdy, T., Raabe, J., & Harding, J. S. (2014). Student-athletes' perceptions of an extrinsic reward program: A mixed-methods exploration of self-determination theory in the context of college football. *Journal of Applied Sport Psychology, 26*(2), 157–71.

Rees, T., Ingledew, D. K., & Hardy, L. (2005). Attribution in sport psychology: Seeking congruence between theory, research, and practice. *Psychology of Sport and Exercise, 6*, 189–204.

Richter, C. P. (1927). Animal behavior and internal drives. *The Quarterly Review of Biology, 2*(3), 307–43.

Richter, C. P., & Wislocki, G. B. (1928). Activity studies on castrated male and female rate with testicular grafts, in correlation with histological of the grafts. *American Journal of Physiology, 86*(3), 651–60.

Roberts, G. C., Treasure, D., & Conroy, D. E. (2007). Understanding the dynamics of motivation in sport and physical activity: An achievement goal interpretation. In G. Tenenbaum, & R. Eklund (Eds.), *Handbook of sport psychology* (3rd ed., pp. 3–30). Hoboken, NJ: Wiley. https://doi.org/10.1002/9781118270011.ch1

Rose, E. A., Parfitt, G., & Williams, S. (2005). Exercise causality orientations, behavioural regulation for exercise and stage of change for exercise: Exploring their relationships. *Psychology of Sport and Exercise, 6*(4), 399–414.

Rowland, T. W. (1998). The biological basis of physical activity. *Medicine and Science in Sports and Exercise, 30*(3), 392–9. Retrieved from www.ncbi.nlm.nih.gov/pubmed/9526885

Rundquist, E. A. (1933). Inheritance of spontaneous activity in rats. *Journal of Comparative Psychology, 16*(3), 415–38.

Ryan, R. M., & Deci, E. L. (2000). Self-determination theory and the facilitation of intrinsic motivation, social development, and well-being. *American Psychologist, 55*(1), 68–78.

Ryan, R. M., & Deci, E. L. (2002). An overview of self-determination theory. In E. L. Deci & R. M. Ryan (Eds.), *Handbook of self-determination research* (pp. 3–33). Rochester, NY: University of Rochester Press.

Ryan, R. M., & Deci, E. L. (2017). *Self-determination theory: Basic psychological needs in motivation, development, and wellness*. New York, NY: Guilford Press.

Salamone, J. D., Cousins, M. S., & Bucher, S. (1994). Anhedonia or anergia? Effects of haloperidol and nucleus accumbens dopamine depletion on instrumental response selection in a T-maze cost/benefit procedure. *Behavioural Brain Research, 65*(2), 221–9. Retrieved from www.ncbi.nlm.nih.gov/pubmed/7718155

Salamone, J. D., Cousins, M. S., McCullough, L. D., Carriero, D. L., & Berkowitz, R. J. (1994). Nucleus accumbens dopamine release increases during instrumental lever pressing for food but not free food consumption. *Pharmacology, Biochemistry, and Behavior, 49*(1), 25–31. Retrieved from www.ncbi.nlm.nih.gov/pubmed/7816884bbc

Salamone, J. D., Keller, R. W., Zigmond, M. J., & Stricker, E. M. (1989). Behavioral activation in rats increases striatal dopamine metabolism measured by dialysis perfusion. *Brain Research, 487*(2), 215–24. Retrieved from www.ncbi.nlm.nih.gov/pubmed/2786443

Schüler, J., Sheldon, K. M., & Fröhlich, S. M. (2010). Implicit need for achievement moderates the relationship between competence need satisfaction and subsequent motivation. *Journal of Research in Personality, 44*(1), 1–12. http://dx.doi.org/10.1016/j.jrp.2009.09.002

Schüler, J., Sheldon, K. M., Prentice, M., & Halusic, M. (2016). Do some people need autonomy more than others? Implicit dispositions toward autonomy moderate the effects of felt autonomy on well-being. *Journal of Personality, 84*(1), 5–20.

Smith, K. S., Tindell, A. J., Aldridge, J. W., & Berridge, K. C. (2009). Ventral pallidum roles in reward and motivation. *Behavioural Brain Research, 196*(2), 155–67. https://doi.org/10.1016/j.bbr.2008.09.038

Standage, M., Duda, J. L., & Pensgaard, A. M. (2005). The effect of competitive outcome and task-involving, ego-involving, and cooperative structures on the psychological well-being of individuals engaged in a co-ordination task: A self-determination approach. *Motivation and Emotion, 29*(1), 41–68. https://doi.org/10.1007/s11031-005-4415-z

Standage, M., & Ryan, R. M. (2012). Self-determination theory and exercise motivation: Facilitating self-regulatory processes to support and maintain health and well-being. In

G. C. Roberts & D. C. Treasure (Eds.), *Advances in motivation in sport and exercise* (3rd ed., pp. 233–70). Champaign, IL: Human Kinetics.

Standage, M., & Ryan, R. M. (2018). Self-determination theory in sport and exercise. In G. Tenenbaum & R. C. Eklund (Eds.), *Handbook of sport psychology* (4th ed.). New York, NY: John Wiley & Sons, Inc.

Standage, M., Sebire, S. J., & Loney, T. (2008). Does exercise motivation predict engagement in objectively assessed bouts of moderate-intensity exercise? A self-determination theory perspective. *Journal of Sport and Exercise Psychology, 30*(4), 337–52.

Stubbe, J. H., & de Geus, E. J. C. (2009). Genetics of exercise behavior. In Y. K. Kim (Ed.), *Handbook of behavior genetics* (pp. 343–58). New York, NY: Springer.

Suchankova, P., Baghaei, F., Rosmond, R., Holm, G., Anckarsäter, H., & Ekman, A. (2011). Genetic variability within the S100B gene influences the personality trait self-directedness. *Psychoneuroendocrinology, 36*(6), 919–23. https://doi.org/10.1016/j.psyneuen.2010.10.017

Thompson, J., Thomas, N., Singleton, A., Piggott, M., Lloyd, S., Perry, E. K., … Court, J. A. (1997). D2 dopamine receptor gene (DRD2) Taq1 A polymorphism: Reduced dopamine D2 receptor binding in the human striatum associated with the A1 allele. *Pharmacogenetics, 7*(6), 479–84. Retrieved from www.ncbi.nlm.nih.gov/pubmed/9429233

Tuvblad, C., Gao, Y., Wang, P., Raine, A., Botwick, T., & Baker, L. A. (2013). The genetic and environmental etiology of decision-making: A longitudinal twin study. *Journal of Adolescence, 36*(2), 245–55. https://doi.org/10.1016/j.adolescence.2012.10.006

Vallerand, R. J. (1997). Toward a hierarchical model of intrinsic and extrinsic motivation. *Advances in Experimental Social Psychology, 29*, 271–360.

Vallerand, R. J. (2007). A hierarchical model of intrinsic and extrinsic motivation for sport and physical activity. In M. S. Hagger & N. L. D. Chatzisarantis (Eds.), *Intrinsic motivation and self-determination in exercise and sport* (pp. 255–79, 356–63). Champaign, IL: Human Kinetics.

Vallerand, R. J., Blanchard, C., Mageau, G. A., Koestner, R., Ratelle, C., Leonard, M., … Marsolais, J. (2003). Les passions de l'ame: On obsessive and harmonious passion. *Journal of Personality and Social Psychology, 85*(4), 756–67.

Vallerand, R. J., Deci, E. L., & Ryan, R. M. (1987). Intrinsic motivation in sport. In K. B. Pandolf (Ed.), *Exercise and sport sciences reviews* (Vol. 15, pp. 389–425). New York, NY: Macmillan.

Vallerand, R. J., Gauvin, L. I., & Halliwell, W. R. (1986). Negative effects of competition on children's intrinsic motivation. *The Journal of Social Psychology, 126*, 649–57.

Vallerand, R. J., & Losier, G. F. (1999). An integrative analysis of intrinsic and extrinsic motivation in sport. *Journal of Applied Sport Psychology, 11*(1), 142–69.

Vallerand, R. J., Mageau, G. A., Elliot, A. J., Dumais, A., Demers, M.-A., & Rousseau, F. (2008). Passion and performance attainment in sport. *Psychology of Sport and Exercise, 9*(3), 373–92. http://dx.doi.org/10.1016/j.psychsport.2007.05.003

Velasco, M., Contreras, F., Cabezas, G. A., Bolívar, A., Fouillioux, C., & Hernández, R. (2002). Dopaminergic receptors: A new antihypertensive mechanism. *Journal of Hypertension. Supplement: Official Journal of the International Society of Hypertension, 20*(Suppl. 3), S55–8. Retrieved from www.ncbi.nlm.nih.gov/pubmed/12184056

Waaktaar, T., & Torgersen, S. (2013). Self-efficacy is mainly genetic, not learned: A multiple-rater twin study on the causal structure of general self-efficacy in young people. *Twin Research and Human Genetics: The Official Journal of the International Society for Twin Studies, 16*(3), 651–60. https://doi.org/10.1017/thg.2013.25

Weiner, B. (1971). *Perceiving the causes of success and failure*. New York, NY: General Learning Press.

Weiner, B. (1979). A theory of motivation for some classroom experiences. *Journal of Educational Psychology, 71*(1), 3–25. http://dx.doi.org/10.1037/0022-0663.71.1.3

Weinstein, N., Deci, E. L., & Ryan, R. M. (2011). Motivational determinants of integrating positive and negative past identities. *Journal of Personality and Social Psychology, 100*(3), 527–44.

Williams, D. M., Dunsiger, S., Ciccolo, J. T., Lewis, B. A., Albrecht, A. E., & Marcus, B. H. (2008). Acute affective response to a moderate-intensity exercise stimulus predicts physical activity participation 6 and 12 months later. *Psychology of Sport and Exercise, 9*(3), 231–45. https://doi.org/10.1016/j.psychsport.2007.04.002

Williams, D. M., Dunsiger, S., Jennings, E. G., & Marcus, B. H. (2012). Does affective valence during and immediately following a 10-min walk predict concurrent and future physical activity? *Annals of Behavioral Medicine: A Publication of the Society of Behavioral Medicine, 44*(1), 43–51. https://doi.org/10.1007/s12160-012-9362-9

Williams, N., Whipp, P. R., Jackson, B., & Dimmock, J. A. (2013). Relatedness support and the retention of young female golfers. *Journal of Applied Sport Psychology, 25*(4), 412–30.

7 Genetics and perceptual-cognitive skills

Expert athletes competing in open-task types of sport must possess an array of perceptual-cognitive skills to successfully execute an appropriate action in often short periods of time. Efficient decision-making starts with anticipation and perception of the situation based on past experience. Then, attention is paid to relevant cues in the environment. With these data in mind, the performer can generate a range of ideas from which the most appropriate solution will be chosen to be executed. This process not only allows the athlete to correctly execute specific strategies, but also to exhibit creative solutions which are of outstanding relevance to success in high-performance sport. Since many cognitive abilities depend on the plasticity of neuronal connections, the regulation of neural plasticity is controlled by genes. Therefore, a full understanding of cognitive processes requires the study of its genomic underpinnings. Moreover, evidence indicates that some of the influences of exercise in the brain can reach the genome with the potential to promote epigenetic modifications.

A cognitive perspective on performance

Athletes, or other performers such as surgeons, soldiers, law-enforcement officers, and actors, must frequently perform under high workload conditions that tax perceptual, cognitive, motor, and emotional resources. While performing, actions are generated from a *response selection sequence* aimed at optimizing the selected actions for the current environmental demands. The effectiveness of these operations depends on several perceptual information mechanisms (see Figure 7.1) processed at that given time, allowing the biological system to encode (store and represent) and access (retrieve) relevant information to the task being performed (Tenenbaum, 2003). Under pressure, changes occur in the perceptual, cognitive, and motor systems, which ultimately affect human performance.

Extensive research which was carried out on twins, family, and adoption data has documented that more than half of the striking individual differences in adult cognitive skills are due to genetic factors (Boomsma, 1993; Bouchard & McGue, 1981; Devlin, Daniels, & Roeder, 1997; McClearn et al., 1997; Plomin, 1999; Wright et al., 2001). This finding was generated across many countries and the entire adult age range. However, in spite of the evidence for the existence of

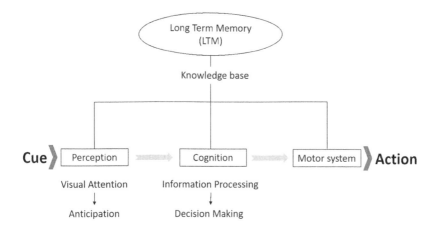

Figure 7.1 Mechanisms underlying response selection and action sequence.

"genes of cognitive ability," actual identification of such genes is an intricate task, though several Mendelian genetic mutations related to severe cognitive effects were identified (Flint, 1999). However, the polygenes (or QTLs) that influence the normal range of cognitive ability are still obscure, though they are probably related to neural function, especially neurotransmission (de Geus, Wright, Martin, & Boomsma, 2001).

Long-term memory: the mind behind the action

Learning and memory are two of the most magical capabilities of the mind. Learning is the biological process of acquiring new knowledge about the world, and memory is the process of retaining and reconstructing that knowledge over time (Kandel, Dudai, & Mayford, 2014). Well-practiced voluntary movements are stored in long-term stable memory structures termed *neural schemas*, which maintain information about anticipated consequences and action plans, and are ready to be retrieved. Neural schemas store information which has been highly rehearsed and utilized by the performer.

When the neural schema is retrieved and activated, it enables one to quickly make decisions and act, with little need to tax central processing executive controls. Therefore, the performer may divert workload resources to other task areas that may require more focused attention and thought. Thus, neural pathways which store schemas are of extreme importance to the control of movement production in well-practiced domains (Schack & Tenenbaum, 2004). Accordingly, the sensory system is automatically guided by the neural schema through long-term working memory structures (Ericsson & Kintsch, 1995), which in turn enable efficient visual attention search and anticipatory decisions to be placed. In other words, access to long-term working memory may be attained via two distinct pathways: a *knowledge-based pathway*, and a *retrieval-based pathway* (Ericsson & Kintsch, 1995). These pathways enable the cognitive system to efficiently control and guide visual attention through eye locations and fixations in the external environment.

Human memory is a heritable and polygenic behavioral trait, with a heritability estimate of ~0.50 (Bouchard & McGue, 1981; McClearn et al., 1997). Long-term memory (i.e., the ability to retain information for several hours, days and even years) depends on de novo protein synthesis and long-term changes in the molecular components of the neuronal synapse (Kandel, 2001), including pre- and postsynaptic processes, extracellular matrix, glia cells, and more (see Anderson, Bell, & Awh, 2012 for review). According to the synaptic plasticity and memory hypothesis, information storage is defined as a change in the pattern of synaptic strength in a specific neuronal circuit involved in the learned behavior (Martin, Grimwood, & Morris, 2000).

Neurons in memory relevant areas are highly plastic, meaning that specific activity patterns can modify neuronal function and structure. Especially prominent to learning and memory events are processes of synaptic plasticity, which include activity-dependent alterations of the efficacy of synaptic transmission (functional plasticity), and changes in the structure and number of synaptic connections (i.e., structural plasticity). The storage of information is also influenced by activity patterns and the timing of neuronal networks, and the history of prior events, which influences the propensity of neurons to be plastic and by this means to change its input-output characteristic (M. Korte & Schmitz, 2016).

Experiments in yeast and Aplysia suggest that a prion-like protein switch might help to maintain long-term synaptic changes required for the formation of long-term memory. Specifically, it has been shown that a neuronal isoform of the cytoplasmic polyadenylation element binding protein (CPEB) regulates local protein synthesis and stabilizes synapse-specific long-term facilitation in Aplysia (Si et al., 2003). CREB is an evolutionarily conserved transcription factor (TF). TFs are critical components in the cellular response to the environment. The human genome encodes roughly 1,500 TFs (Vaquerizas, Kummerfeld, Teichmann, & Luscombe, 2009), with roles in diverse biological processes, including long-term memory (Mayr & Montminy, 2001). Figure 7.2 is a simplified diagram showing generalized molecular pathways that induce long-term changes in neuronal activity via CREB. This diagram focuses on extracellular signals that activate membrane proteins commonly found in neurons. Membrane proteins activate various second messenger and intracellular signaling pathways, which eventually target CREB, promoting transcription and translation of target proteins that change neuronal mechanisms in the long term. The image shows three receptors: G-protein-coupled receptor (GPCR), a calcium channel (such as NMDAR), and a receptor tyrosine kinase channel (TRK). The GPCR acts through a heterotrimeric g-protein to activate adenylate cyclase (AC), increasing intracellular cyclic AMP (cAMP), which acts through phosphorylation cascades and protein kinase A (PKA) to target CREB (Chrivia et al., 1993; Conkright et al., 2003). The calcium channel increases intracellular calcium ions (Ca2+),

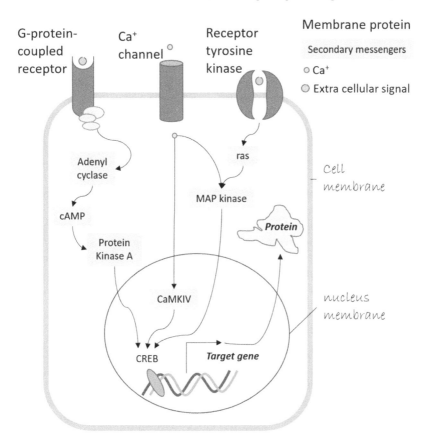

Figure 7.2 CREB cAMP neuron pathway.

which can act through CaMKIV to target CREB. The TRK can act through RAS and MAP kinase to target CREB. CREB promotes transcription and translation of target proteins, and these proteins disperse throughout the neuron to effect long-term changes. CREB is a conserved regulator of long-term memory in a variety of organisms, including humans (Silva, Kogan, Frankland, & Kida, 1998; Yin, Del Vecchio, Zhou, & Tully, 1995).

Several animal models identified CREB-related "memory genes." A microarray study of transgenic mice expressing a constitutively active form of CREB in the hippocampus revealed four potential "memory genes" including *BDNF* (Barco et al., 2005). In vitro stimulation of long-term potentiation in hippocampal slices uncovered 41 "plasticity-associated genes" in the mouse dentate gyrus (Ploski, Park, Ping, Monsey, & Schafe, 2010). In C. elegans, neuronal expression of CREB reduces the long-term memory ability of CREB null worms, and neuronal CREB overexpression increases the duration of long-term memory (Kauffman, Ashraf, Corces-Zimmerman, Landis, & Murphy, 2010). Using a combined approach of memory training with genome-wide transcriptional analysis of *C. elegans* CREB mutants, Lakhina et al. (2015) identified 757 direct and indirect CREB target genes expressed in the basal, resting state, and those induced upon long-term memory training. Many of these identified genes possess mammalian orthologs, providing a unique resource for investigators to explore the roles of these memory genes in higher organisms.

In humans, the only protein with well-characterized prion properties is the prion protein PrP, encoded by the *PRNP* gene on the short arm of chromosome 20. The common methionine/valine *PRNP* polymorphism at codon 129 (M129V) modulates the folding behavior of the protein (Petchanikow et al., 2001; Tahiri-Alaoui, Gill, Disterer, & James, 2004). This polymorphism was found to be associated with long-term memory (LTM) among 354 healthy young subjects (Papassotiropoulos et al., 2005).

Neural schemas not only allow efficient control over decision-making and action, they also enable the perception-cognition-motion processes to anticipate and adjust to unexpected changes in the environment. If matching neural schemas do not exist for the given environmental conditions, corresponding decisions and actions may be slow, inappropriate, or unsuccessful altogether (references).

From cue to action: the perceptual-cognitive sequence

The sequential decision-making process consists of two main systems which consistently interact with each other. The first system is the *perceptual system*, which relies on *fast paced visual cues* occurring within the visual field. The second system consists of *cognitive operations* that process the information gathered by the perceptual system and feeds forward that information through working memory for response selection. The neural schema supervises the performance of the two systems. Neural schemas are also defined by their cyclical nature of taking in information from the perceptual system to guide cognitive processing for motor response selection. The performer must pass several decision junctures when environmental conditions change over the course of these cycles. Each choice made in the decision sequence relates to a general plan stored in LTM. However, consequences may differ if a problem is inappropriately matched to a neural schema. The first decision that must be made relates to the *perceptual system*, whose goal is to direct visual attention to the task-essential cues in the environment. When the perceptually-critical cues are fed forward to the cognitive system, the neural schema allows the system to anticipate upcoming events by utilizing a precomputed estimate of likelihood for consequences, based upon the number of times similar situations have led down attached action paths in the performer's history (Tenenbaum & Lidor, 2005). The final decision of the cycle relates to the timing of the motor response, which is crucial in dynamic environments for actions to be successful. For instance, if a correct decision has been made, but activates actions in the motor system at the wrong time, the result may be system failure.

Anticipation is the most crucial component in the decision-making sequence, because it activates alternative and competing solutions from LTM to help the performer select the most appropriate action response. At this juncture, the motor system activates and remains "on alert" to prepare for possible environmental alterations, to respond swiftly and sufficiently to change.

Biological mechanisms and genetic factors of the perceptual-cognitive sequence

Heritability estimation of cognition approximates 0.50–0.70 percent of the variance, meaning that genetic differences among people account for 0.50–0.70 percent of the variation in performance on tests of cognitive abilities, such as reasoning, memory, processing speed, mental rotation, and knowledge (Bouchard & McGue, 1981). Molecular genetic studies also support the significant role of genetic factors in cognition (Davies et al., 2011). However, uncovering genetic loci underlying cognitive ability is very challenging due to two reasons: (1) the relative heterogeneity in the measurement of the cognitive phenotypes, and (2) the overlapping and the lack of knowledge regarding the biological mechanism which underlies cognitive abilities such as working memory, attention, cognitive flexibility, and impulse control. General cognitive ability (g) has been defined as a latent trait underlying shared variance across multiple subdomains of cognitive performance, psychometrically obtained as the first principal component of several distinct neuropsychological test scores (Johnson, Edmonds, Carlos Moraes, Medeiros Filho, & Tenenbaum, 2007).

There are two complementary approaches aimed at uncovering genetic contributions to multifactorial traits, such as cognition: the *candidate gene (CG) approach* and the *GWAS* approach. CG approach centers on investigating the validity of an "educated guess" about the genetic basis of a trait. This approach involves assessing the association between a particular allele (or set of alleles) of a gene that may be involved in the trait. The selected genes are usually related to the biological mechanisms underlying the trait, and therefore, this approach usually requires a fundamental knowledge of these biologic mechanisms. The GWAS approach can pinpoint genes regardless of whether their function was known before. These studies typically genotype thousands of people for 300,000 to 1 million SNPs. Each approach has its own limitations (A. Korte & Farlow, 2013), and combined methods also exist (Xu & Taylor, 2009).

Genetic factors of cognition uncovered by the GC approach

Cognitive abilities are largely mediated by prefrontal cortex (PFC) function and are modulated by dopaminergic, noradrenergic, serotonergic, and cholinergic input. Therefore, changes in these systems can also have a grave impact on cognitive abilities. Indeed, polymorphisms in genes associated with these neurotransmitters are associated with phenotypic differences in cognitive abilities. The PFC includes several distinct areas that can be grouped to form sub-regions: the medial prefrontal cortex (mPFC) and orbital frontal cortex (OFC) (Groenewegen & Uylings, 2000; Robbins, 2000; Teffer & Semendeferi, 2012). The mPFC and OFC receive input from the dopamine, norepinephrine, serotonin, and acetylcholine neurotransmitter systems and differ slightly in the origin of afferent projections and destination of efferent communication. Theses neurotransmitters can influence the efficiency of neural transmission (Berridge et al., 2006; MacDonald, Nyberg, & Bäckman, 2006).

Based on animal models it was found that the mPFC is responsible for attentional processing and for cognitive flexibility requiring set-shifting, whereas the OFC regulates the cognitive flexibility required for reversal learning and response inhibition (Logue & Gould, 2014).

Polymorphisms in genes associated with dopaminergic systems

Three dopaminergic genes have been associated with executive function (see Figure 2.4 in Chapter 2 for a detailed list of dopaminergic genes): the *COMT* gene, the *DRD2*, and the *DRD4*. COMT is the enzyme that degrades DA in PFC thereby regulating synaptic levels of DA (Malhotra et al., 2002). The Val allele of the Val158Met COMT polymorphism is associated with a high activity state of COMT which increases the rate of DA degradation leading to a lower level of DA in PFC. The Met allele, however, produces COMT with a low activity state, which slows the rate of degradation resulting in higher levels of DA. With the crucial role mPFC DA plays in set-shifting and attention, these genetic-related differences in levels of mPFC DA are associated with different performances in these executive function tasks. In normal adult subjects, met/met-carriers demonstrated superior sustained attention, decreased activity in the anterior cingulate cortex (Blasi et al., 2005; Stefanis et al., 2005), and better performance in cognitive flexibility (Barnett, Jones, Robbins, & Müller, 2007; Wishart et al., 2011) compared to val/val carriers. Although most studies using normal adult subjects detect an advantage of the met allele on sustained attention, there are some conflicting results. For example, Maksimov, Vaht, Murd, Harro, & Bachmann, (2015) reported that val homozygotes showed relatively higher levels of correct target perception with a longer target/mask time interval than with a shorter time interval. The majority of conflicting results regarding the role of *COMT* Val158Met polymorphism on sustained attention come from research using younger and older subjects (Logue & Gould, 2014). Wishart et al. (2011) also identified an interaction between *COMT* Val158Met genotype and the *DRD2* rs1800497 (A1+/-) polymorphism. Individuals carrying the *COMT* Val allele who were homozygous for the T allele of the *DRD2* gene, exhibited significantly reduced cognitive flexibility.

DRD2 receptors are most prominently expressed in the striatum but some are expressed in the PFC as well (Markett, Montag, Walter, Plieger, & Reuter, 2011). The striatal density of DRD2 receptors is determined by a SNP rs1800497. Reduced striatal DRD2 density is found in individuals carrying at least one A1 allele (Ritchie & Noble, 2003). The A1+ genotype has also been associated with improved cognitive flexibility (Markett et al., 2011; Stelzel, Basten, Montag, Reuter, & Fiebach, 2010). Relative to A1+ carriers of the A1 allele exhibited higher striatal density of DRD2, decreased flexibility in a task-switching assay, and increased functional connectivity in dorsal frontostriatal circuits (Stelzel et al., 2010).

Several different polymorphisms of the dopamine D4 receptor have been identified and one in particular, a 48-base pair variable number tandem repeat in exon 3, has variants associated with attentional function (DiMaio, Grizenko, & Joober, 2003). The 7-repeat variant of *DRD4* was shown to be half as potent in its ability to inhibit the synthesis of cyclic adenosine monophosphate (cAMP), thereby decreasing the sensitivity to DA in this variant. In healthy adults, the 7-repeat variant allele was associated with improved cognitive flexibility (Müller et al., 2007), and relatively higher levels of correct target perception with a longer target/mask time interval than with a shorter time interval (Maksimov et al., 2015). In addition, homozygous 7-repeat carriers were more accurate in a go/no-go task compared to homozygous 4-repeat carriers (Krämer et al., 2009).

The dopamine beta-hydroxylase (DBH) enzyme is involved in the conversion of dopamine to norepinephrine. Plasma levels of this enzyme are under genetic control by the *DBH* gene, which is known to have several polymorphisms. One of these polymorphisms, a G-to-A substitution at position 444, exon 2 (G444A) on chromosome 9, affects DBH levels in plasma and cerebrospinal fluid (CSF), with the A allele associated with lower levels of the enzyme (Cubells et al., 2000). Increasing gene dose of the G allele of the DBH gene was associated with increased working memory accuracy at a high memory load (Parasuraman, Greenwood, Kumar, & Fossella, 2005).

DAT1 encodes to dopamine transporter (DAT), which plays a crucial role in determining the duration and amplitude of dopamine action by rapidly recapturing extracellular dopamine into presynaptic terminals after release. The *DAT1* gene (*SLC6A3*) includes 15 exons, with a VNTR polymorphism in the fifteenth exon, a region encoding the transcript's 3′ UTR (Vandenbergh et al., 1992). The 40-bp VNTR element is repeated between 3 and 13 times but occurs with greatest frequency in the 9- and 10-repeat forms. The *DAT1* 10-repeat allele, associated with increased expression of the gene, presumably leads to relatively decreased extra-synaptic striatal dopamine levels, consistent with a human single-photon-emission computed tomography report of increased striatal DAT availability in 9-repeat carriers relative to 10-repeat carriers (Heinz et al., 2000; Jacobsen et al., 2000). During reward anticipation, *DAT1* 9-repeat carriers activated the ventral striatum more than 10-repeat individuals (Dreher, Kohn, Kolachana, Weinberger, & Berman, 2009), likely reflecting lower extra-synaptic striatal dopamine levels in 10-repeat carriers in whom *DAT1* gene expression is greater both in vitro and in vivo (Dreher et al., 2009; Mill, Asherson, Browes, D'Souza, & Craig, 2002).

Polymorphisms in genes associated with noradrenergic neurotransmission

In noradrenergic neurons, the *DBH* gene codes for the enzyme dopamine β-hydroxylase which catalyzes the conversion of DA to NE and plays a critical role in maintaining the balance of DA and NE in the cortex. Polymorphisms in the *DBH* gene are associated with variations in *DBH* activity. Specifically, a C/T SNP at 1021 in the promoter region of the gene accounts for up to 50 percent of the variation in *DBH* activity (Chen et al., 2010; Tang, Anderson, Zabetian, Köhnke, & Cubells, 2005; Zabetian et al., 2001). The T allele, which decreases gene transcription and slows the rate of DA conversion to NE, was associated with poor performance in a sustained attention task (Greene, Bellgrove, Gill, & Robertson, 2009).

Polymorphism in BDNF

BDNF is a secreted protein encoded by the BDNF gene (Jones & Reichardt, 1990; Maisonpierre et al., 1991). BDNF is a member of the "neurotrophin" family of growth factors, which have pivotal roles in the process of neurogenesis (the growing of new neurons from neural stem cells) (Benraiss, Chmielnicki, Lerner, Roh, & Goldman, 2001; Pencea, Bingaman, Wiegand, & Luskin, 2001; Zigova, Pencea, Wiegand, & Luskin, 1998), and support the survival of existing neurons (Acheson et al., 1995; Huang & Reichardt, 2001). In the brain, it is active in the hippocampus, cerebral cortex, and basal forebrain; areas vital to learning, memory, and higher thinking (Yamada & Nabeshima, 2003). BDNF itself is important for LTM (Bekinschtein et al., 2008). BDNF activity is correlated with increased long-term potentiation and neurogenesis, which can be induced by physical activity (Vaynman & Gomez-Pinilla, 2006). In addition to its production and functions in the brain and nervous system, BDNF secreted by contracting skeletal muscle has been found to play a role in muscle repair, regeneration, and differentiation. Therefore, BDNF plays a role in peripheral metabolism, myogenesis, and muscle regeneration (Pedersen, 2013).

Polymorphisms in genes associated with serotonergic system

The 1438 polymorphism in the *5-HT2A* gene has been associated with expression levels of functional 5-HT2A receptors in the cortex. Individuals with the A-1438A allele of the 5-HT2A receptor performed poorer on a go/no-go task than did subjects with the G-1438G allele (Nomura et al., 2006). Although the exact influence of the 1438 polymorphism on the 5-HT2A receptor is unknown, the reduced response inhibition could be due to a decreased expression of 5-HT2A receptors on pyramidal neurons in the cortex. This is consistent with fact that activation of excitatory 5-HT2A receptors in OFC is associated with improved response inhibition.

Multiple studies have demonstrated a link between the serotonin transporter polymorphic region (5-HTTLPR), previously describes in chapters 4 and 5, and cognition. The two variants of the 5-HTTLPR polymorphism, are the short (s) and long (l) alleles, reflecting a variable number of repeats in the polymorphic region of *SLC6A4* (Canli & Lesch, 2007). The s allele is related to lower transcriptional efficiency of the serotonin transporter (Bennett et al., 2002; Glatz, Mössner, Heils, & Lesch, 2003), resulting in lower serotonin transporter function (Lesch et al., 1996). Carriers of the short allele also show a reduction in the density of the serotonin receptor 5-HT1A, which leads to decreased serotonergic transmission (David et al., 2005; Li, Wichems, Heils, Lesch, & Murphy, 2000).

Carriers of the s allele showed (1) enhanced conflict monitoring and updating in working memory (WM) (Strobel et al., 2007), (2) higher WM capacity as indexed by performance in a change detection task (Anderson et al., 2012), (3) intense errors processing (Althaus et al., 2009), (4) higher score in tests of logical reasoning (Madsen et al., 2011), (5) accurate pattern recognition memory and fewer omission errors in a go/no-go task (Roiser, Rogers, Cook, & Sahakian, 2006), (6) greater performance in tests of executive control (Borg et al., 2009; Madsen et al., 2011), (7) accuracy in detection changes during the comparison of two visual images (Paaver et al., 2007), and (8) greater inhibitory motor control (Fallgatter, Jatzke, Bartsch, Hamelbeck, & Lesch, 1999). Overall, performance in various attention-demanding tasks is superior for carriers of the short allele.

A functional genetic variation at the serotonin transporter 30 untranslated region, independent of 5HTTLPR, was associated with errors in reversal learning (Vallender, Lynch, Novak, & Miller, 2009). The polymorphism comprising haplotype (T1970, G1991, and T2327 (T:G:T)) was associated with lower levels of gene expression and monkeys with the T:G:T haplotype made fewer errors in reversal learning than the C:C:C haplotype. If this polymorphism in the serotonin transporter results in decreased reuptake of serotonin, the reversal learning results are consistent with other results showing that increased 5-HT activity in OFC is associated with superior reversal learning.

Polymorphism in a gene associated with cholinergic systems

Cholinergic receptors influence neuronal function in the parietal cortex (Xiang, Huguenard, & Prince, 1998), where they regulate fast synaptic transmission (Alkondon, Pereira, Eisenberg, & Albuquerque, 2000). Although most cholinergic receptors are muscarinic, nicotinic receptors are particularly important (Phillips, McAlonan, Robb, & Brown, 2000). Human cholinergic innervation in the parietal cortex appears to be nicotinic, not muscarinic (Mentis et al., 2001). The *CHRNA4* gene codes for the α4 subunit of the acetylcholine receptors nAChRs. A SNP (rs1044396) has been identified as being involved in a C to T substitution (Steinlein et al., 1997). This SNP is associated with the efficiency of component processes of visuospatial attention (Parasuraman et al., 2005). In an extensive review of the literature, Greenwood, Parasuraman, & Espeseth, (2012) concluded that the T allele is associated with better attention and higher cortical activity.

Genetic factors of cognition uncovered by the GWAS approach

Using this approach, several cognitive GWAS with fewer than 20,000 subjects yielded no genome-wide significant (GWS) effects (Benyamin et al., 2014; Davies et al., 2011; Lencz et al., 2014), while a few GWS loci were identified in larger GWAS of 35,298 (Trampush et al., 2017) and 53,949 (Davies et al., 2015) subjects. The number of the identified cognitive loci is much less than the number of loci that were identified for physiological or anatomical traits such as height (Gudbjartsson et al., 2008; Weedon et al., 2008).

Genome-wide analyses of common SNPs indicate that, over the life course, these SNPs or variants in linkage disequilibrium with these SNPs jointly explain between 26–51 percent of the variance in intelligence (Benyamin et al., 2014; Davies et al., 2011). However, no single polymorphism was reliably associated with variation in intelligence, suggesting that intelligence is highly polygenic, each genetic variant making only a small contribution. These many small effects might be aggregated in networks of functionally linked genes, such as genes in the postsynaptic density and associated complexes (Hill et al., 2014).

Phenotypes implicated in cognitive differences center on the central nervous structures, such as white matter integrity (Lopez et al., 2012; Penke et al., 2012), brain volume (McDaniel, 2005; Stein et al., 2012), and synapse (Hill et al., 2014). The synapse (see Figure 7.3) is a major source of possible genetic variation, since a large number of genes are expressed in the synapse (Schrimpf et al., 2005) and because of direct evidence for the effects of mutations in this system on cognition (Nithianantharajah et al., 2013). A specific component within the synapse is the postsynaptic density (PSD). PSDs are large groups of proteins and cytoskeletal components attached to the postsynaptic membrane of a synapse (Walikonis et al., 2000). Mutations in genes expressed in the PSD have been linked to dozens of neurological and cognitive disorders (Bayés et al., 2011; Collins et al., 2006; Kirov et al., 2012).

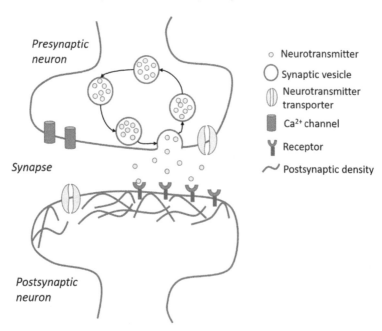

Figure 7.3 The synapse and postsynaptic density.

Scientific evidence suggests that the elaboration of complex learning involved duplication and subsequent divergence of genes in the PSD (Ryan et al., 2013). For example, Hill et al. (2014) tested a network of 1461 genes in the postsynaptic density and associated complexes to test their association with intelligence among 3511 individuals (the Cognitive Ageing Genetics in England and Scotland consortium) phenotyped for general cognitive ability, fluid cognitive ability, crystallized cognitive ability, memory, and speed of processing. The results revealed that genetic variation in the macromolecular machines formed by membrane-associated guanylate kinase (MAGUK) contributes to variation in intelligence.

Recently, Lam et al. (2017) performed a large-scale cognitive GWAS meta-analysis (N = 107,207). They identified 70 independent genomic loci associated with GCA. Results showed significant enrichment for genes causing Mendelian disorders with an intellectual disability phenotype. Competitive pathway analysis implicated the biological processes of neurogenesis and synaptic regulation, as well as the gene targets of two pharmacologic agents: cinnarizine, a T-type calcium channel blocker; and LY97241, a potassium channel inhibitor. Transcriptome-wide and epigenome-wide analysis revealed that the implicated loci were enriched for genes expressed across all brain regions (most strongly in the cerebellum); enrichment was exclusive to genes expressed in neurons, but not oligodendrocytes or astrocytes. Finally, we report genetic correlations between cognitive ability and disparate phenotypes including psychiatric disorders, several autoimmune disorders, longevity, and maternal age at first birth.

Gene-environment consideration in cognition

Gene-environment correlation

Cognition abilities might be subjected to gene-environment correlation, since environmental experiences are themselves heritable (Kendler & Baker, 2007). *Transactional models* posit that these gene-environment correlations are key mechanisms of cognitive development (Tucker-Drob, Briley, & Harden, 2013), and that genetic differences among people matter for cognition because initial genetic differences lead to different environmental experiences. There are two dimensions along which heritability differs: age/development and socioeconomic advantage. People in high-opportunity contexts actively evoke and select positive environmental experiences on the basis of their genetic predispositions; these learning experiences, in turn, reciprocally influence cognition. The net result of this transactional process is increasing genetic influence with increasing age and increasing environmental opportunity (Tucker-Drob et al., 2013).

Exercise as an epigenetic modulator of cognition

Although all neurons carry the same genetic information, they vary in morphology, functions, and response to environment. Such variability results mostly from differences in gene expression (Goldberg, Allis, & Bernstein, 2007;

Jaenisch & Bird, 2003). Epigenetic mechanisms are processes that regulate gene activity (see chapters 1 and 8 for a detailed description). Through these mechanisms, the brain gains high plasticity in response to experience and can integrate and store new information to shape future neuronal and behavioral responses (Stefanelli et al., 2018; Woldemichael, Bohacek, Gapp, & Mansuy, 2014).

The positive actions of exercise on cognition have received abundant support (see Basso & Suzuki, 2017; Browne et al., 2017; R. M. Fernandes et al., 2018; Northey, Cherbuin, Pumpa, Smee, & Rattray, 2018 for review). Several studies showed that exercise regulates the transcription of *BDNF* gene by engaging changes in histone acetylation and DNA methylation (Gomez-Pinilla & Hillman, 2013; Ieraci, Mallei, Musazzi, & Popoli, 2015; Sleiman et al., 2016). It appears that physical exercise activates signaling cascades that trigger a wave of phosphorylation and other post-translational modifications that reach the nucleus, and engage epigenetic mechanisms to alter chromatin conformation and gene expression (J. Fernandes, Arida, & Gomez-Pinilla, 2017). Accumulating scientific evidence in the last few years portrays the capacity of exercise to promote profound alterations in the program of genes and their protein products in the form of epigenomic manifestations. The remarkable capacity of epigenetic mechanisms to regulate synaptic and cognitive plasticity has a fundamental value for the control of neurological and psychological processes. As more studies continue to reveal the details by which exercise influences a varied assortment of gene regulatory mechanisms, it is becoming clear that gene reprogramming is instrumental for transducing the effects of exercise on brain structure and function. Recent developments in the epigenetic field are leading to a paradigm shift in basic and clinical neuroscience to account for how environmental factors can impact long-term brain function (J. Fernandes et al., 2017).

DM and actions under pressure

Under pressure conditions, the perceptual and cognitive systems may shift away from their normal processing modes. A performer can learn and reliably exercise all the instructions and skills given to him/her before engaging in the task, but under extreme conditions (e.g., thoughts and fear of unsuccessful outcomes), his/her performance can suffer badly if the pressures are deemed to be too much to bear (see Chapter 5). It may be the case that affective responses *narrow attention* to the point that relevant perceptual cues are missed, appropriate cognitive responses are not selected, or retrieval of necessary information is blocked (Tenenbaum, 2003). A lack of situational control constrains the cognitive processing system from functioning under normal goal-directed processes, and may develop into interfering thoughts simultaneously and, likely ineffectively, competing for attention (Abernethy, 1993). This results in the failure of the sequential flow of processes between the perceptual, cognitive, and motor systems, and consequences may include delayed response-times, greater response selection errors, or diffuse or non-proficient motor responses. Thus, when pressure is perceived to be debilitating by the performer, otherwise reliable LTM neural schemas may become overwhelmingly ineffective. In contrast, when pressure conditions are perceived as *challenging*, rather than *debilitating*, the perceptual, cognitive, and control systems can function as under optimal conditions, to take in environmental information and select appropriate cognitive responses to enable and plan coordinated motor actions. The interactive effect of these conditions and systems allows the performer to operate at peak performance.

There are substantial individual differences in the cognitive response to stress that are at least partly genetically determined. A variant of the gene encoding the α2-adrenegic receptor (*ADRA2B*), for instance, has been linked to increased emotional memory formation (de Quervain et al., 2007; Rasch et al., 2009), increased amygdala responses to stress (Cousijn et al., 2010), and to a reduced ability to engage the appropriate memory system under stress (Wirz, Wacker, Felten, Reuter, & Schwabe, 2017). This research field is still in its infancy and future studies must address questions related to the actual mechanisms underlying the stress-induced changes in memory (Quaedflieg & Schwabe, 2018).

Neurological foundation of high-level performance

In a summary of research (Tenenbaum et al., 2009) have concluded that high-level performers exhibit quiet activation in non-essential areas of the brain and minimize communication between the thinking and the motor regions which is an indication of neural efficiency. Brain electrical activity maps of novice shooters revealed higher cortical activity (i.e., electroencephalogram (EEG) gamma power) in novice than in expert shooters. High Gamma power is a state which results in greater performance variability and diminished accuracy, which is typically the case with young and/or novice performers. The lower levels of gamma power in the expert reduces neuromotor noise, thus enabling greater consistency of performance. Under psychological stress, experts can reverse to a "noisy neural activation," which usually results in performance decline (see Hatfield, Haufler, Hung, & Spalding, 2004, 2009, for extensive review).

Using the expert-novice paradigm, EEG studies revealed that expert marksmen showed less neural activation in the left temporal region (T3) than in the right homologous region, prior to trigger pulling tasks (Hatfield, Landers, & Ray, 1984). According to the authors these findings indicate that experts suffer less potential interference from left-hemispheric verbal–analytic activity to enable automated motor processes to be managed effectively. Similarly, Haufler, Spalding, Santa Maria and Hatfield, (2000) observed less activation in the frontal, central, temporal, parietal, and occipital regions in expert than novice shooters. The skill difference was of greatest magnitude in the left temporal region and revealed a similar pattern of temporal asymmetry in the experts to that observed earlier by Hatfield et al. (1984). No differences in cortical activation were attributed to skill-level while performing cognitive tasks with which the participants were equally familiar, suggesting that the task-specific EEG differences were attributed to task-specific skills. The findings of the early studies using EEG indicate clearly that excellency in performance of motor task is achieved through maintaining cortical relaxation, while those with "noisy minds" exhibited higher susceptibility to performance decline. These results were also reported in a study where soldiers were required to shoot or inhibit shooting of enemy and friendly soldiers (Kerick, Douglass, & Hatfield, 2004). In addition, the investigators noted a decrease in alpha power as they progressively challenged the study participants with cognitive load (i.e., challenged them with increasing attention demands and decision-making during shooting). Such a negative relationship between demand and alpha power provides a form of concurrent validation for the notion that higher alpha level activation is associated with cortical relaxation.

The relationship between expertise, cortical activation, and order formation in LTM is considered a major challenge. Neurophysiological methods, like EEG-coherence measures (Deeny, Hillman, Janelle, & Hatfield, 2003), and methods for measuring the structure of mental representation (Schack, 1999) are required to gain more information about the link between neural activation and motor performance quality. The simultaneous neurophysiologic findings in Schack's (1999) research on gymnasts indicated that experts' cognitive activation of movement representations is accompanied by activation of several cortical areas. These patterns of activation provide a glimpse of the network of neurophysiologic areas with a high mental economy and a high stability.

Summary

It is very well established that perception and cognition are fundamental psychological structures and procedures in sport performance. Moreover, it is very well established that cognition relies on neurological circuits and anatomical structure, meaning that the biological mechanisms of cognition are very well documented and studied. Yet, the connection between genetic factors (based on biological mechanisms) and the cognition-aspects of sport performance has rarely been studied.

References

Abernethy, B. (1993). Attention. In R. N. Singer, M. Murphey, & L. K. Tennant (Eds.), *Handbook of research in sport psychology* (pp. 127–70). New York, NY: Macmillan.

Acheson, A., Conover, J. C., Fandl, J. P., DeChiara, T. M., Russell, M., Thadani, A., … Lindsay, R. M. (1995). A BDNF autocrine loop in adult sensory neurons prevents cell death. *Nature, 374*(6521), 450–3. https://doi.org/10.1038/374450a0

Alkondon, M., Pereira, E. F., Eisenberg, H. M., & Albuquerque, E. X. (2000). Nicotinic receptor activation in human cerebral cortical interneurons: A mechanism for inhibition and disinhibition of neuronal networks. *The Journal of Neuroscience: The Official Journal of the Society for Neuroscience, 20*(1), 66–75. Retrieved from www.ncbi.nlm.nih.gov/pubmed/10627582

Althaus, M., Groen, Y., Wijers, A. A., Mulder, L. J. M., Minderaa, R. B., Kema, I. P., … Hoekstra, P. J. (2009). Differential effects of 5-HTTLPR and DRD2/ANKK1 polymorphisms on electrocortical measures of error and feedback processing in children. *Clinical Neurophysiology, 120*(1), 93–107. https://doi.org/10.1016/j.clinph.2008.10.012

Anderson, D. E., Bell, T. A., & Awh, E. (2012). Polymorphisms in the 5-HTTLPR gene mediate storage capacity of visual working memory. *Journal of Cognitive Neuroscience, 24*(5), 1069–76. https://doi.org/10.1162/jocn_a_00207

Barco, A., Patterson, S., Alarcon, J. M., Gromova, P., Mata-Roig, M., Morozov, A., … Kandel, E. R. (2005). Gene expression profiling of facilitated L-LTP in VP16-CREB mice reveals that BDNF is critical for the maintenance of LTP and its synaptic capture. *Neuron, 48*(1), 123–37. https://doi.org/10.1016/j.neuron.2005.09.005

Barnett, J. H., Jones, P. B., Robbins, T. W., & Müller, U. (2007). Effects of the catechol-O-methyltransferase Val158Met polymorphism on executive function: A meta-analysis of the Wisconsin Card Sort Test in schizophrenia and healthy controls. *Molecular Psychiatry, 12*(5), 502–9. https://doi.org/10.1038/sj.mp. 4001973

Basso, J. C., & Suzuki, W. A. (2017). The effects of acute exercise on mood, cognition, neurophysiology, and neurochemical pathways: A review. *Brain Plasticity, 2*(2), 127–52. https://doi.org/10.3233/BPL-160040

Bayés, À., van de Lagemaat, L. N., Collins, M. O., Croning, M. D. R., Whittle, I. R., Choudhary, J. S., & Grant, S. G. N. (2011). Characterization of the proteome, diseases and evolution of the human postsynaptic density. *Nature Neuroscience, 14*(1), 19–21. https://doi.org/10.1038/nn.2719

Bekinschtein, P., Cammarota, M., Katche, C., Slipczuk, L., Rossato, J. I., Goldin, A., … Medina, J. H. (2008). BDNF is essential to promote persistence of long-term memory storage. *Proceedings of the National Academy of Sciences of the United States of America, 105*(7), 2711–6. https://doi.org/10.1073/pnas.0711863105

Bennett, A. J., Lesch, K. P., Heils, A., Long, J. C., Lorenz, J. G., Shoaf, S. E., … Higley, J. D. (2002). Early experience and serotonin transporter gene variation interact to influence primate CNS function. *Molecular Psychiatry, 7*(1), 118–22. https://doi.org/10.1038/sj/mp/4000949

Benraiss, A., Chmielnicki, E., Lerner, K., Roh, D., & Goldman, S. A. (2001). Adenoviral brain-derived neurotrophic factor induces both neostriatal and olfactory neuronal recruitment from endogenous progenitor cells in the adult forebrain. *The Journal of Neuroscience: The Official Journal of the Society for Neuroscience, 21*(17), 6718–31. Retrieved from www.ncbi.nlm.nih.gov/pubmed/11517261

Benyamin, B., Pourcain, B. St., Davis, O. S., Davies, G., Hansell, N. K., Brion, M.-J., … Visscher, P. M. (2014). Childhood intelligence is heritable, highly polygenic and associated with FNBP1L. *Molecular Psychiatry, 19*(2), 253–8. https://doi.org/10.1038/mp. 2012.184

Berridge, C. W., Devilbiss, D. M., Andrzejewski, M. E., Arnsten, A. F. T., Kelley, A. E., Schmeichel, B., … Spencer, R. C. (2006). Methylphenidate preferentially increases catecholamine neurotransmission within the prefrontal cortex at low doses that enhance cognitive function. *Biological Psychiatry, 60*(10), 1111–20. https://doi.org/10.1016/j.biopsych.2006.04.022

Blasi, G., Mattay, V. S., Bertolino, A., Elvevåg, B., Callicott, J. H., Das, S., … Weinberger, D. R. (2005). Effect of catechol-o-methyltransferase val158met genotype on attentional control. *Journal of Neuroscience, 25*(20), 5038–45. https://doi.org/10.1523/JNEUROSCI.0476-05.2005

Boomsma, D. I. (1993). Current status and future prospects in twin studies of the development of cognitive abilities, infancy to old age. In T. J. Bouchard & P. Propping (Eds.), *Twins as a tool of behavioral genetics* (pp. 67–82). Chichester, England: Wiley and Sons.

Borg, J., Henningsson, S., Saijo, T., Inoue, M., Bah, J., Westberg, L., … Farde, L. (2009). Serotonin transporter genotype is associated with cognitive performance but not regional 5-HT1A receptor binding in humans. *The International Journal of Neuropsychopharmacology, 12*(6), 783–92. https://doi.org/10.1017/S1461145708009759

Bouchard, T. J., & McGue, M. (1981). Familial studies of intelligence: A review. *Science,* *212*(4498), 1055–9. Retrieved from www.ncbi.nlm.nih.gov/pubmed/7195071

Browne, S. E., Flynn, M. J., O'Neill, B. V., Howatson, G., Bell, P. G., & Haskell-Ramsay, C. F. (2017). Effects of acute high-intensity exercise on cognitive performance in trained individuals: A systematic review. *Progress in Brain Research, 234,* 161–87. https://doi.org/10.1016/BS.PBR.2017.06.003

Canli, T., & Lesch, K.-P. (2007). Long story short: The serotonin transporter in emotion regulation and social cognition. *Nature Neuroscience, 10*(9), 1103–9. https://doi.org/10.1038/nn1964

Chen, Y., Wen, G., Rao, F., Zhang, K., Wang, L., Rodriguez-Flores, J. L., … O'Connor, D. T. (2010). Human dopamine beta-hydroxylase (DBH) regulatory polymorphism that influences enzymatic activity, autonomic function, and blood pressure. *Journal of Hypertension, 28*(1), 76–86. https://doi.org/10.1097/HJH.0b013e328332bc87

Chrivia, J. C., Kwok, R. P. S., Lamb, N., Hagiwara, M., Montminy, M. R., & Goodman, R. H. (1993). Phosphorylated CREB binds specifically to the nuclear protein CBP. *Nature, 365*(6449), 855–9. https://doi.org/10.1038/365855a0

Collins, M. O., Husi, H., Yu, L., Brandon, J. M., Anderson, C. N. G., Blackstock, W. P., … Grant, S. G. N. (2006). Molecular characterization and comparison of the components and multiprotein complexes in the postsynaptic proteome. *Journal of Neurochemistry, 97*(Suppl. 1), S16–23. https://doi.org/10.1111/j.1471-4159.2005.03507.x

Conkright, M. D., Canettieri, G., Screaton, R., Guzman, E., Miraglia, L., Hogenesch, J. B., & Montminy, M. (2003). TORCs: Transducers of regulated CREB activity. *Molecular Cell, 12*(2), 413–23. Retrieved from www.ncbi.nlm.nih.gov/pubmed/ 14536081

Cousijn, H., Rijpkema, M., Qin, S., van Marle, H. J. F., Franke, B., Hermans, E. J., … Fernandez, G. (2010). Acute stress modulates genotype effects on amygdala processing in humans. *Proceedings of the National Academy of Sciences, 107*(21), 9867–72. https://doi.org/10.1073/pnas.1003514107

Cubells, J. F., Kranzler, H. R., McCance-Katz, E., Anderson, G. M., Malison, R. T., Price, L. H., & Gelernter, J. (2000). A haplotype at the DBH locus, associated with low plasma dopamine beta-hydroxylase activity, also associates with cocaine-induced paranoia. *Molecular Psychiatry, 5*(1), 56–63. Retrieved from www.ncbi.nlm.nih.gov/ pubmed/10673769

David, S. P., Murthy, N. V., Rabiner, E. A., Munafò, M. R., Johnstone, E. C., Jacob, R., … Grasby, P. M. (2005). A functional genetic variation of the serotonin (5-ht) transporter affects 5-HT1A receptor binding in humans. *Journal of Neuroscience, 25*(10), 2586–90. https://doi.org/10.1523/JNEUROSCI.3769-04.2005

Davies, G., Armstrong, N., Bis, J. C., Bressler, J., Chouraki, V., Giddaluru, S., … Deary, I. J. (2015). Genetic contributions to variation in general cognitive function: A meta-analysis of genome-wide association studies in the charge consortium (n=53 949). *Molecular Psychiatry, 20*(2), 183–92. https://doi.org/10.1038/mp. 2014.188

Davies, G., Tenesa, A., Payton, A., Yang, J., Harris, S. E., Liewald, D., … Deary, I. J. (2011). Genome-wide association studies establish that human intelligence is highly heritable and polygenic. *Molecular Psychiatry, 16*(10), 996–1005. https://doi.org/10.1038/mp. 2011.85

de Geus, E. J., Wright, M. J., Martin, N. G., & Boomsma, D. I. (2001). Genetics of brain function and cognition. *Behavior Genetics, 31*(6), 489–95. Retrieved from www.ncbi.nlm.nih.gov/pubmed/11838528

de Quervain, D. J.-F., Kolassa, I.-T., Ertl, V., Onyut, P. L., Neuner, F., Elbert, T., & Papassotiropoulos, A. (2007). A deletion variant of the alpha2b-adrenoceptor is related to emotional memory in Europeans and Africans. *Nature Neuroscience, 10*(9), 1137–9. https://doi.org/10.1038/nn1945

Deeny, S. P., Hillman, C. H., Janelle, C. M., & Hatfield, B. D. (2003). Cortico-cortical communication and superior performance in skilled marksmen: An EEG coherence analysis. *Journal of Sport and Exercise Psychology, 25*(2), 188–204. https://doi.org/10.1123/jsep.25.2.188

Devlin, B., Daniels, M., & Roeder, K. (1997). The heritability of IQ. *Nature, 388*(6641), 468–71. https://doi.org/10.1038/41319

DiMaio, S., Grizenko, N., & Joober, R. (2003). Dopamine genes and attention-deficit hyperactivity disorder: A review. *Journal of Psychiatry and Neuroscience: JPN, 28*(1), 27–38. Retrieved from www.ncbi.nlm.nih.gov/pubmed/12587848

Dreher, J. C., Kohn, P., Kolachana, B., Weinberger, D. R., & Berman, K. F. (2009). Variation in dopamine genes influences responsivity of the human reward system. *Proceedings of the National Academy of Sciences of the United States of America, 106*(2), 617–22.

Ericsson, K. A., & Kintsch, W. (1995). Long-term working memory. *Psychological Review, 102*(2), 211–45. Retrieved from www.ncbi.nlm.nih.gov/pubmed/7740089

Fallgatter, A. J., Jatzke, S., Bartsch, A. J., Hamelbeck, B., & Lesch, K. P. (1999). Serotonin transporter promoter polymorphism influences topography of inhibitory motor control. *The International Journal of Neuropsychopharmacology, 2*(Suppl. 2), S1461145799001455. https://doi.org/10.1017/S1461145799001455

Fernandes, J., Arida, R. M., & Gomez-Pinilla, F. (2017). Physical exercise as an epigenetic modulator of brain plasticity and cognition. *Neuroscience and Biobehavioral Reviews, 80*, 443–56. https://doi.org/10.1016/j.neubiorev.2017.06.012

Fernandes, R. M., Correa, M. G., Dos Santos, M. A. R., Almeida, A. P. C. P. S. C., Fagundes, N. C. F., Maia, L. C., & Lima, R. R. (2018). The effects of moderate physical exercise on adult cognition: A systematic review. *Frontiers in Physiology, 9*, 667. https://doi.org/10.3389/fphys.2018.00667

Flint, J. (1999). The genetic basis of cognition. *Brain: A Journal of Neurology, 122*(Pt. 11), 2015–32. Retrieved from www.ncbi.nlm.nih.gov/pubmed/10545388

Glatz, K., Mössner, R., Heils, A., & Lesch, K. P. (2003). Glucocorticoid-regulated human serotonin transporter (5-HTT) expression is modulated by the 5-HTT gene-promotor-linked polymorphic region. *Journal of Neurochemistry, 86*(5), 1072–8. Retrieved from www.ncbi.nlm.nih.gov/pubmed/12911615

Goldberg, A. D., Allis, C. D., & Bernstein, E. (2007). Epigenetics: A landscape takes shape. *Cell, 128*(4), 635–8. https://doi.org/10.1016/j.cell.2007.02.006

Gomez-Pinilla, F., & Hillman, C. (2013). The influence of exercise on cognitive abilities. *Comprehensive Physiology, 3*(1), 403–28. https://doi.org/10.1002/cphy.c110063

Greene, C. M., Bellgrove, M. A., Gill, M., & Robertson, I. H. (2009). Noradrenergic genotype predicts lapses in sustained attention. *Neuropsychologia, 47*(2), 591–4. https://doi.org/10.1016/j.neuropsychologia.2008.10.003

Greenwood, P. M., Parasuraman, R., & Espeseth, T. (2012). A cognitive phenotype for a polymorphism in the nicotinic receptor gene CHRNA4. *Neuroscience and Biobehavioral Reviews, 36*(4), 1331–41. https://doi.org/10.1016/j.neubiorev.2012.02.010

Groenewegen, H. J., & Uylings, H. B. M. (2000). The prefrontal cortex and the integration of sensory, limbic and autonomic information. *Progress in Brain Research, 126*, 3–28. https://doi.org/10.1016/S0079-6123(00)26003-2

Gudbjartsson, D. F., Walters, G. B., Thorleifsson, G., Stefansson, H., Halldorsson, B. V., Zusmanovich, P., … Stefansson, K. (2008). Many sequence variants affecting diversity of adult human height. *Nature Genetics, 40*(5), 609–15. https://doi.org/10.1038/ng.122

Hatfield, B. D., Haufler, A. J., Hung, T.-M., & Spalding, T. W. (2004). Electroencephalographic studies of skilled psychomotor performance. *Journal of Clinical Neurophysiology: Official Publication of the American Electroencephalographic Society, 21*(3), 144–56. Retrieved from www.ncbi.nlm.nih.gov/pubmed/15375345

Hatfield, B. D., Landers, D. M., & Ray, W. J. (1984). Cognitive processes during self-paced motor performance: An electroencephalographic profile of skilled marksmen. *Journal of Sport Psychology, 6*(1), 42–59. https://doi.org/10.1123/jsp.6.1.42

Haufler, A. J., Spalding, T. W., Santa Maria, D. L., & Hatfield, B. D. (2000). Neuro-cognitive activity during a self-paced visuospatial task: Comparative EEG profiles in marksmen and novice shooters. *Biological Psychology, 53*(2–3), 131–60. Retrieved from www.ncbi.nlm.nih.gov/pubmed/10967230

Heinz, A., Goldman, D., Jones, D. W., Palmour, R., Hommer, D., Gorey, J. G., ... Weinberger, D. R. (2000). Genotype influences in vivo dopamine transporter availability in human striatum. *Neuropsychopharmacology, 22*, 133–9.

Hill, W. D., Davies, G., van de Lagemaat, L. N., Christoforou, A., Marioni, R. E., Fernandes, C. P. D., ... Deary, I. J. (2014). Human cognitive ability is influenced by genetic variation in components of postsynaptic signalling complexes assembled by NMDA receptors and MAGUK proteins. *Translational Psychiatry, 4*(1), e341–e341. https://doi.org/10.1038/tp. 2013.114

Huang, E. J., & Reichardt, L. F. (2001). Neurotrophins: Roles in neuronal development and function. *Annual Review of Neuroscience, 24*, 677–736. https://doi.org/10.1146/annurev.neuro.24.1.677

Ieraci, A., Mallei, A., Musazzi, L., & Popoli, M. (2015). Physical exercise and acute restraint stress differentially modulate hippocampal brain-derived neurotrophic factor transcripts and epigenetic mechanisms in mice. *Hippocampus, 25*(11), 1380–92. https://doi.org/10.1002/hipo.22458

Jacobsen, L., Staley, L., Zoghbi, S., Seibyl, J., Kosten, T., & Innis, R. (2000). Prediction of dopamine transporter binding availability by genotype: A preliminary report. *American Journal of Psychiatry, 157*, 1700–3.

Jaenisch, R., & Bird, A. (2003). Epigenetic regulation of gene expression: How the genome integrates intrinsic and environmental signals. *Nature Genetics, 33*(Suppl. 3), S245–54. https://doi.org/10.1038/ng1089

Johnson, M. B., Edmonds, W. A., Carlos Moraes, L., Medeiros Filho, E. S., & Tenenbaum, G. (2007). Linking affect and performance of an international level archer incorporating an idiosyncratic probabilistic method. *Psychology of Sport and Exercise, 8*(3), 317–35. https://doi.org/10.1016/j.psychsport.2006.05.004

Jones, K. R., & Reichardt, L. F. (1990). Molecular cloning of a human gene that is a member of the nerve growth factor family. *Proceedings of the National Academy of Sciences of the United States of America, 87*(20), 8060–4. Retrieved from www.pubmedcentral.nih.gov/articlerender.fcgi?artid=54892&tool=pmcentrez&rendertype=abstract

Kandel, E. R. (2001). The molecular biology of memory storage: A dialogue between genes and synapses. *Science, 294*(5544), 1030–8. https://doi.org/10.1126/science.1067020

Kandel, E. R., Dudai, Y., & Mayford, M. R. (2014). The molecular and systems biology of memory. *Cell, 157*(1), 163–86. https://doi.org/10.1016/j.cell.2014.03.001

Kauffman, A. L., Ashraf, J. M., Corces-Zimmerman, M. R., Landis, J. N., & Murphy, C. T. (2010). Insulin signaling and dietary restriction differentially influence the decline of learning and memory with age. *PloS Biology, 8*(5), e1000372. https://doi.org/10.1371/journal.pbio.1000372

Kendler, K. S., & Baker, J. H. (2007). Genetic influences on measures of the environment: A systematic review. *Psychological Medicine, 37*(5), 615. https://doi.org/10.1017/S0033291706009524

Kerick, S. E., Douglass, L. W., & Hatfield, B. D. (2004). Cerebral cortical adaptations associated with visuomotor practice. *Medicine and Science in Sports and Exercise, 36*(1), 118–29. https://doi.org/10.1249/01.MSS.0000106176.31784.D4

Kirov, G., Pocklington, A. J., Holmans, P., Ivanov, D., Ikeda, M., Ruderfer, D., … Owen, M. J. (2012). De novo CNV analysis implicates specific abnormalities of postsynaptic signalling complexes in the pathogenesis of schizophrenia. *Molecular Psychiatry, 17*(2), 142–53. https://doi.org/10.1038/mp. 2011.154

Korte, A., & Farlow, A. (2013). The advantages and limitations of trait analysis with GWAS: A review. *Plant Methods, 9*(1), 29. https://doi.org/10.1186/1746-4811-9-29

Korte, M., & Schmitz, D. (2016). Cellular and system biology of memory: Timing, molecules, and beyond. *Physiological Reviews, 96*(2), 647–93. https://doi.org/10.1152/physrev.00010.2015

Krämer, U. M., Rojo, N., Schüle, R., Cunillera, T., Schöls, L., Marco-Pallarés, J., … Münte, T. F. (2009). ADHD candidate gene (DRD4 exon III) affects inhibitory control in a healthy sample. *BMC Neuroscience, 10*(1), 150. https://doi.org/10.1186/1471-2202-10-150

Lakhina, V., Arey, R. N., Kaletsky, R., Kauffman, A., Stein, G., Keyes, W., … Murphy, C. T. (2015). Genome-wide functional analysis of CREB/long-term memory-dependent transcription reveals distinct basal and memory gene expression programs. *Neuron, 85*(2), 330–45. https://doi.org/10.1016/j.neuron.2014.12.029

Lam, M., Trampush, J. W., Yu, J., Knowles, E., Davies, G., Liewald, D. C., … Lencz, T. (2017). Large-scale cognitive GWAS meta-analysis reveals tissue-specific neural expression and potential nootropic drug targets. *Cell Reports, 21*(9), 2597–613. https://doi.org/10.1016/j.celrep. 2017.11.028

Lencz, T., Knowles, E., Davies, G., Guha, S., Liewald, D. C., Starr, J. M., … Malhotra, A. K. (2014). Molecular genetic evidence for overlap between general cognitive ability and risk for schizophrenia: A report from the Cognitive Genomics consorTium (COGENT). *Molecular Psychiatry, 19*(2), 168–74. https://doi.org/10.1038/mp. 2013.166

Lesch, K. P., Bengel, D., Heils, A., Sabol, S. Z., Greenberg, B. D., Petri, S., … Murphy, D. L. (1996). Association of anxiety-related traits with a polymorphism in the serotonin transporter gene regulatory region. *Science, 274*(5292), 1527–31. Retrieved from www.ncbi.nlm.nih.gov/pubmed/8929413

Li, Q., Wichems, C., Heils, A., Lesch, K. P., & Murphy, D. L. (2000). Reduction in the density and expression, but not G-protein coupling, of serotonin receptors (5-HT1A) in 5-HT transporter knock-out mice: Gender and brain region differences. *The Journal of Neuroscience: The Official Journal of the Society for Neuroscience, 20*(21), 7888–95. Retrieved from www.ncbi.nlm.nih.gov/pubmed/11050108

Logue, S. F., & Gould, T. J. (2014). The neural and genetic basis of executive function: Attention, cognitive flexibility, and response inhibition. *Pharmacology, Biochemistry, and Behavior, 123*, 45–54. https://doi.org/10.1016/j.pbb.2013.08.007

Lopez, L. M., Bastin, M. E., Maniega, S. M., Penke, L., Davies, G., Christoforou, A., … Deary, I. J. (2012). A genome-wide search for genetic influences and biological pathways related to the brain's white matter integrity. *Neurobiology of Aging, 33*(8), 1847. e1–14. https://doi.org/10.1016/j.neurobiolaging.2012.02.003

MacDonald, S. W. S., Nyberg, L., & Bäckman, L. (2006). Intra-individual variability in behavior: Links to brain structure, neurotransmission and neuronal activity. *Trends in Neurosciences, 29*(8), 474–80. https://doi.org/10.1016/j.tins.2006.06.011

Madsen, K., Erritzoe, D., Mortensen, E. L., Gade, A., Madsen, J., Baaré, W., … Hassel-balch, S. G. (2011). Cognitive function is related to fronto-striatal serotonin transporter levels – A brain PET study in young healthy subjects. *Psychopharmacology, 213*(2–3), 573–81. https://doi.org/10.1007/s00213-010-1926-4

Maisonpierre, P. C., Le Beau, M. M., Espinosa, R., Ip, N. Y., Belluscio, L., de la Monte, S. M., … Yancopoulos, G. D. (1991). Human and rat brain-derived neurotrophic factor and neurotrophin-3: Gene structures, distributions, and chromosomal localizations. *Genomics, 10*(3), 558–68. Retrieved from www.ncbi.nlm.nih.gov/pubmed/1889806

Maksimov, M., Vaht, M., Murd, C., Harro, J., & Bachmann, T. (2015). Brain dopaminergic system related genetic variability interacts with target/mask timing in metacontrast masking. *Neuropsychologia, 71*, 112–18. https://doi.org/10.1016/J.NEUROPSYCHO LOGIA.2015.03.022

Malhotra, A. K., Kestler, L. J., Mazzanti, C., Bates, J. A., Goldberg, T., & Goldman, D. (2002). A functional polymorphism in the COMT gene and performance on a test of prefrontal cognition. *American Journal of Psychiatry, 159*(4), 652–4. https://doi. org/10.1176/appi.ajp. 159.4.652

Markett, S., Montag, C., Walter, N. T., Plieger, T., & Reuter, M. (2011). On the molecular genetics of flexibility: The case of task-switching, inhibitory control and genetic variants. *Cognitive, Affective, and Behavioral Neuroscience, 11*(4), 644–51. https://doi. org/10.3758/s13415-011-0058-6

Martin, S. J., Grimwood, P. D., & Morris, R. G. (2000). Synaptic plasticity and memory: An evaluation of the hypothesis. *Annual Review of Neuroscience, 23*(1), 649–711. https://doi.org/10.1146/annurev.neuro.23.1.649

Mayr, B., & Montminy, M. (2001). Transcriptional regulation by the phosphorylation-dependent factor CREB. *Nature Reviews Molecular Cell Biology, 2*(8), 599–609. https://doi.org/10.1038/35085068

McClearn, G. E., Johansson, B., Berg, S., Pedersen, N. L., Ahern, F., Petrill, S. A., & Plomin, R. (1997). Substantial genetic influence on cognitive abilities in twins 80 or more years old. *Science, 276*(5318), 1560–3. Retrieved from www.ncbi.nlm.nih.gov/ pubmed/9171059

McDaniel, M. A. (2005). Big-brained people are smarter: A meta-analysis of the relationship between in vivo brain volume and intelligence. *Intelligence, 33*(4), 337–46. https:// doi.org/10.1016/J.INTELL.2004.11.005

Mentis, M., Sunderland, T., Lai, J., Connolly, C., Krasuski, J., Levine, B., … Rapoport, S. I. (2001). Muscarinic versus nicotinic modulation of a visual task: A pet study using drug probes. *Neuropsychopharmacology, 25*(4), 555–64. https://doi.org/10.1016/ S0893-133X(01)00264-0

Mill, J., Asherson, P., Browes, C., D'Souza, U., & Craig, I. (2002). Expression of the dopamine transporter gene is regulated by the 3' UTR VNTR: Evidence from brain and lymphocytes using quantitative RT-PCR. *American Journal of Medical Genetics, 114*(8), 975–9.

Müller, J., Dreisbach, G., Brocke, B., Lesch, K.-P., Strobel, A., & Goschke, T. (2007). Dopamine and cognitive control: The influence of spontaneous eyeblink rate, DRD4 exon III polymorphism and gender on flexibility in set-shifting. *Brain Research, 1131*(1), 155–62. https://doi.org/10.1016/j.brainres.2006.11.002

Nithianantharajah, J., Komiyama, N. H., McKechanie, A., Johnstone, M., Blackwood, D. H., St Clair, D., … Grant, S. G. N. (2013). Synaptic scaffold evolution generated components of vertebrate cognitive complexity. *Nature Neuroscience, 16*(1), 16–24. https:// doi.org/10.1038/nn.3276

Nomura, M., Kusumi, I., Kaneko, M., Masui, T., Daiguji, M., Ueno, T., … Nomura, Y. (2006). Involvement of a polymorphism in the 5-HT2A receptor gene in impulsive behavior. *Psychopharmacology, 187*(1), 30–5. https://doi.org/10.1007/s00213-006-0398-z

Northey, J. M., Cherbuin, N., Pumpa, K. L., Smee, D. J., & Rattray, B. (2018). Exercise interventions for cognitive function in adults older than 50: A systematic review with meta-analysis. *British Journal of Sports Medicine, 52*(3), 154–60. https://doi. org/10.1136/bjsports-2016-096587

Paaver, M., Nordquist, N., Parik, J., Harro, M., Oreland, L., & Harro, J. (2007). Platelet MAO activity and the 5-HTT gene promoter polymorphism are associated with impulsivity and cognitive style in visual information processing. *Psychopharmacology, 194*(4), 545–54. https://doi.org/10.1007/s00213-007-0867-z

Papassotiropoulos, A., Wollmer, M. A., Aguzzi, A., Hock, C., Nitsch, R. M., & de Quervain, D. J.-F. (2005). The prion gene is associated with human long-term memory. *Human Molecular Genetics, 14*(15), 2241–6. https://doi.org/10.1093/hmg/ddi228

Parasuraman, R., Greenwood, P. M., Kumar, R., & Fossella, J. (2005). Beyond heritability: Neurotransmitter genes differentially modulate visuospatial attention and working memory. *Psychological Science, 16*(3), 200–7. https://doi.org/10.1111/ j.0956-7976.2005.00804.x

Pedersen, B. K. (2013). Muscle as a secretory organ. *Comprehensive Physiology, 3*(3), 1337–62. https://doi.org/10.1002/cphy.c120033

Pencea, V., Bingaman, K. D., Wiegand, S. J., & Luskin, M. B. (2001). Infusion of brain-derived neurotrophic factor into the lateral ventricle of the adult rat leads to new neurons in the parenchyma of the striatum, septum, thalamus, and hypothalamus. *The Journal of Neuroscience: The Official Journal of the Society for Neuroscience, 21*(17), 6706–17. Retrieved from www.ncbi.nlm.nih.gov/pubmed/11517260

Penke, L., Maniega, S. M., Bastin, M. E., Valdés Hernández, M. C., Murray, C., Royle, N. A., … Deary, I. J. (2012). Brain white matter tract integrity as a neural foundation for general intelligence. *Molecular Psychiatry, 17*(10), 1026–30. https://doi.org/ 10.1038/mp. 2012.66

Petchanikow, C., Saborio, G. P., Anderes, L., Frossard, M. J., Olmedo, M. I., & Soto, C. (2001). Biochemical and structural studies of the prion protein polymorphism. *FEBS Letters, 509*(3), 451–6. Retrieved from www.ncbi.nlm.nih.gov/pubmed/11749972

Phillips, J. M., McAlonan, K., Robb, W. G., & Brown, V. J. (2000). Cholinergic neurotransmission influences covert orientation of visuospatial attention in the rat. *Psychopharmacology, 150*(1), 112–6. Retrieved from www.ncbi.nlm.nih.gov/pubmed/ 10867983

Plomin, R. (1999). Genetics and general cognitive ability. *Nature, 402*(Suppl. 6761), C25–9. https://doi.org/10.1038/35011520

Ploski, J. E., Park, K. W., Ping, J., Monsey, M. S., & Schafe, G. E. (2010). Identification of plasticity-associated genes regulated by Pavlovian fear conditioning in the lateral amygdala. *Journal of Neurochemistry, 112*(3), 636–50. https://doi.org/10.1111/ j.1471-4159.2009.06491.x

Quaedflieg, C. W. E. M., & Schwabe, L. (2018). Memory dynamics under stress. *Memory, 26*(3), 364–76. https://doi.org/10.1080/09658211.2017.1338299

Rasch, B., Spalek, K., Buholzer, S., Luechinger, R., Boesiger, P., Papassotiropoulos, A., & de Quervain, D. J.-F. (2009). A genetic variation of the noradrenergic system is related to differential amygdala activation during encoding of emotional memories. *Proceedings of the National Academy of Sciences of the United States of America, 106*(45), 19191–6. https://doi.org/10.1073/pnas.0907425106

Ritchie, T., & Noble, E. P. (2003). Association of seven polymorphisms of the D2 dopamine receptor gene with brain receptor-binding characteristics. *Neurochemical Research, 28*(1), 73–82. Retrieved from www.ncbi.nlm.nih.gov/pubmed/12587665

Robbins, T. W. (2000). From arousal to cognition: The integrative position of the prefrontal cortex. *Progress in Brain Research, 126*, 469–83. https://doi.org/10.1016/ S0079-6123(00)26030-5

Roiser, J. P., Rogers, R. D., Cook, L. J., & Sahakian, B. J. (2006). The effect of polymorphism at the serotonin transporter gene on decision-making, memory and executive function in ecstasy users and controls. *Psychopharmacology, 188*(2), 213–27. https:// doi.org/10.1007/s00213-006-0495-z

Ryan, T. J., Kopanitsa, M. V., Indersmitten, T., Nithianantharajah, J., Afinowi, N. O., Pettit, C., … Komiyama, N. H. (2013). Evolution of GluN2A/B cytoplasmic domains diversified vertebrate synaptic plasticity and behavior. *Nature Neuroscience, 16*(1), 25–32. https://doi.org/10.1038/nn.3277

Schack, T. (1999). Dynamic topographic spectral analysis of cognitive processes. In C. Uhl (Ed.), *Analysis of neuro-physiological brain functioning.* New York, NY: Academic Press.

Schack, T., & Tenenbaum, G. (2004). The cognitive architecture of complex movement. [Special issue part II: The construction of action-new perspectives in movement science]. *International Journal of Sport and Exercise Psychology, 2,* 403–38.

Schrimpf, S. P., Meskenaite, V., Brunner, E., Rutishauser, D., Walther, P., Eng, J., … Sonderegger, P. (2005). Proteomic analysis of synaptosomes using isotope-coded affinity tags and mass spectrometry. *Proteomics, 5*(10), 2531–41. https://doi.org/10.1002/pmic.200401198

Si, K., Giustetto, M., Etkin, A., Hsu, R., Janisiewicz, A. M., Miniaci, M. C., … Kandel, E. R. (2003). A neuronal isoform of CPEB regulates local protein synthesis and stabilizes synapse-specific long-term facilitation in aplysia. *Cell, 115*(7), 893–904. Retrieved from www.ncbi.nlm.nih.gov/pubmed/14697206

Silva, A. J., Kogan, J. H., Frankland, P. W., & Kida, S. (1998). Creb and memory. *Annual Review of Neuroscience, 21*(1), 127–48. https://doi.org/10.1146/annurev.neuro.21.1.127

Sleiman, S. F., Henry, J., Al-Haddad, R., El Hayek, L., Abou Haidar, E., Stringer, T., … Chao, M. V. (2016). Exercise promotes the expression of brain derived neurotrophic factor (BDNF) through the action of the ketone body β-hydroxybutyrate. *ELife, 5.* https://doi.org/10.7554/eLife.15092

Stefanelli, G., Walters, B. J., Ramzan, F., Narkaj, K., Tao, C., & Zovkic, I. B. (2018). Epigenetic mechanisms of learning and memory. *Molecular-Genetic and Statistical Techniques for Behavioral and Neural Research,* 345–82. https://doi.org/10.1016/B978-0-12-804078-2.00015-5

Stefanis, N. C., van Os, J., Avramopoulos, D., Smyrnis, N., Evdokimidis, I., & Stefanis, C. N. (2005). Effect of COMT Val158 met polymorphism on the continuous performance test, identical pairs version: Tuning rather than improving performance. *American Journal of Psychiatry, 162*(9), 1752–4. https://doi.org/10.1176/appi.ajp.162.9.1752

Stein, J. L., Medland, S. E., Vasquez, A. A., Hibar, D. P., Senstad, R. E., Winkler, A. M., … Enhancing Neuro Imaging Genetics through Meta-Analysis Consortium. (2012). Identification of common variants associated with human hippocampal and intracranial volumes. *Nature Genetics, 44*(5), 552–61. https://doi.org/10.1038/ng.2250

Steinlein, O. K., Deckert, J., Nothen, M. M., Franke, P., Maier, W., Beckmann, H., & Propping, P. (1997). Neuronal nicotinic acetylcholine receptor alpha 4 subunit (CHRNA4) and panic disorder: An association study. *American Journal of Medical Genetics, 74,* 199–201.

Stelzel, C., Basten, U., Montag, C., Reuter, M., & Fiebach, C. J. (2010). Frontostriatal involvement in task switching depends on genetic differences in D2 receptor density. *Journal of Neuroscience, 30*(42), 14205–12. https://doi.org/10.1523/jneurosci.1062-10.2010

Strobel, A., Dreisbach, G., Müller, J., Goschke, T., Brocke, B., & Lesch, K.-P. (2007). Genetic variation of serotonin function and cognitive control. *Journal of Cognitive Neuroscience, 19*(12), 1923–31. https://doi.org/10.1162/jocn.2007.19.12.1923

Tahiri-Alaoui, A., Gill, A. C., Disterer, P., & James, W. (2004). Methionine 129 variant of human prion protein oligomerizes more rapidly than the valine 129 variant: Implications for disease susceptibility to Creutzfeldt-Jakob disease. *The Journal of Biological Chemistry, 279*(30), 31390–7. https://doi.org/10.1074/jbc.M401754200

Tang, Y., Anderson, G. M., Zabetian, C. P., Köhnke, M. D., & Cubells, J. F. (2005). Haplotype-controlled analysis of the association of a non-synonymous single nucleotide polymorphism atDBH (+ 1603C → T) with plasma dopamine β-hydroxylase activity. *American Journal of Medical Genetics Part B: Neuropsychiatric Genetics, 139B*(1), 88–90. https://doi.org/10.1002/ajmg.b.30220

Teffer, K., & Semendeferi, K. (2012). Human prefrontal cortex. *Progress in Brain Research, 195,* 191–218. https://doi.org/10.1016/B978-0-444-53860-4.00009-X

Tenenbaum, G. (2003). Expert athletes: An integrated approach to decision making. In J. L. Starkes & K. A. Ericsson (Eds.), *Expert performance in sports* (pp. 191–218). Champaign, IL: Human Kinetics.

Tenenbaum, G., Hatfield, B., Eklund, R. C., Land, W., Camielo, L., Razon, S., & Schack, K. A. (2009). Conceptual framework for studying emotions-cognitions-performance linkage under conditions which vary in perceived pressure. In M. Raab, J. G. Johnson, & H. Heekeren (Eds.), *Progress in brain research: Mind and motion – The bidirectional link between thought and action* (pp. 159–78). Amsterdam, the Netherlands: Elsevier.

Tenenbaum, G., & Lidor, R. (2005). Research on decision making and the use of cognitive strategies in sport setting. In D. Hackfort, J. Duda, & R. Lidor (Eds.), *Handbook of research on applied sport psychology* (pp. 75–91). Morgantown WV: Fitness Information Technology.

Trampush, J. W., Yang, M. L. Z., Yu, J., Knowles, E., Davies, G., Liewald, D. C., … Lencz, T. (2017). GWAS meta-analysis reveals novel loci and genetic correlates for general cognitive function: A report from the COGENT consortium. *Molecular Psychiatry, 22*(3), 336–45. https://doi.org/10.1038/mp. 2016.244

Tucker-Drob, E. M., Briley, D. A., & Harden, K. P. (2013). Genetic and environmental influences on cognition across development and context. *Current Directions in Psychological Science, 22*(5), 349–55. https://doi.org/10.1177/0963721413485087

Vallender, E. J., Lynch, L., Novak, M. A., & Miller, G. M. (2009). Polymorphisms in the 3′ UTR of the serotonin transporter are associated with cognitive flexibility in rhesus macaques. *American Journal of Medical Genetics Part B: Neuropsychiatric Genetics, 150B*(4), 467–75. https://doi.org/10.1002/ajmg.b.30835

Vandenbergh, D. J., Persico, A. M., Hawkins, A. L., Griffin, C. A., Li, X., Jabs, E. W., & Uhl, G. R. (1992). Human dopamine transporter gene (DAT1) maps to chromosome 5p15.3 and displays a VNTR. *Genomics, 14*(4), 1104–6.

Vaquerizas, J. M., Kummerfeld, S. K., Teichmann, S. A., & Luscombe, N. M. (2009). A census of human transcription factors: Function, expression and evolution. *Nature Reviews Genetics, 10*(4), 252–63. https://doi.org/10.1038/nrg2538

Vaynman, S., & Gomez-Pinilla, F. (2006). Revenge of the "sit": How lifestyle impacts neuronal and cognitive health through molecular systems that interface energy metabolism with neuronal plasticity. *Journal of Neuroscience Research, 84*(4), 699–715. https://doi.org/10.1002/jnr.20979

Walikonis, R. S., Jensen, O. N., Mann, M., Provance, D. W., Mercer, J. A., & Kennedy, M. B. (2000). Identification of proteins in the postsynaptic density fraction by mass spectrometry. *The Journal of Neuroscience: The Official Journal of the Society for Neuroscience, 20*(11), 4069–80. Retrieved from www.ncbi.nlm.nih.gov/pubmed/10818142

Weedon, M. N., Lango, H., Lindgren, C. M., Wallace, C., Evans, D. M., Mangino, M., … Frayling, T. M. (2008). Genome-wide association analysis identifies 20 loci that influence adult height. *Nature Genetics, 40*(5), 575–83. https://doi.org/10.1038/ng.121

Wirz, L., Wacker, J., Felten, A., Reuter, M., & Schwabe, L. (2017). A deletion variant of the α2b-adrenoceptor modulates the stress-induced shift from "cognitive" to "habit" memory. *The Journal of Neuroscience: The Official Journal of the Society for Neuroscience, 37*(8), 2149–60. https://doi.org/10.1523/jneurosci.3507-16.2017

Wishart, H. A., Roth, R. M., Saykin, A. J., Rhodes, C. H., Tsongalis, G. J., Pattin, K. A., … McAllister, T. W. (2011). COMT Val158Met genotype and individual differences in executive function in healthy adults. *Journal of the International Neuropsychological Society, 17*(1), 174–80. https://doi.org/10.1017/S1355617710001402

Woldemichael, B. T., Bohacek, J., Gapp, K., & Mansuy, I. M. (2014). Epigenetics of memory and plasticity. *Progress in Molecular Biology and Translational Science, 122*, 305–40. https://doi.org/10.1016/B978-0-12-420170-5.00011-8

Wright, M., De Geus, E., Ando, J., Luciano, M., Posthuma, D., Ono, Y., … Boomsma, D. (2001). Genetics of cognition: Outline of a collaborative twin study. *Twin Research: The Official Journal of the International Society for Twin Studies, 4*(1), 48–56. Retrieved from www.ncbi.nlm.nih.gov/pubmed/11665325

Xiang, Z., Huguenard, J. R., & Prince, D. A. (1998). Cholinergic switching within neocortical inhibitory networks. *Science, 281*(5379), 985–8. Retrieved from www.ncbi.nlm.nih.gov/pubmed/9703513

Xu, Z., & Taylor, J. A. (2009). SNPinfo: Integrating GWAS and candidate gene information into functional SNP selection for genetic association studies. *Nucleic Acids Research, 37*(Suppl. 2), W600–5. https://doi.org/10.1093/nar/gkp290

Yamada, K., & Nabeshima, T. (2003). Brain-derived neurotrophic factor/TrkB signaling in memory processes. *Journal of Pharmacological Sciences, 91*(4), 267–70. Retrieved from www.ncbi.nlm.nih.gov/pubmed/12719654

Yin, J. C., Del Vecchio, M., Zhou, H., & Tully, T. (1995). CREB as a memory modulator: Induced expression of a dCREB2 activator isoform enhances long-term memory in Drosophila. *Cell, 81*(1), 107–15. Retrieved from www.ncbi.nlm.nih.gov/pubmed/7720066

Zabetian, C. P., Anderson, G. M., Buxbaum, S. G., Elston, R. C., Ichinose, H., Nagatsu, T., … Cubells, J. F. (2001). A quantitative-trait analysis of human Plasma–dopamine β-hydroxylase activity: Evidence for a major functional polymorphism at the DBH locus. *The American Journal of Human Genetics, 68*(2), 515–22. https://doi.org/10.1086/318198

Zigova, T., Pencea, V., Wiegand, S. J., & Luskin, M. B. (1998). Intraventricular administration of BDNF increases the number of newly generated neurons in the adult olfactory bulb. *Molecular and Cellular Neurosciences, 11*(4), 234–45. https://doi.org/10.1006/mcne.1998.0684

8 The gene-environment paradigm for capturing motor behavior and proficiency

Psychologists have long been interested in how people become experts. According to the deliberate-practice framework, it requires more than a decade of investment in highly structured training to develop the necessary expertise. However, recent evidence has shown that individual differences in accumulated amounts of deliberate practice accounted for about one-third of the reliable variance in performance; leaving most of the variance unaccounted for. The present chapter contributes to the ongoing nature-nurture debate by emphasizing the role of genetics in expertise development.

In the year 1896, Gregor Mandel, also known as the founding father of modern genetics, had been deceased for more than a decade. His revolutionary study (originally published in 1866) was lost for approximately three decades, only to be rediscovered in 1900 by Hugo de Vries, Carl Correns, and Erich von Tschermak, who had reached similar conclusions from their own research. In 1896, the term "gene" had not yet been coined. The term entered the mainstream in 1905 via Wilhelm Johannsen. In 1896, scientific phrases such as DNA, Chromosomes, Heritability, and gene expression were nonexistent. However, in 1896, at the opening ceremony for the Olympic games, people stood and cheered at the sight of the human body at its finest: flexible, strong, quick, and magnificent. By 2016, 120 years later, genetic knowledge is vastly developed, the human genome is decoded, mechanisms have been studied and analyzed, and advanced applications in the fields of genetic engineering tried and tested. Moreover, advanced methods for gene editing such as "Crispr" are already used. Despite all these marvelous accomplishments, 120 years after the Olympic games of 1896 we still stand, befuddled by the intricacies of the human body and still ask ourselves: what makes a person a performer?

Scientists have been interested in how people become "performers" or "experts" for a long time. This issue can be approached in two, or more, perspectives: the *conceptual perspective*, and the *molecular perspective*. At the conceptual level the questions center mainly on the components which determine one's performance/expertise, the performer's genetic predisposition, which was determined the moment he/she was conceived, or the environment he/she was raised in, or the combination/interaction of these two components. These issues are discussed in the first section of this chapter. At the molecular level, the questions about these issues focus on gene expression and regulation. From this perspective, stimuli (be it external or internal, physiological or psychological) can lead to a cascade of molecular events, that finally lead to phenotypes – related to performance. The questions raised herein pertain to the mechanisms that relate stimuli to phenotype, turn a cue into an action. Within this framework effort is directed toward explaining people's variability in response to stimuli; a variation that divides people into high vs. low responders.

The nature vs. nurture debate

The term *Tabula Rasa* ("blank slate"), coined by John Locke in 1690, represents the view that human behavioral traits develop almost exclusively from environmental influences. The "blank slate view" was widely held during much of the twentieth century, and the debate between this view, which denies the influence of genetics (and the view admitting that genetic factors also contribute to human behavior) was and still is at the core of an ideological dispute over research agendas. This debate is usually described by the famous phrase "nature vs. nurture," which is attributed to Sir Francis Galton in 1874. Galton, the founding father of eugenics and behavioral genetics (Gillham, 2001), was influenced by the book *On the Origin of Species* written by his half-cousin, Charles Darwin (Fancher, 2009). The book, dealing with diversity of life, made Galton interested in the factors that determine what he called human "talent and character" and its hereditary basis. He constructed his own theory of inheritance in which nature and not nurture plays the leading role. Ironically, Galton and Darwin were not aware that their contemporary, Gregor Mendel, solved (with iconic experimental design) the problem that bothered Darwin the most – the lack of an explanation for heredity.

According to the "nature" point of view, experts are "born" but training is necessary to reach a high level of performance. However, innate ability limits the ultimate level of performance a person can achieve. Galton argued for this position on the basis of his finding that eminence in science, music, art, sports, and other domains tends to run in families. The opposing view is that experts are "made" – that either talent does not exist or its effects on performance are over-shadowed by the effect of training. Watson (1930), the founder of behaviorism, captured this view when he stated that "practicing more intensively than others … is probably the most reasonable explanation we have today not only for success in any line, but even for genius" (p. 212).

More recently, in the spirit of Watson, Ericsson, Krampe, and Tesch-Römer (1993) proposed their influential deliberate-practice view of expert performance. This view holds that expert performance largely reflects accumulated amounts of deliberate practice, which Ericsson et al. defined as engagement in structured activities created specifically to improve performance in a domain. Ericsson et al. (1993) concluded that "high levels of deliberate practice are necessary to attain expert level performance" (p. 392) and that "the differences between expert performers and normal adults reflect a lifelong period of deliberate effort to improve performance in a specific domain" (p. 400). Ericsson (2007) reiterated this perspective when he claimed that "the distinctive characteristics of elite performers are adaptations to extended and intense practice activities that selectively activate dormant genes that all healthy children's DNA contain[s]" (p. 4).

The deliberate-practice view has inspired a great deal of interest in expert performance. The article by Ericsson et al. (1993) has been cited more than 8,700 times by July 2018 and their research has been discussed in a number of popular books. Ericsson et al.'s findings were also the inspiration for what Gladwell (2008) termed the "10,000-hour rule" – the idea that it takes approximately 10,000 hours of practice to become an expert. At the same time, the deliberate-practice view has been sharply criticized in scientific literature with arguments that deliberate practice ignores psychological theorizing (Gardner, 1995); correlates with success because it is a proxy for ability (Gardner, 1995); does not establish the case that a great deal of practice is sufficient for great talent (Anderson, 2000); and that the importance of practice does not project on the lack of the importance of talent (Marcus, 2012).

Furthermore, although deliberate practice is important, growing evidence indicates that it is not as important as Ericsson and colleagues (Ericsson 2007; Ericsson et al., 1993; Ericsson & Moxley, 2012) have argued. Gobet and Campitelli (2007) found a large amount of variability in the total amount of deliberate practice even among master-level chess players. Hambrick et al. (2014) found that deliberate practice accounted for about one-third of the reliable variance in performance in chess and music. One of the most persuasive pieces of evidence about the (lack of) importance of deliberate practice is the meta-analysis conducted by Macnamara, Hambrick, and Oswald (2014), in which they found that deliberate practice explained 26 percent of the variance in performance for games, 21 percent for music, 18 percent for sports, 4 percent for education, and less than 1 percent for professions.

While the supporters of the "nurture" point of view, of which deliberate practice is the extreme representation, deny the importance of genetic factors, the supporters of the "nature" point of view acknowledge the importance of both genetic and environmental factors. Nature vs. nurture, nowadays, is more of "nature *and* nurture." The importance of genetic factors to motor performance and expertise is not questionable anymore, and is described in several reviews (see for example: Davids & Baker, 2007; Johnson & Tenenbaum, 2006; Klissouras, 2001; Yan, Papadimitriou, Lidor, & Eynon, 2016). However, while genetic factors related to performance were extensively studied in physiological domains (see for example, Eynon et al., 2013; Lippi, Longo, & Maffulli, 2010; Macarthur & North, 2005; Ostrander, Huson, & Ostrander, 2009; Pérusse et al., 2013; Roth et al., 2012), the role of genetic factors in psychological traits related to motor performance were studied mainly in non-sport domains, as described in the previous chapters.

The nature vs. nurture debate in sport was also reviewed (see for example Davids & Baker, 2007; Johnson & Tenenbaum, 2006; Klissouras, 2001), and several models were suggested for the relative role of genetic and environmental factors. According to Guilherme, Tritto, North, Lancha, & Artioli (2014), quantitative sport performances such as swimming, running, jumping, etc., are more influenced by genetic factors than sports in which performance "per se" is not of a quantitative nature (team sports, surfing, combat sports). Their model (presented in Figure 8.1) describes how some performance-relevant quantitative traits strongly influenced by genetic factors relate to "predictable sports," while "unpredictable sports" are less influenced by genetic factors, and, therefore, genotype-phenotype relationships are less likely to be established.

According to Tucker and Collins (2012), performance results from the complex relationship between intrinsic (nature and nurture) and extrinsic factors (nurture) (see Figure 8.2). Only a few intrinsic factors have been well studied, though many others are also relevant. Many of the intrinsic factors are multifactorial traits determined by both nature and nurture. Sex (male) differentiation is totally controlled by genes such as SRY, SOX9, and DHTR. The number of SNPs which contribute together with the relative contribution toward the trait is indicated. The correct combination of intrinsic factors determines an inherently talented athlete. Inherently talented athletes must be exposed to the correct combination of extrinsic factors to become elite athletes. Winning an elite athletic event produces a champion. Exposure of athletes to extrinsic factors can result in injury, illness, or burnout. A similar concept was suggested by Ferec (2014).

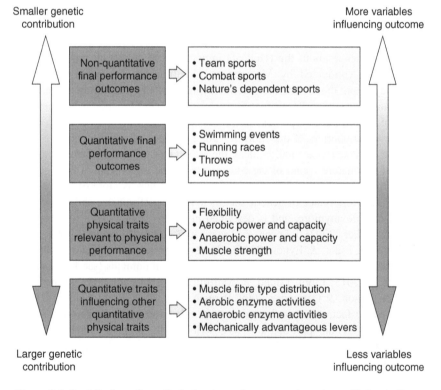

Figure 8.1 Contribution of genetic factors to performance-relevant quantitative traits.

Source: from Guilherme et al. (2014).

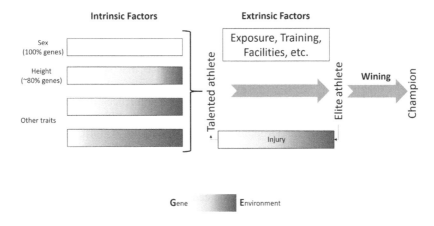

Figure 8.2 The complex relationship between intrinsic (nature and nurture) and extrinsic factors (nurture) that determine elite athletics (from Tucker & Collins, 2012).

Gene-environment relations: a conceptual perspective

The models described in the previous section emphasize the importance of both genetic and environmental factors to motor performance, but do not capture the full complex relations, correlations, and interactions between genes and environment in sport and performance. Gene-environment interactions usually refer to a situation in which the effect of an environmental exposure on behavior/health/performance is dependent on a person's genotype, or, conversely, when environmental exposure moderates genes' effects. All-human multifactorial traits result from complex interplay between genetic and environmental factors. Specific genetic make-up does not necessarily ensure elite athletic performance. It will always result from the gene-environment interactions.

The term *gene-environment interaction* has two main meanings: *substantial meaning* and *statistical meaning*. The substantial meaning implies that when it comes to psychological, physiological, and other traits, both genes and environments are important. In statistical terms, it means that there are main effects of the environment and main effects of genes, but the effect of one variable cannot be understood without taking into account the other variable, since their effects are not independent.

Genes and environment are interconnected/dependent/related entities. Although some environmental influences may be largely random, such as experiencing a natural disaster, many environmental influences are not entirely random (Kendler, Neale, Kessler, Heath, & Eaves, 1993). Three specific gene-environment interactions have been suggested (Plomin, DeFries, & Loehlin, 1977; Scarr & McCartney, 1983): *Passive gene-environment correlation* refers to the fact that biologically related relatives share both genes and environment;

Evocative gene-environment correlation refers to the idea that individuals' geno-types influence the responses they receive from the environment; and *Active gene-environment correlation* refers to the fact that individuals actively select and influence their environment.

Evidence exists in the literature for each of these processes. The important point is that many sources of behavioral influence that we might consider "environmental" are actually under a degree of genetic influence (Kendler & Baker, 2007); so often genetic and environmental influences do not represent independent sources of influence. This also makes it difficult to determine whether the genes or the environment is the causal agent. If, for example, indi-viduals are genetically predisposed toward sensation seeking, and this makes them more likely to spend time in bars (a gene-environment correlation), and this increases their risk of alcohol addiction, are the predisposing sensation-seeking genes or the bar environment the causal agent? In actuality, the question is debatable – they both play a role; it is much more informative to try to under-stand the pathways of risk than to ask whether the genes or the environment were the critical factor in outcomes and behaviors.

Gene-environment correlation refers to the situations in which genes and environment are correlated, or interdependent. In this respect, three specific cor-relations have been suggested (Plomin et al., 1977; Scarr & McCartney, 1983):

- **Passive gene-environment correlation** refers to the fact that biologically related relatives share both genes and environment. According to this model, athletic parents will pass to their offspring both "athletic personality" and "athletic environment."
- **Evocative gene-environment correlation** refers to the idea that indi-viduals' genotypes influence the responses they receive from the environ-ment. According to this model, a person with specific "athletic personality" will attract specific attitudes from the environment.
- **Active gene-environment correlation** refers to the fact that individuals act-ively select and influence their environment. According to this model, a person with specific "athletic personality" will choose a specific environ-ment that best fits his/her personality. For example, a person with a genetic predisposition toward sensation seeking might choose to participate in high-risk sport (Baretta, Greco, & Steca, 2017).

Gene-environment interaction refers to situations in which the effect of genes depends on the environment, and/or the effect of the environment depends on genotype (Halldorsdottir & Binder, 2017; Krueger et al., 2008; Manuck & McCaffery, 2014). Gene-environment interactions account for the reason people respond differently to environmental factors. In motor proficiency, gene-environment interactions account for people's variation in responding to exercise (Bouchard & Rankinen, 2001). Though this phenomenon is quite well known in sport, it is usually attributed to physiological genetic predisposition.

Gene-environment relations: molecular perspective

From molecular perspective, the term "Gene-environment relations" refer to the mechanisms that lead from genetic information to a pronounced trait. These mechanisms include biological and environmental forces working together in a complex, yet very well-choreographed manner. The complexity of these mechanisms makes it almost impossible to simplify it into two separate forces: "Gene" and "Environment."

The central dogma of molecular biology is an explanation of the flow of genetic information within a biological system. The idea was first described in 1958 by Francis Crick (most noted for the discovery of the structure of the DNA molecule in 1953 with James Watson) (Crick, 1958):

> This states that once "information" has passed into protein it cannot get out again. In more detail, the transfer of information from nucleic acid to nucleic acid, or from nucleic acid to protein may be possible, but transfer from protein to protein, or from protein to nucleic acid is impossible. Information means here the precise determination of sequence, either of bases in the nucleic acid or of amino acid residues in the protein.

The central dogma as described by Crick is presented in Figure 8.3. The gray arrows represent a simplified two-steps version of this dogma (DNA → RNA → protein), suggested by Crick's colleague, James Watson (Thieffry & Sarkar, 1998). Both versions have been criticized (Biro, 2004; Klein & Klein, 2016; Morange, 2006; Strasser, 2006) mainly because they do not capture the complexity of information flows in biological systems, and since they could not explain later discoveries.

While the term "the central dogma" refers to the flow of information in biological systems, the term "gene expression" refers to the mechanisms by which information from a gene is used in the synthesis of a functional gene product. These products are often proteins, but in non-protein coding genes the product is a functional RNA. These mechanisms are often referred to as "the machinery of life" and are described in detail in molecular biology text books.

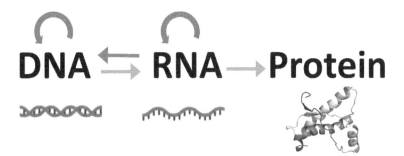

Figure 8.3 The central dogma of the flow of information in biological systems.

The expression of genes is highly regulated at each stage of the gene expression process (Figure 8.4): at the DNA level, these are the mechanisms, named "chromatin remodelling," that make the gene "readable"; at the RNA level, these mechanisms include the transcription of RNA from DNA, the processing of pre-RNA to mature RNA, and the release of the RNA to the cytoplasm, the stability of the RNA in the cytoplasm and RNA translation; at the protein level these mechanisms include the post-translational modification of a protein. These sophisticated and complex mechanisms are used to trigger developmental pathways, respond to stimuli, or adapt to new environments.

The gene regulation mechanisms constantly react with the environment, either in an "acute" form, as a response to stimuli, or in "chronic" form as an adaptation. For example, a physiological or psychological stimuli will lead to a cascade of events that will result in a production of protein(s). This happened at a specific time point. However, adaptations to an ever-changing environment involve long-lasting modifications, with a long-lasting effect on physiological and psychological aspects of human health and behavior. In the next section we will center on basic mechanisms which direct the expression of genes based on

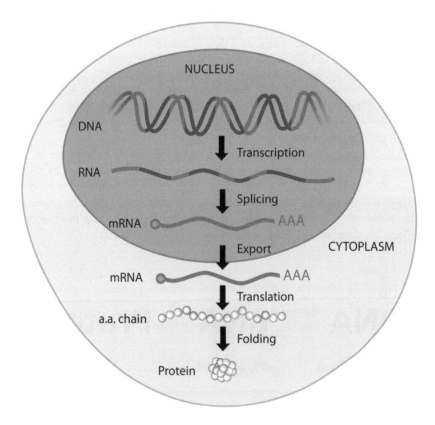

Figure 8.4 Gene regulation mechanisms.

environmental changes and developmental status, also known as "epigenetic mechanisms." Epigenetic mechanisms are the mechanisms related to changes in gene expression without alterations in the DNA sequence (Deans & Maggert, 2015; Mann, 2014; Nagy & Turecki, 2015; Nicoglou & Merlin, 2017; Van Speybroeck, 2002). The main epigenetic mechanisms are: DNA methylation, histone modification, and non-coding RNA action.

DNA methylation. It is the most frequently occurring epigenetic mechanism, that make genes more or less "readable." The DNA molecule wraps around small proteins, named "histone," forming a "beads on a string" structure, named nucleosome (Figure 8.5a). This DNA-protein complex is named "chromatin." The chromatin has two forms: the compact form, heterochromatin, in which the genes are unreadable, and the loose form, euchromatin, in which the genes are readable (Figure 8.5b).

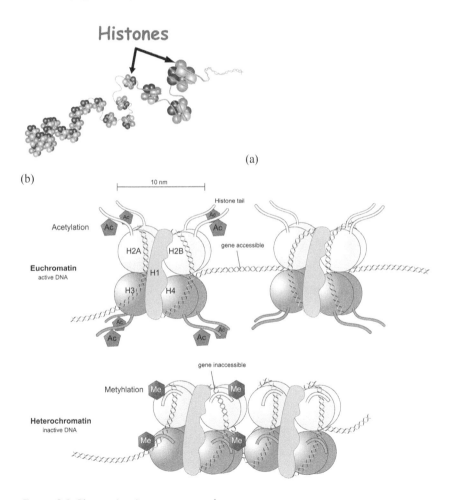

Figure 8.5 Chromatin, chromosome, nucleosome.

DNA methylation refers to an addition of a methyl group to the DNA strand at specific sites of cytosines that precede guanines, called CpG islands (D'Urso & Brickner, 2014). CpG islands are often located around the promoters of house-keeping genes or other genes frequently expressed in a cell (56 percent of genes) (Antequera & Bird, 1993). Unmethylated CpG islands are the target of TFs to start the transcription. By contrast, the CpG sequences in inactive genes are usually methylated to suppress their expression.

Histone modification. The basic repeating unit of chromatin, the nucleosome, consists of 146 bp of DNA wrapped around an octameric histone core formed by two copies each of histones H2A, H2B, H3, and H4. Histones, beside possessing a definite structural function, have a specific role in modulating the physical access of nuclear factors to DNA. It is now clear that post-translational modifications of charged aminoacids of histone tails that protrude from the core structure of the nucleosome can alter chromatin conformation and create binding sites for TFs playing a direct regulatory role in gene expression (Felsenfeld & Groudine, 2003). Both DNA methylation and histone modification are presented in Figure 8.6.

ncRNAs. Another mechanism of gene regulation is mediated by small, non-coding RNAs. Among these small RNAs are the microRNAs (miRNAs) and short interfering RNAs (siRNAs); they are both 20–30 nucleotide-long double-stranded RNA molecules, encoded by their own set of genes (miRNAs) or introduced into the cell from outside sources (siRNAs) (Carthew & Sontheimer, 2009; Grimm, 2009). The siRNAs are more often produced by long, linear,

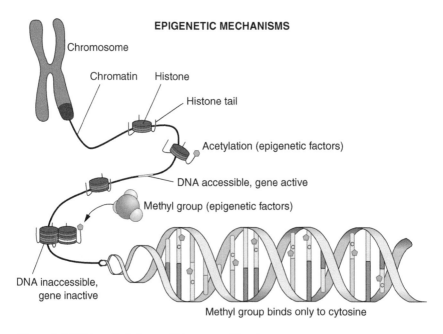

Figure 8.6 DNA methylation and histone modification.

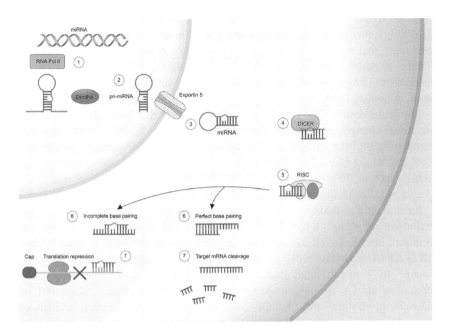

Figure 8.7 miRNA formation.

perfectly base paired double strand RNA (dsRNAs) precursors introduced into the cell by virus, taken up from the environment or experimentally or clinically induced. The miRNAs are typically expressed in the nucleus in the form of longer precursors which are subsequently exported into the cytoplasm and processed by the enzyme Dicer into ~22 nucleotide-long miRNA. One single strand of these short RNAs, the mature guide or antisense strand, will next be loaded into the RNA-induced silencing complex RISC together with one or more Ago (Argonaute) protein, which will allow it to bind to its mRNA target and induce silencing (Figure 8.7).

Epigenetic mechanisms in mental and cognitive domains

Although the critical role for epigenetic mechanisms in development and cell differentiation has long been appreciated, recent evidence reveals that these mechanisms are also employed in post-mitotic neurons as a means of consolidating and stabilizing cognitive-behavioral memories (Day & Sweatt, 2011). Epigenetics plays an essential role in neural reorganization, including those that govern the brain plasticity (Deibel, Zelinski, Keeley, Kovalchuk, & McDonald, 2015).

Histone modifications in the CNS are essential components of memory formation and consolidation. Indeed, multiple types of behavioral experiences, such as contextual fear conditioning, are capable of inducing histone modifications in several brain regions (see, among others for examples: Bredy et al., 2007; Chwang, Arthur, Schumacher, & Sweatt, 2007; Gupta et al., 2010; Koshibu et al., 2009; Levenson et al., 2004). Importantly, interference with the molecular machinery that regulates histone acetylation, phosphorylation, and methylation disrupts associative learning and long-term potentiation (LTP; a cellular correlate of memory) (Day & Sweatt, 2011; Ieraci, Mallei, Musazzi, & Popoli, 2015; Levenson & Sweatt, 2005).

Physical exercise (PE) is a strong gene modulator that induces structural and functional changes in the brain, determining enormous effect on both cognitive functioning and mental status (Mandolesi et al., 2018). Moreover, epigenetic mechanisms are strongly influenced by different biological and environmental factors, such as PE (Grazioli et al., 2017), which determine the nature and mode of epigenetic mechanisms activation.

Several animal studies reveal how motor activity is able to improve cognitive performances acting on epigenetic mechanisms and influencing the expression of those genes involved in neuroplasticity (Fernandes, Arida, & Gomez-Pinilla, 2017). DNA methylation plays a key role in LTM (Deibel et al., 2015; Kim & Kaang, 2017). In particular, mechanisms related to DNA methylation relieve the repressive effects of memory-suppressor genes to favor the expression of plasticity-promoting and memory consolidation genes. Several evidences showed that PE is able to coordinate the action of the genes involved in synaptic plasticity that regulate memory consolidation (Ding, Vaynman, Akhavan, Ying, & Gomez-Pinilla, 2006; Molteni, Ying, & Gomez-Pinilla, 2002).

Histone modifications are post-translational chemical changes in histone proteins. They include histone methylation/demethylation, acetylation/deacetylation, and phosphorylation, all due to the activity of specific enzymes, which modify the chromatin structure, thereby regulating gene expression. It has been demonstrated that histone acetylation is a requisite for LTM (Barrett & Wood, 2008; Fernandes et al., 2017). In animals, motor activity increases these genetic mechanisms in the hippocampus and the frontal cortex, improving memory performances in behavioral tasks (Cechinel et al., 2016). Recently, following four weeks of motor exercise, there has been evidence of an increasing of the activity of enzymes involved in histone acetylation/deacetylation, the epigenetic mechanisms that determine an enhancing in the expression of BDNF (Maejima, Kanemura, Kokubun, Murata, & Takayanagi, 2018).

MicroRNAs (miRNAs) are small, single stranded RNA molecules able to inhibit the expression of target genes. They are widely expressed in the brain, participating in epigenetic mechanisms and acting as regulators of numerous biological processes in the brain, ranging from cell proliferation, differentiation, apoptosis, synaptic plasticity, and memory consolidation (Saab & Mansuy, 2014). Recent evidences demonstrate that PE can mitigate the harmful effects of traumatic brain injury and aging on cognitive function by regulating the hippocampal expression of miR21(Hu et al., 2015) and miR-34a (Kou et al., 2017). Furthermore, PE contributes to attenuating the effects of stress-related increases in miR-124, involved in neurogenesis and memory formation (Pan-Vazquez et al., 2015).

Interpersonal variation in response to the environment

The twenty-first century has been characterized by a constant push toward making medicine more personalized (Ginsburg & Willard, 2009; Hamburg & Collins, 2010). Researchers have made great strides in achieving this goal through pharma-cogenomics, a field that explores the impact of genomic variability on drug respon-siveness (Wang, McLeod, & Weinshilboum, 2011), but little data exists regarding the heterogeneity in responsiveness to exercise training (Guyatt, Juniper, Walter, Griffith, & Goldstein, 1998), a major component in performance variability.

The vast majority of studies dealing with physical activity have emphasized main effects and group differences, while paying little attention to individual differences, and the contributions at the level of a group may not fully apply to each member of that group (Bouchard & Rankinen, 2001). Indeed, even well-controlled studies using homogenous populations have demonstrated significant heterogeneity in training responses. Hubal et al. (2005) reported that 1-repetition maximum (1RM) strength of the elbow flexors increased between 0 percent and 250 percent following 12 weeks of training. Similarly, Bamman, Petrella, Kim, Mayhew and Cross (2007), categorized participants as extreme, moderate, or low responders to a resistance-training regimen. These authors demonstrated that despite similar adherence to a resistance-training program, mean changes in muscle fiber size among response clusters varied from 0 percent to 60 percent.

Despite the accumulating evidence on heterogeneity in exercise responsiveness (Booth & Laye, 2010; Bouchard, 1983, 1995; Church et al., 2009; Hubal et al., 2005; Kohrt et al., 1991; Sisson et al., 2009), only a small number of studies have been conducted to identify factors responsible for variability in exercise responses. The HERITAGE (HEalth, RIsk factors, exercise Training And GEnetics) family study (Bouchard et al., 1995), the FAMuSS (Functional single nucleotide poly-morphisms Associated with MUscle Size and Strength) study, and others provided key data regarding the genomic contribution to exercise responsiveness.

The goal of any training program is to maximize the dose/response specific to the long-term objective(s) (e.g., reestablishing energy balance, improving cardiorespiratory capacity, increasing muscle mass/strength, etc.). This presents three major challenges: (1) knowing exactly what to measure, (2) knowing when to make the measurement, and (3) connecting that measurement to a well-defined health outcome. A number of studies have documented post-exercise increases in transcription rate and/or mRNA content of genes related to muscle function and metabolism (Louis, Raue, Yang, Jemiolo, & Trappe, 2007; Mahoney, Parise, Melov, Safdar, & Tarnopolsky, 2005; Perry et al., 2010; Pilegaard, Ordway, Saltin, & Neufer, 2000; Pilegaard, Saltin, & Neufer, 2003). While this approach has revealed important aspects of how cells respond to exercise, very little is known as to how these molecular responses ultimately translate to the individual's molecular and related cellular mechanisms; this in turn limits the ability to prescribe the desired dose required for optimal long-term outcomes. Nevertheless, the variation in psychological aspects related training responsiveness is usually ignored, though it is well established that

both cognition and mental factors contribute to performance. Possible responsiveness and reaction interaction that might exist between specific genetic
endowment and performance is presented in Figure 8.8.

"low," "medium," and "high" represent different levels of specific psychological trait, corresponding to different genetic make-ups. **A** describes responsiveness interaction, in which people with high-trait score respond to

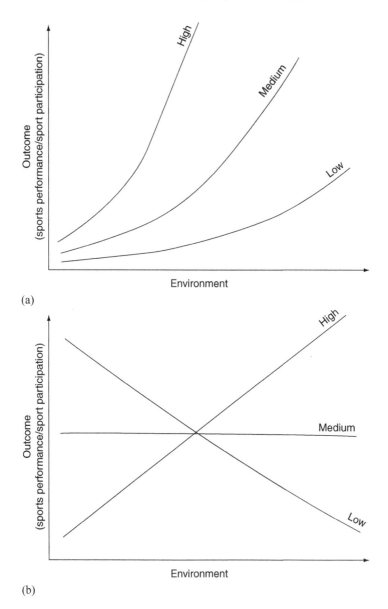

(a)

(b)

Figure 8.8 Possible interactions between environment and different levels of trait.

environment abruptly compared to medium and low trait scored. **B** describes reaction interaction, in which each personality trait level prospers at different environment extremes.

Summary: gene-environment model for motor performance

It seems that it is almost impossible to capture the complexity and multidimensionality of motor performance in a simplified model. The illustrative model presented in Figure 8.9 is composed of four layers. The first layer is the genotype space. This layer represents the *genetic predisposition* determined at fertilization and is stable and unchanged during life. The second layer represents the level of *specific trait* (out of many traits) related to performance, such as self-efficacy, coping with stress, emotion regulation capacity, exertion/pain tolerance, and such. The level of the trait represents gene-environment interaction and might vary over time. The third layer represents the *nurturing environment*. It can be described on a continuum ranging from supportive to non-supportive environment. The last layer represents the *performance level*, which is the outcome of the other levels. The colorful lines represent different patterns of performance development. For example, the red line represents a specific genetic profile related to the moderate level of the trait, moderate nurturing environment, and moderate-high level of performance. At another time point it might reach a higher level of trait, go through another nurturing environment and lead to a different level of performance (the red dashed line). Other combinations (the

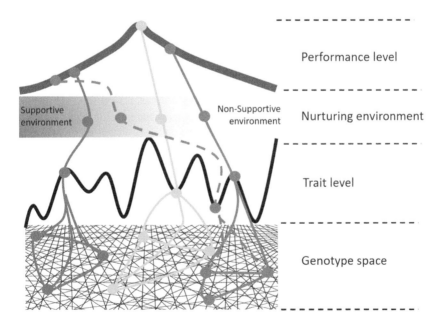

Figure 8.9 Gene-environment model determining motor performance.

green line and the yellow line) might follow another path and might end up at different levels of performance. According to the model, high levels of specific traits (e.g., motivation) and/or the existence of a supportive environment do not always ensure a high level of performance. This is relevant especially in sports where the level of "unknown" factors is high, such as where the performance depends on environmental conditions (sailing, surfing) or where the performance depends on opponent performance (team and combat sports).

Any study on the genetic basis of motor performance must incorporate the psychological domain and the complicated interaction between psychological and physiological traits as well as the continuous interaction with the environment.

References

Anderson, J. R. (2000). *Learning and memory: An integrated approach.* New York, NY: John Wiley and Sons.

Antequera, F., & Bird, A. (1993). Number of CpG islands and genes in human and mouse. *Proceedings of the National Academy of Sciences of the United States of America, 90*(24), 11995–9. Retrieved from www.ncbi.nlm.nih.gov/pubmed/7505451

Bamman, M. M., Petrella, J. K., Kim, J., Mayhew, D. L., & Cross, J. M. (2007). Cluster analysis tests the importance of myogenic gene expression during myofiber hypertrophy in humans. *Journal of Applied Physiology, 102*(6), 2232–9. https://doi.org/10.1152/japplphysiol.00024.2007

Barrett, R. M., & Wood, M. A. (2008). Beyond transcription factors: The role of chromatin modifying enzymes in regulating transcription required for memory. *Learning and Memory, 15*(7), 460–7. https://doi.org/10.1101/lm.917508

Baretta, D., Greco, A., & Steca, P. (2017). Understanding performance in risky sport: The role of self-efficacy beliefs and sensation seeking in competitive freediving. *Personality and Individual Differences, 117*, 161–5.

Biro, J. C. (2004). Seven fundamental, unsolved questions in molecular biology. *Medical Hypotheses, 63*(6), 951–62. https://doi.org/10.1016/j.mehy.2004.06.024

Booth, F. W., & Laye, M. J. (2010). The future: Genes, physical activity and health. *Acta Physiologica, 199*(4), 549–56. https://doi.org/10.1111/j.1748-1716.2010.02117.x

Bouchard, C. (1983). Human adaptability may have a genetic basis. In: Proceedings of the 18th Annual Meeting of the Society of Prospective Medicine. Canadian Public Health Association, Otta. In F. Landry (Ed.), *Health Risk Estimation, Risk Reduction and Health Promotion* (pp. 463–76). Ottawa, Canada: Canadian Public Health Association.

Bouchard, C. (1995). Individual differences in the response to regular exercise. *International Journal of Obesity and Related Metabolic Disorders: Journal of the International Association for the Study of Obesity, 19*(Suppl. 4), S5–8. Retrieved from www.ncbi.nlm.nih.gov/pubmed/8581095

Bouchard, C., Leon, A. S., Rao, D. C., Skinner, J. S., Wilmore, J. H., & Gagnon, J. (1995). The heritage family study. Aims, design, and measurement protocol. *Medicine and Science in Sports and Exercise, 27*(5), 721–9. Retrieved from www.ncbi.nlm.nih.gov/pubmed/7674877

Bouchard, C., & Rankinen, T. (2001). Individual differences in response to regular physical activity. *Medicine and Science in Sports and Exercise, 33*(Suppl. 6), S446–51; Discussion S452–3. Retrieved from www.ncbi.nlm.nih.gov/pubmed/11427769

Bredy, T. W., Wu, H., Crego, C., Zellhoefer, J., Sun, Y. E., & Barad, M. (2007). Histone modifications around individual BDNF gene promoters in prefrontal cortex are associated with extinction of conditioned fear. *Learning and Memory, 14*(4), 268–76. https://doi.org/10.1101/lm.500907

Carthew, R. W., & Sontheimer, E. J. (2009). Origins and mechanisms of miRNAs and siRNAs. *Cell, 136*(4), 642–55. https://doi.org/10.1016/j.cell.2009.01.035

Cechinel, L. R., Basso, C. G., Bertoldi, K., Schallenberger, B., de Meireles, L. C. F., & Siqueira, I. R. (2016). Treadmill exercise induces age and protocol-dependent epigenetic changes in prefrontal cortex of Wistar rats. *Behavioural Brain Research, 313*, 82–7. https://doi.org/10.1016/j.bbr.2016.07.016

Church, T. S., Martin, C. K., Thompson, A. M., Earnest, C. P., Mikus, C. R., & Blair, S. N. (2009). Changes in weight, waist circumference and compensatory responses with different doses of exercise among sedentary, overweight postmenopausal women. *PloS One, 4*(2), e4515. https://doi.org/10.1371/journal.pone.0004515

Chwang, W. B., Arthur, J. S., Schumacher, A., & Sweatt, J. D. (2007). The nuclear kinase mitogen- and stress-activated protein kinase 1 regulates hippocampal chromatin remodeling in memory formation. *The Journal of Neuroscience: The Official Journal of the Society for Neuroscience, 27*(46), 12732–42. https://doi.org/10.1523/jneurosci. 2522-07.2007

Crick, F. H. (1958). On protein synthesis. *Symposia of the Society for Experimental Biology, 12*, 138–63. Retrieved from www.ncbi.nlm.nih.gov/pubmed/13580867

Davids, K., & Baker, J. (2007). Genes, environment and sport performance: Why the nature-nurture dualism is no longer relevant. *Sports Medicine, 37*(11), 691–80. Retrieved from https://link.springer.com/content/pdf/10.2165%2F00007256-20073711 0-00004.pdf

Day, J. J., & Sweatt, J. D. (2011). Epigenetic mechanisms in cognition. *Neuron, 70*(5), 813–29. https://doi.org/10.1016/j.neuron.2011.05.019

Deans, C., & Maggert, K. A. (2015). What do you mean, "epigenetic"? *Genetics, 199*(4), 887–96. https://doi.org/10.1534/genetics.114.173492

Deibel, S. H., Zelinski, E. L., Keeley, R. J., Kovalchuk, O., & McDonald, R. J. (2015). Epigenetic alterations in the suprachiasmatic nucleus and hippocampus contribute to age-related cognitive decline. *Oncotarget, 6*(27), 23181–203. https://doi.org/10.18632/oncotarget.4036

Ding, Q., Vaynman, S., Akhavan, M., Ying, Z., & Gomez-Pinilla, F. (2006). Insulin-like growth factor I interfaces with brain-derived neurotrophic factor-mediated synaptic plasticity to modulate aspects of exercise-induced cognitive function. *Neuroscience, 140*(3), 823–33. https://doi.org/10.1016/j.neuroscience.2006.02.084

D'Urso, A., & Brickner, J. H. (2014). Mechanisms of epigenetic memory. *Trends in Genetics, 30*(6), 230–6. https://doi.org/10.1016/j.tig.2014.04.004

Ericsson, K. A. (2007). Deliberate practice and the modifiability of body and mind: Toward a science of the structure and acquisition of expert and elite performance. *International Journal of Sport Psychology, 38*(1), 4–34. Retrieved from http://psycnet.apa.org/record/2007-06716-002

Ericsson, K. A., Krampe, R. T., & Tesch-Römer, C. (1993). The role of deliberate practice in the acquisition of expert performance. *Psychological Review, 100*(3), 363–406. Retrieved from http://projects.ict.usc.edu/itw/gel/EricssonDeliberatePracticePR93.PDF

Ericsson, K. A., & Moxley, J. H. (2012). The expert performance approach and deliberate practice: Some potential implications for studying creative performance in organizations. In M. D. Mumford (Ed.), *The handbook of organizational creativity* (pp. 141–67). London, England: Academic Press.

Eynon, N., Hanson, E. D., Lucia, A., Houweling, P. J., Garton, F., North, K. N., & Bishop, D. J. (2013). Genes for elite power and sprint performance: ACTN3 leads the way. *Sports Medicine, 43*(9), 803–17. https://doi.org/10.1007/s40279-013-0059-4

Fancher, R. E. (2009). Scientific cousins: The relationship between Charles Darwin and Francis Galton. *American Psychologist, 64*(2), 84–92. https://doi.org/10.1037/a0013339

Felsenfeld, G., & Groudine, M. (2003). Controlling the double helix. *Nature, 421*(6921), 448–53. https://doi.org/10.1038/nature01411

Ferec, A. (2014). *Genetics for trainers: Decoding the sports genes* [Kindle edition]. Retrieved from www.amazon.com/genetics-trainers-decoding-sports-genes-ebook/dp/B00IB32V1O

Fernandes, J., Arida, R. M., & Gomez-Pinilla, F. (2017). Physical exercise as an epigenetic modulator of brain plasticity and cognition. *Neuroscience and Biobehavioral Reviews, 80*, 443–56. https://doi.org/10.1016/j.neubiorev.2017.06.012

Gardner, H. (1995). Expert performance: Its structure and acquisition: Comment. *American Psychologist, 50*(9), 802–3. https://doi.org/10.1037/0003-066X.50.9.802

Gillham, N. W. (2001). Sir Francis Galton and the birth of eugenics. *Annual Review of Genetics, 35*(1), 83–101. https://doi.org/10.1146/annurev.genet.35.102401.090055

Ginsburg, G. S., & Willard, H. F. (2009). Genomic and personalized medicine: Foundations and applications. *Translational Research, 154*(6), 277–87. https://doi.org/10.1016/j.trsl.2009.09.005

Gladwell, M. (2008). *Outliers: The story of success*. New York, NY: Little, Brown. Retrieved from www.HachetteBookGroup.com

Gobet, F., & Campitelli, G. (2007). The role of domain-specific practice, handedness, and starting age in chess. *Developmental Psychology, 43*(1), 159–72. Retrieved from http://psycnet.apa.org/buy/2006-23020-013

Grazioli, E., Dimauro, I., Mercatelli, N., Wang, G., Pitsiladis, Y., Di Luigi, L., & Caporossi, D. (2017). Physical activity in the prevention of human diseases: Role of epigenetic modifications. *BMC Genomics, 18*(S8), 802. https://doi.org/10.1186/s12864-017-4193-5

Grimm, D. (2009). Small silencing RNAs: State-of-the-art. *Advanced Drug Delivery Reviews, 61*(9), 672–703. https://doi.org/10.1016/j.addr.2009.05.002

Guilherme, J. P. L. F., Tritto, A. C. C., North, K. N., Lancha, J. R. A. H., & Artioli, G. G. (2014). Genetics and sport performance: Current challenges and directions to the future. *Revista Brasileira de Educação Física e Esporte, 28*(1), 177–93. https://doi.org/10.1590/S1807-55092014000100177

Gupta, S., Kim, S. Y., Artis, S., Molfese, D. L., Schumacher, A., Sweatt, J. D., … Lubin, F. D. (2010). Histone methylation regulates memory formation. *Journal of Neuroscience, 30*(10), 3589–99. https://doi.org/10.1523/jneurosci.3732-09.2010

Guyatt, G. H., Juniper, E. F., Walter, S. D., Griffith, L. E., & Goldstein, R. S. (1998). Interpreting treatment effects in randomised trials. *BMJ (Clinical Research Ed.), 316*(7132), 690–3. Retrieved from www.ncbi.nlm.nih.gov/pubmed/9522799

Halldorsdottir, T., & Binder, E. B. (2017). Gene × environment interactions: From molecular mechanisms to behavior. *Annual Review of Psychology, 3*(68), 215–41.

Hambrick, D. Z., Oswald, F. L., Altmann, E. M., Meinz, E. J., Gobet, F., & Campitelli, G. (2014). Deliberate practice: Is that all it takes to become an expert? *Intelligence, 45*(1), 34–45. https://doi.org/10.1016/j.intell.2013.04.001

Hamburg, M. A., & Collins, F. S. (2010). The path to personalized medicine. *New England Journal of Medicine, 363*(4), 301–4. https://doi.org/10.1056/NEJMp1006304

Hu, T., Zhou, F.-J., Chang, Y.-F., Li, Y.-S., Liu, G.-C., Hong, Y., … Bao, T. (2015). MIR21 is associated with the cognitive improvement following voluntary running wheel exercise in TBI mice. *Journal of Molecular Neuroscience: MN, 57*(1), 114–22. https://doi.org/10.1007/s12031-015-0584-8

Hubal, M. J., Gordish-Dressman, H., Thompson, P. D., Price, T. B., Hoffman, E. P., Angelopoulos, T. J., … Clarkson, P. M. (2005). Variability in muscle size and strength gain after unilateral resistance training. *Medicine and Science in Sports and Exercise, 37*(6), 964–72. Retrieved from www.ncbi.nlm.nih.gov/pubmed/15947721

Ieraci, A., Mallei, A., Musazzi, L., & Popoli, M. (2015). Physical exercise and acute restraint stress differentially modulate hippocampal brain-derived neurotrophic factor transcripts and epigenetic mechanisms in mice. *Hippocampus, 25*(11), 1380–92. https://doi.org/10.1002/hipo.22458

Johnson, M., & Tenenbaum, G. (2006). The roles of nature and nurture in expertise in sport. In D. Hackfort & G. Tenenbaum (Eds.), *Essential processes for attaining peak performance* (pp. 26–52). Oxford, England; Aachen, Germany: Meyer and Meyer Sport.

Kendler, K. S., & Baker, J. H. (2007). Genetic influences on measures of the environment: A systematic review. *Psychological Medicine, 37*(5), 615. https://doi.org/10.1017/S0033291706009524

Kendler, K. S., Neale, M. C., Kessler, R. C., Heath, A. C., & Eaves, L. J. (1993). A longitudinal twin study of personality and major depression in women. *Archives of General Psychiatry, 50*, 853–62.

Kim, S., & Kaang, B.-K. (2017). Epigenetic regulation and chromatin remodeling in learning and memory. *Experimental and Molecular Medicine, 49*(1), e281–e281. https://doi.org/10.1038/emm.2016.140

Klein, G., & Klein, E. (2016). The rise and fall of central dogmas. *OncoImmunology, 5*(10), e1043071. https://doi.org/10.1080/2162402X.2015.1043071

Klissouras, V. (2001). The nature and nurture of human performance. *European Journal of Sport Science, 1*(2), 1–10. Retrieved from https://pdfs.semanticscholar.org/0186/1e9 3b6aa0e0fdff28b5197f2a4535839d253.pdf

Kohrt, W. M., Malley, M. T., Coggan, A. R., Spina, R. J., Ogawa, T., Ehsani, A. A., … Holloszy, J. O. (1991). Effects of gender, age, and fitness level on response of VO2max to training in 60–71 yr olds. *Journal of Applied Physiology, 71*(5), 2004–11. Retrieved from www.ncbi.nlm.nih.gov/pubmed/1761503

Koshibu, K., Gräff, J., Beullens, M., Heitz, F. D., Berchtold, D., Russig, H., … Mansuy, I. M. (2009). Protein phosphatase 1 regulates the histone code for long-term memory. *The Journal of Neuroscience: The Official Journal of the Society for Neuroscience, 29*(41), 13079–89. https://doi.org/10.1523/JNEUROSCI.3610-09.2009

Kou, X., Li, J., Liu, X., Chang, J., Zhao, Q., Jia, S., … Chen, N. (2017). Swimming attenuates d-galactose-induced brain aging via suppressing miR-34a-mediated autophagy impairment and abnormal mitochondrial dynamics. *Journal of Applied Physiology, 122*(6), 1462–9. https://doi.org/10.1152/japplphysiol.00018.2017

Krueger, R. F., South, S., Johnson, W., & Iacono, W. (2008). The heritability of personality is not always 50%: Gene-environment interactions and correlations between personality and parenting. *Journal of Personality, 76*(6), 1485–522.

Levenson, J. M., O'Riordan, K. J., Brown, K. D., Trinh, M. A., Molfese, D. L., & Sweatt, J. D. (2004). Regulation of histone acetylation during memory formation in the hippocampus. *Journal of Biological Chemistry, 279*(39), 40545–9. https://doi.org/10.1074/jbc.M402229200

Levenson, J. M., & Sweatt, J. D. (2005). Epigenetic mechanisms in memory formation. *Nature Reviews Neuroscience, 6*(2), 108–18. https://doi.org/10.1038/nrn1604

Lippi, G., Longo, U. G., & Maffulli, N. (2010). Genetics and sports. *British Medical Bulletin, 93*, 27–47. https://doi.org/10.1093/bmb/ldp007

Louis, E., Raue, U., Yang, Y., Jemiolo, B., & Trappe, S. (2007). Time course of proteolytic, cytokine, and myostatin gene expression after acute exercise in human skeletal muscle. *Journal of Applied Physiology, 103*(5), 1744. https://doi.org/10.1152/japplphysiol.00679.2007

Macarthur, D. G., & North, K. N. (2005). Genes and human elite athletic performance. *Human Genetics, 116*(5), 331–9. https://doi.org/10.1007/s00439-005-1261-8

Macnamara, B. N., Hambrick, D. Z., & Oswald, F. L. (2014). Deliberate practice and performance in music, games, sports, education, and professions: A meta-analysis. *Psychological Science, 25*(8), 1608–18.

Maejima, H., Kanemura, N., Kokubun, T., Murata, K., & Takayanagi, K. (2018). Exercise enhances cognitive function and neurotrophin expression in the hippocampus accompanied by changes in epigenetic programming in senescence-accelerated mice. *Neuroscience Letters, 665*, 67–73. https://doi.org/10.1016/j.neulet.2017.11.023

Mahoney, D. J., Parise, G., Melov, S., Safdar, A., & Tarnopolsky, M. A. (2005). Analysis of global mRNA expression in human skeletal muscle during recovery from endurance exercise. *FASEB Journal: Official Publication of the Federation of American Societies for Experimental Biology, 19*(11), 1498–500. https://doi.org/10.1096/fj.04-3149fje

Mandolesi, L., Polverino, A., Montuori, S., Foti, F., Ferraioli, G., Sorrentino, P., & Sorrentino, G. (2018). Effects of physical exercise on cognitive functioning and well-being: Biological and psychological benefits. *Frontiers in Psychology, 9*, 509. https://doi.org/10.3389/fpsyg.2018.00509

Mann, J. R. (2014). Epigenetics and memigenetics. *Cellular and Molecular Life Sciences, 71*(7), 1117–22. https://doi.org/10.1007/s00018-014-1560-0

Manuck, S. B., & McCaffery, J. M. (2014). Gene–environment interaction. *Annual Review of Psychology, 65*(1), 41–70.

Marcus, G. (2012). *Guitar zero: The science of becoming musical at any age.* New York, NY: Penguin.

Molteni, R., Ying, Z., & Gomez-Pinilla, F. (2002). Differential effects of acute and chronic exercise on plasticity-related genes in the rat hippocampus revealed by microarray. *The European Journal of Neuroscience, 16*(6), 1107–16. Retrieved from www.ncbi.nlm.nih.gov/pubmed/12383240

Morange, M. (2006). The protein side of the central dogma: Permanence and change. *History and Philosophy of the Life Sciences, 28*(4), 513–24. Retrieved from www.ncbi.nlm.nih.gov/pubmed/18351049

Nagy, C., & Turecki, G. (2015). Transgenerational epigenetic inheritance: An open discussion. *Epigenomics, 7*(5), 781–90. https://doi.org/10.2217/epi.15.46

Nicoglou, A., & Merlin, F. (2017). Epigenetics: A way to bridge the gap between biological fields. *Studies in History and Philosophy of Science Part C: Studies in History and Philosophy of Biological and Biomedical Sciences, 66*, 73–82. https://doi.org/10.1016/j.shpsc.2017.10.002

Ostrander, E. A., Huson, H. J., & Ostrander, G. K. (2009). Genetics of athletic performance. *Annual Review of Genomics and Human Genetics, 10*(1), 407–29. https://doi.org/10.1146/annurev-genom-082908-150058

Pan-Vazquez, A., Rye, N., Ameri, M., McSparron, B., Smallwood, G., Bickerdyke, J., ... Toledo-Rodriguez, M. (2015). Impact of voluntary exercise and housing conditions on hippocampal glucocorticoid receptor, miR-124 and anxiety. *Molecular Brain, 8*, 40. https://doi.org/10.1186/s13041-015-0128-8

Perry, C. G. R., Lally, J., Holloway, G. P., Heigenhauser, G. J. F., Bonen, A., & Spriet, L. L. (2010). Repeated transient mRNA bursts precede increases in transcriptional and mitochondrial proteins during training in human skeletal muscle. *The Journal of Physiology, 588*(Pt. 23), 4795–810. https://doi.org/10.1113/jphysiol.2010.199448

Pérusse, L., Rankinen, T., Hagberg, J. M., Loos, R. J. F., Roth, S. M., Sarzynski, M. A., … Bouchard, C. (2013). Advances in exercise, fitness, and performance genomics in 2012. *Medicine and Science in Sports and Exercise, 45*(5), 824–31. https://doi.org/10.1249/MSS.0b013e31828b28a3

Pilegaard, H., Ordway, G. A., Saltin, B., & Neufer, P. D. (2000). Transcriptional regulation of gene expression in human skeletal muscle during recovery from exercise. *American Journal of Physiology, Endocrinology and Metabolism, 279*(4), e806–14. Retrieved from www.ncbi.nlm.nih.gov/pubmed/11001762

Pilegaard, H., Saltin, B., & Neufer, P. D. (2003). Exercise induces transient transcriptional activation of the PGC-1alpha gene in human skeletal muscle. *The Journal of Physiology, 546*(Pt. 3), 851–8. Retrieved from www.ncbi.nlm.nih.gov/pubmed/12563009

Plomin, R., DeFries, J. C., & Loehlin, J. C. (1977). Genotype-environment interaction and correlation in the analysis of human behavior. *Psychological Bulletin, 84*(2), 309–22. Retrieved from www.ncbi.nlm.nih.gov/pubmed/557211

Roth, S. M., Rankinen, T., Hagberg, J. M., Loos, R. J. F., Pérusse, L., Sarzynski, M. A., … Bouchard, C. (2012). Advances in exercise, fitness, and performance genomics in 2011. *Medicine and Science in Sports and Exercise, 44*(5), 809–17. https://doi.org/10.1249/MSS.0b013e31824f28b6

Saab, B. J., & Mansuy, I. M. (2014). Neuroepigenetics of memory formation and impairment: The role of microRNAs. *Neuropharmacology, 80*, 61–9. https://doi.org/10.1016/j.neuropharm.2014.01.026

Scarr, S., & McCartney, K. (1983). How people make their own environments: A theory of genotype greater than environment effects. *Child Development, 54*(2), 424–35. Retrieved from www.ncbi.nlm.nih.gov/pubmed/6683622

Sisson, S. B., Katzmarzyk, P. T., Ernest, C. P., Bouchard, C., Blair, S. N., & Church, T. S. (2009). Volume of exercise and fitness nonresponse in sedentary, postmenopausal women. *Medicine and Science in Sports and Exercise, 41*(3), 539–45. https://doi.org/10.1249/MSS.0b013e3181896c4e

Strasser, B. J. (2006). A world in one dimension: Linus Pauling, Francis Crick and the central dogma of molecular biology. *History and Philosophy of the Life Sciences, 28*(4), 491–512. Retrieved from www.ncbi.nlm.nih.gov/pubmed/18351048

Thieffry, D., & Sarkar, S. (1998). Forty years under the central dogma. *Trends in Biochemical Sciences, 23*(8), 312–6. Retrieved from www.ncbi.nlm.nih.gov/pubmed/9757833

Tucker, R., & Collins, M. (2012). What makes champions? A review of the relative contribution of genes and training to sporting success. *British Journal of Sports Medicine, 46*(8), 555–61. https://doi.org/10.1136/bjsports-2011-090548

Van Speybroeck, L. (2002). From epigenesis to epigenetics: The case of C. H. Waddington. *Annals of the New York Academy of Sciences, 981*, 61–81. Retrieved from www.ncbi.nlm.nih.gov/pubmed/12547674

Wang, L., McLeod, H. L., & Weinshilboum, R. M. (2011). Genomics and drug response. *New England Journal of Medicine, 364*(12), 1144–53. https://doi.org/10.1056/NEJMra1010600

Watson, J. B. (1930). *Behaviorism* (Rev. ed.). New York, NY: W. W. Norton and Co.
Yan, X., Papadimitriou, I., Lidor, R., & Eynon, N. (2016). Nature versus nurture in determining athletic ability. In *Medicine and Sport Science, 61*, 15–28. https://doi.org/10.1159/000445238

Index

Page numbers in **bold** denote tables, those in *italics* denote figures.

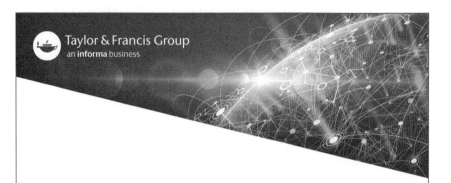

Taylor & Francis eBooks

www.taylorfrancis.com

A single destination for eBooks from Taylor & Francis
with increased functionality and an improved user
experience to meet the needs of our customers.

90,000+ eBooks of award-winning academic content in
Humanities, Social Science, Science, Technology, Engineering,
and Medical written by a global network of editors and authors.

TAYLOR & FRANCIS EBOOKS OFFERS:

A streamlined
experience for
our library
customers

A single point
of discovery
for all of our
eBook content

Improved
search and
discovery of
content at both
book and
chapter level

REQUEST A FREE TRIAL

support@taylorfrancis.com

 Routledge
Taylor & Francis Group

 CRC Press
Taylor & Francis Group

For Product Safety Concerns and Information please contact our
EU representative GPSR@taylorandfrancis.com Taylor & Francis
Verlag GmbH, Kaufingerstraße 24, 80331 München, Germany